Pancreatic Neuroendocrine Neoplasms

Stefano La Rosa • Fausto Sessa
Editors

Pancreatic Neuroendocrine Neoplasms

Practical Approach to Diagnosis, Classification, and Therapy

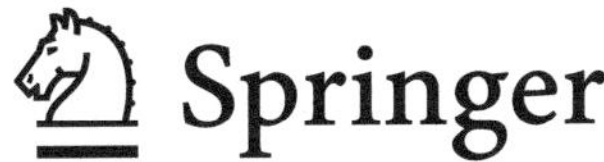 Springer

Editors
Stefano La Rosa
Department of Pathology
Ospedale di Circolo
Varese, Italy

Fausto Sessa
Department of Surgical
and Morphological Sciences
University of Insubria
Varese, Italy

ISBN 978-3-319-36004-1   ISBN 978-3-319-17235-4   (eBook)
DOI 10.1007/978-3-319-17235-4

Springer Cham Heidelberg New York Dordrecht London

Printed on acid-free paper

Springer International Publishing AG Switzerland is part of Springer Science+Business Media
(www.springer.com)

Preface

Since the early 2000s, the advances in imaging technologies and the wide diffusion of endoscopic ultrasound-guided fine needle aspiration have led to an increased detection of pancreatic neuroendocrine neoplasms compelling radiologists, pathologists, and nuclear medicine physicians to manage these diseases at an earlier stage. The increased surgical expertise together with new pharmacological options has also changed the therapeutic approach. At the same time, the refined WHO classification of 2010, increased experience of pathologists in this field, better knowledge of the clinicopathological features, and the availability of new molecular technologies have all increased our understanding of the pathogenesis and progression of such neoplasms. For all these reasons, the field of pancreatic neuroendocrine neoplasms has rapidly grown in the last 10 years and the aim of this book is to capture these dynamic changes providing a broad overview of this topic.

After a historical and epidemiological overview, four chapters attempt to capture the technical advances in diagnostic procedures providing insights for a critical evaluation of the new diagnostic options. The chapters on the immunohistochemical approach to diagnosis and on the criteria now used to classify pancreatic neuroendocrine neoplasm in different prognostic categories represent the bridge between the diagnostic step and the full characterization of the different entities. These are treated in 11 chapters which cover the epidemiology, diagnosis, morphology, and prognosis of each tumor type. A specific chapter is also dedicated to hyperplastic and microadenomatous neuroendocrine lesions, which may represent a diagnostic challenge for pathologists and clinicians.

Careful consideration is given to the molecular features of various tumors and a specific chapter gives a critical overview of the most important knowledge which has contributed to our understanding of the pathogenesis of such neoplasms and may have potential implications for new therapeutic pathways. The final chapters consider the surgical and medical approaches to therapy, providing a practical and analytical overview of the available options.

The book is written by a multidisciplinary team of worldwide-recognized experts and is addressed to radiologists, nuclear medicine physicians, endocrinologists, pathologists, surgeons, and oncologists interested in endocrine tumors of the pancreas.

The editors wish to thank the contributing authors and hope the readers will find all the information they need for their daily practice.

Varese, Italy

Varese, Italy

Stefano La Rosa

Fausto Sessa

Contents

Historical Background and Epidemiology

1

Fausto Sessa and Roberta Maragliano

1.1 Historical Background

The pancreas is a deeply located organ, which had been neglected for centuries until 1543 when the anatomist Andries van Wesel, better known *as Andreas Vesalius* (1514–1564), gave his description in the fifth book of "De Humani Corporis Fabrica Libri Septem." However, Rufus of Ephesus (circa 100 A.D.) first gave the name pancreas to the organ, which had previously been described by Herophilus of Chalcedon (circa 300 B.C.). For several centuries, this organ was forgotten probably because the canons of ancient medicine had not linked the theories of body fluids to any pancreatic diseases.

In 1642, Johann Georg Wirsung (1589–1643) described the main pancreatic duct when he was a prosector in Padua, Italy, where he performed autopsies under the guidance of his mentor, Ioannes Veslingius (Johann Vesling, 1598–1649). In 1720, the German anatomist Abraham Vater described the site of conjunction between the bile duct and the pancreatic duct, now known as the ampulla of Vater. The physiologist Albrecht Von Haller (1708–1777) noted that the pancreatic duct entered the small bowel in conjunction with

the bile duct and suggested that the pancreatic juice could act by diluting and softening the bile. Thomas Wharton observed the similarity between the structure of the pancreas and that of the submaxillary gland from which Samuel Thomas *von* Sömmerring (1755–1830) employed the term "Bauchspeicheldrüse" or "abdominal salivary gland." This terminology was used until the beginning of the last century [1–4].

In February 1869, Paul Langerhans (1847–1888) first described the pancreatic islets, which make up the 1–2 % of the mass of the pancreas (average weight 70–100 g) (Fig. 1.1a). At the end of his medical studies, he presented a thesis entitled "Contributions to the microscopic anatomy of the pancreas," in which he refers to *islands of clear cells* throughout the gland, staining differently than the surrounding tissue (Fig. 1.1b) [5].

In 1893, E. Laguesse named these clusters of clear cells "Islands of Langerhans" and suggested that they were the pancreatic units involved in diabetes mellitus [6]. In 1902, he described in detail the histological characteristics of the islets in dogs after ligation of the duct. After that, E. Lindsay Opie (1873–1971) described the hyaline changes of pancreatic islets in diabetic patients. At the beginning of the last century, F.G. Banting and C.H. Best, working at the University of Toronto under the supervision of the physiologist J.J. R. Macleod, obtained "isletin" from Ringer's solution containing pancreatic juice from dogs (Fig. 1.2). Insulin was not

F. Sessa (✉) • R. Maragliano
Department of Surgical and Morphological Sciences,
University of Insubria, Via O. Rossi 9,
21100 Varese, Italy
e-mail: fausto.sessa@uninsubria.it

S. La Rosa, F. Sessa (eds.), *Pancreatic Neuroendocrine Neoplasms: Practical Approach to Diagnosis,*
Classification, and Therapy, DOI 10.1007/978-3-319-17235-4_1,
© Springer International Publishing Switzerland 2015

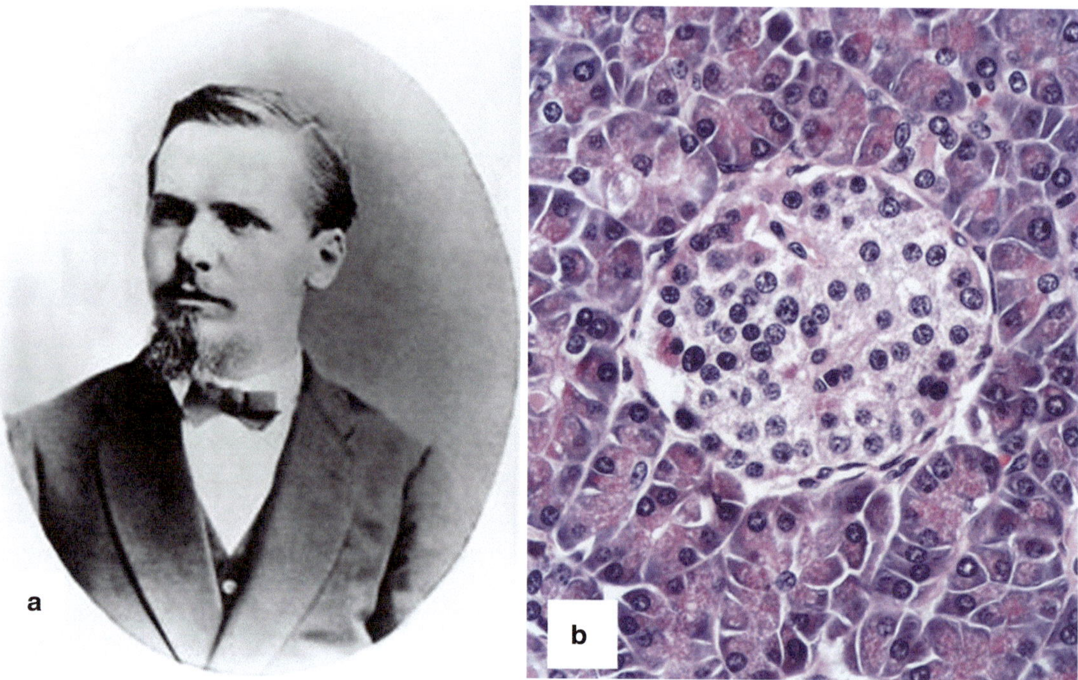

Fig. 1.1 (**a**) Paul Langerhans (1847–1888) in 1873 (© Bildarchiv Preußischer Kulturbesitz, Berlin, 1873, Photographer: Ruf und Dilger [85]) (**b**) Histological appearance of the islet of Langerhans (hematoxylin-eosin)

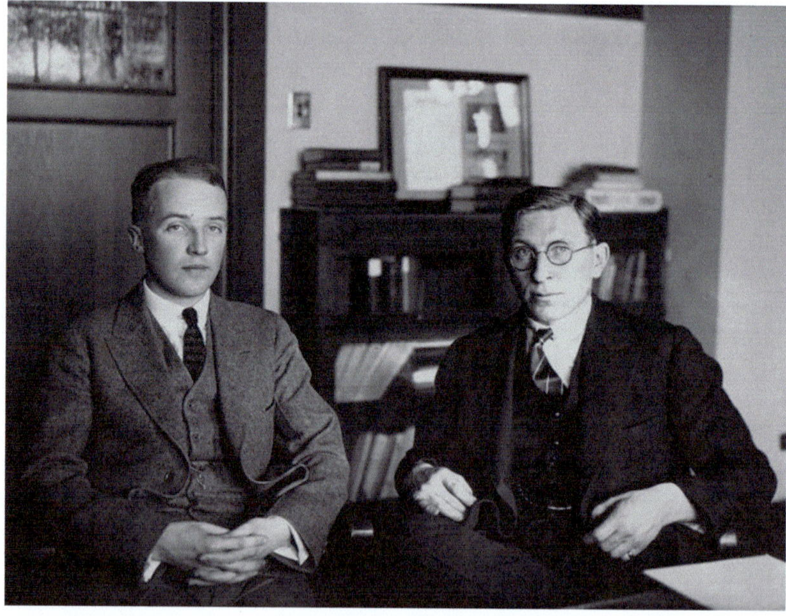

Fig. 1.2 Frederick Grant Banting (1891–1941) (*right*) and Charles Herbert Best (1899–1978) (*left*) in 1924 (Courtesy of the Thomas Fisher Rare Book Library, University of Toronto)

successfully isolated until December 1921 with the aid of the biochemist, J. B. Collip [7].

C.P. Kimball and J.R. Murlin first postulated the existence of a second pancreatic hormone in 1923, when they found that acetone precipitated a fraction of aqueous extracts of the pancreas soluble in 95 % alcohol, allowing the separation of an unknown substance from insulin. The

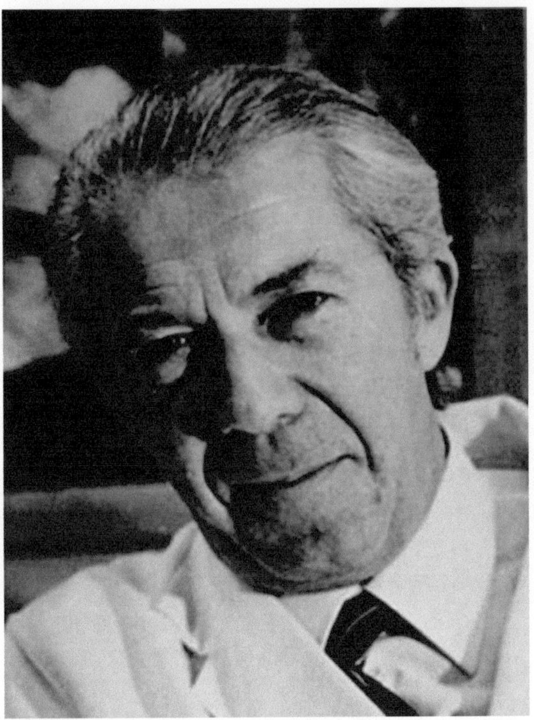

Fig. 1.3 Christian René de Duve (1917–2013) in 1974 [86]

injection of this fraction into dogs and rabbits caused a rapid rise in blood glucose levels. They inferred from these results that the preparation contained a second pancreatic hormone and named it "*gluc*ose *agon*ist," hence the term glucagon also known as the H-G or hyperglycemic-glycogenolytic factor. The H-G factor was subsequently dismissed as a contaminant [8]. However, E. Sutherland and C. de Duve who found the H-G factor in the pancreas and gastric mucosa of the dog (Fig. 1.3) speculated that the new factor might be a second hormone involved in glucose metabolism, so the name glucagon was reintroduced, probably by de Duve, to replace that of the H-G factor [9].

Nonetheless, E. Laguesse was the first to suggest the endocrine function of islet cells, while V. Diamare distinguished two types of endocrine cells that M. Lane, in 1907, had called A cells and beta cells, defined B cells by Bensley in 1911 [10, 11]. W. Bloom described the third cell type in 1931, and then J.F. Deconinck identified type

IV and type V cells, using electron microscopy [12–14].

The use of immunohistochemistry has allowed the localization of glucagon in A cells, insulin in B cells, somatostatin in D cells, and pancreatic polypeptide (PP) in type V cells, in addition to recognizing the topography of endocrine cells within the islets (see Fig. 7.1).

In 1902, A.G. Nicholls described the first adenoma arising from islet cells, while performing an autopsy. The tumor was small, round, encapsulated, and probably represented the first nonfunctioning pancreatic neuroendocrine tumor (PanNET) [15]. In 1927, 5 years after the discovery of insulin, R. M. Wilder reported the first case of hyperinsulinism associated with an islet cell tumor that was metastatic to the liver and lymph node [16]. The alcoholic extracts from the neoplastic tissue of the liver that looked like pancreatic islet cells acted like insulin when injected into rabbits. R. R. Graham (1890–1948) first removed an insulinoma at the Toronto General Hospital in 1929. In 1938, A.O. Whipple (1881–1963) described for the first time the classical triad (shakiness, syncope, and sweating) associated with an insulin-producing islet cell tumor alias insulinoma [17].

In 1955, R.M. Zollinger and E.H. Ellison suggested that a non-beta cell pancreatic adenoma might have a functional role in producing an ulcerogenic factor, which was isolated by R.A. Gregory and named "gastrin" [18, 19]. Subsequently, in 1958, J.V. Verner and A.B. Morrison described a diarrheogenic syndrome due to a non-beta cell tumor (WDHA syndrome: water diarrhea, hypokalemia, and achlorhydria) (see Chap. 11). In addition, PanNETs have been reported in association with other types of endocrine tumors. In 1927, H.W. Cushing and then C.W. Lloyd described an association between PanNETs and parathyroid and pituitary tumors. In 1953, L.O. Underdahl and M.P. Moldawer both described multiple endocrine adenomas involving the pancreas, parathyroid, and pituitary [20, 21]. A year later, P. Wermer suggested a genetic basis of inheritance for the syndrome now called MEN1. However, PanNETs have also been observed, although less frequently, in von Hippel-Lindau (VHL) disease and in association with the type 1 neurofibromatosis (NF-1) and tuberous sclerosis complex (TSC).

Over the years, the terminology and classification of PanNETs have undergone multiple changes. In 1938, G. F. Laidlaw proposed the term "nesidioblastoma" and "nesiodioblasts" for cells that differentiate from the secretory duct epithelium to form islets. R.F. Weichert and L.M. Roth instead suggested "carcinoid-islet cell tumor" to stress the morphological similarity of islet tumors to intestinal carcinoids that were described for the first time in September 1907, by S. Oberndorfer, who then published his seminal paper entitled "Carcinoid tumors of the small intestine" in the *Frankfurt Journal of Pathology*. He described and characterized the tumor that had previously been referred to as a "benign carcinoma." Successively, I. Sziji introduced the term "apudomas," in 1969, to refer to APUD characteristic of pancreatic endocrine cells. Nonetheless, the term "islet cell tumors" was used most often [22–25].

From the 2000 WHO Histological Typing of Endocrine Tumours to the 2004 WHO Classifications of Tumours of the Endocrine Organs, PanNETs have been divided into two main categories: well- and poorly differentiated neuroendocrine tumors. Well-differentiated tumors were subsequently divided into benign neuroendocrine tumors, neuroendocrine tumors of uncertain malignant potential, and well-differentiated neuroendocrine carcinomas [26, 27]. The last WHO Classification of Tumours of the Digestive System, published in 2010, introduced a three-tiered classification separating Grade 1 and Grade 2 PanNETs and Grade 3 pancreatic neuroendocrine carcinomas (PanNECs) of large cell and small cell type [28].

In 2011 the complete exomes of ten PanNETs were sequenced, followed by the screening for mutations of the most commonly found altered genes in a cohort of 58 tumors. MEN1 was found to be the most frequently mutated gene as it was altered in 44 % of PanNETs, but the most striking discovery was the identification of additional somatic mutations in 43 % of PanNETs. They harbored mutations in two subunits of a transcription/chromatin remodeling complex, the death domain-associated protein (DAXX) and the thalassemia/mental retardation syndrome X-linked (ATRX), while 14 % harbored mutations in the mammalian target of the rapamycin (mTOR) pathway. In addition, PanNETs seem to have a degree of genetic complexity lower than that of ductal adenocarcinomas (DAC) because they harbor a median of 16 somatic mutations versus 66 somatic mutations in DAC. This may explain the different behavior of the two pancreatic entities [29, 30].

1.2 Epidemiology

PanNETs account for less than 3 % of pancreatic neoplasms, but their incidence has been increasing over the past 20 years. Based on the Surveillance, Epidemiology, and End Results (SEER) data, the incidence of all neuroendocrine tumors (NETs) in the USA increased nearly fivefold over the past three decades from 1.09 per 100,000 in 1973 to 5.25 per 100,000 in 2004. The same data suggest a sex and race difference in the site of origin (gastrointestinal tract, pancreas, lung, thyroid, adrenal gland, adenohypophysis, parathyroid) and in the incidence of these tumors. Male patients are more likely to develop PanNETs (0.38 per 100,000) than female ones (0.27 per 100,000), and African-Americans (0.36 per 100,000) are more susceptible than American Indians/Alaskan Natives (0.20 per 100,000) [31]. Nevertheless, SEER data show that PanNETs represent about 7 % of all gastroenteropancreatic (GEP)-NETs and have an incidence of 0.43 per 100,000 in 2007, a twofold increase in the incidence since 1980 [32]. In addition, SEER data showed that exocrine pancreatic cancers tended to decrease over time, whereas the incidence rates of endocrine neoplasms increased. From the period 1977–1981 to 2002–2005, the incidence of exocrine cancers decreased by approximately 11 %, while the incidence of endocrine cancers rose 90 % for younger adults (<60 years) and 149 % in older adults (>60 years) [33].

Although most PanNETs occur sporadically, nearly 10 % are associated with genetic syndromes. These include MEN1, VHL, NF-1, and TSC.

However, published epidemiological studies on PanNETs are poorly comparable for several reasons:

(a) In the past, there was no consensus among pathologists on the diagnostic criteria of PanNETs or the criteria to establish their malignant potential.

(b) PanNETs may be functioning or nonfunctioning, depending on the cell type and hormone hypersecretion and on the lack of clinical syndromes.

(c) PanNETs have been included in several epidemiological studies together with gastrointestinal neuroendocrine tumors (GI-NETs), or studies only reported data from single referral centers.

(d) The national registries of tumors started at different times in different countries, for example, 1953 in Norway and 1973 in the USA. This means that they utilize different histological criteria and different tools for diagnoses.

(e) Tumor registries generally only recorded malignant tumors. This explains why they do not reflect the real incidence of PanNETs, since "benign" tumors were omitted from many national registries.

(f) Healthcare systems could affect the incidence results because not all the people could benefit from them; hence, the tumor registry may include only the records of a fraction of the population.

In addition, the widespread use of abdominal imaging, like computer tomography (CT) and ultrasound scans in the last 20 years, is altering the time of discovery and has increased the number of pancreatic lesions in asymptomatic patients with an increase of the so-called pancreatic incidentalomas. This may in part explain the different incidence of PanNETs between countries with public or private healthcare services. In a series of 475 pancreatectomies (January 1995–June 2007), 64 out of 475 (13.5 %) were performed for lesions found incidentally ("pan-

creatic incidentalomas"), 10 of which (15,6 %) were diagnosed as PanNETs. In the remaining 411 pancreatectomies performed for symptomatic patients, only 23 cases were PanNETs (5,6 %) ($p < 0.05$). Interestingly, more than 90 % of the incidentally found PanNETs were observed after the year 2000 [34]. Crippa et al. in a series of 355 nonfunctioning PanNETs (NF-PanNETs) (124 incidentally found and 235 detected because of symptoms) reported that the frequency of incidental NF-PanNETs increased from 9 % during the period 1992–1996 to 40 % in the period 2002–2006. They also reclassified all cases according to the WHO 2010 criteria and found that most of the incidentally found NF-PanNETs were G1 (73 %) and had a lower tumor stage, smaller size, and better survival, whereas only 42 % of symptomatic NF-PanNETs were G1 [35].

1.2.1 Autopsy Studies

In the first part of the last century, the epidemiological studies were based on autopsy findings, frequently reporting "incidentalomas" which probably represented NF-PanNETs. A.G. Nicholls reported the first case of a PanNET detected among 1,514 autopsies [15]. In a series of 34,079 autopsies focusing on a search for PanNETs, 170 cases were reported, corresponding to a frequency of 0.5 %. The studies were not always informative regarding the patients' status and the symptoms of excessive hormone secretion. However the autopsy series showed a PanNET frequency ranging from 0.1 % to 2.5 %. For instance, B. Korpassy found four cases (0.8 %) of macroscopically evident PanNETs among 500 autopsies [36]. Twenty-four cases (0.3 %) of "benign islet cell neoplasms" were observed by V.K. Frantz in a series of 9,158 consecutive autopsies [37]. S. Warren et al. reported 42 PanNETs that they defined "islet cell tumors" among 4,666 autopsies corresponding to a frequency of 0.9 % [38]. V. Becker who observed 62 PanNETs in his autopsy series reported a similar frequency of 1.4 % [39]. In two studies performed by L. Grimelius and W. Kimura [40, 41], 11 PanNETs were found among 1,366 Swedish autopsy cases (0.8 %) and 20 PanNETs were found among 800 consecutive Japanese autopsies (2.5 %). Furthermore, K.Y. Lam and C.Y. Lo described 13 PanNETs in a series of 11,472 Chinese autopsies (0.11 %) where only 4 patients were endocrinologically symptomatic [42]. The last autopsy series in which the presence of PanNETs had systematically been investigated was reported by S. Kishi et al. who identified 6 (1.2 %) cases in a series of 413 autopsies [43].

1.2.2 Study Population

Several studies have been performed on the incidence of GEP-NETs in defined populations [31, 32, 42, 44–54] including East Asia, North and South America, and West Europe. No or a few information is available from Africa and East Europe.

In 2014, Ito reported a second nationwide survey analysis of GEP-NETs in Japan which had been performed in 2010. The results were compared with the first nationwide survey analysis performed in 2005. The incidence of PanNETs was 1.27 per 100,000, and the prevalence was 2.69 per 100,000. A total of 3,379 PanNETs were treated in 2010 compared to 2,845 treated in 2005, a 1.2-fold increase. NF-PanNETs comprised 65.5 % of cases followed by insulinomas (20.9 %) and gastrinomas (8.2 %) [54]. In 2005, NF-PanNETs were 47.4 % followed by insulinomas (38.2 %) and gastrinomas (7.9 %) [50]. The study by Ito et al. reported for the first time the grading of PanNETs according to the 2010 WHO classification and showed that NECs represented 7.5 % of pancreatic neuroendocrine neoplasms (PanNENs). The frequency of NECs among NF-PanNENs was 9.7 % compared with 3.2 % among functioning ones. In Taiwan, a nationwide cancer registry-based study on NETs was performed from January 1996 to December 2008. The annual incidence increased from 0.30 per 100,000 in 1996 to 0.55 per 100,000 in 2000 to 1.51 per 100,000 in 2008 signifying the incidence rate increased by 83 % from 1996 to 2000 and by 175 % from 2000 to 2008. The pancreas was the fourth primary site, representing 6 % of all the

NETs. The incidence of PanNETs increased from 0.02 per 100,000 in 1996 to 0.13 per 100,000 in 2008, which is lower than the Japanese data, probably because only malignant PanNETs were recorded as in the SEER database [55].

From South America, O'Connor reported an observational study on GEP and bronchial NETs in Argentina. A total of 532 NETs were found, which included 71 bronchial NETs and 461 GEP-NETs, 116 of which were pancreatic (25.2 %). In this PanNET series, the lymph node involvement was detected in 44 (37.9 %) cases and liver metastases in 74 (63.8 %) cases. In this study the 2010 WHO grading system was applied independently of the site of origin to 457 GEP-NENs with NEC representing the 9 %. In Brazil, a study published in 2011 by Estrozi et al. reported 773 GEP-NETs that included 126 PanNETs (16.4 %) found in *Consultoria em Patologia* from January 1997 to December 2009. The grading in this study was also done according to the 2010 WHO classification criteria and reported that the majority (64.5 %) were G1 PanNETs, followed by G2 PanNETs (27.5 %) and NECs (8 %). In these two South American studies, no data about the incidence was given although Estrozi noted an increase in the percentage of GEP-NETs out of the total number of surgical pathology cases from 0.18 % to 0.50 %.

In Spain, a national registry of GEP-NETs started in 2001, thanks to GETNE (Spanish Society of Neuroendocrine Tumors). From January 2001 to December 2008, 837 NETs with follow-up were registered, including 288 PanNETs (33.7 %), 171 of which were NF-PanNETs and 67 insulinomas. No information about incidence was given in relationship to the population of this multi-institutional academic and community registry [51].

In 2013, a study by Scherübl et al. reported that the number of GEP-NETs increased about fivefold between 1976 and 2006 in Germany [52]. A total of 2,821 GEP-NETs were documented with an incidence of 4.65 per 100,000 in comparison to 0.3 per 100,000 in 1976. The incidence of PanNETs was 0.11 per 100,000 in 1976 and 0.5 per 100,000 in 2006. At the same time, the authors reported that the survival of GEP-

NETs patients had improved significantly. A prospective study was done in Austria from May 2004 to April 2005 documenting 285 GEP-NETs, which means an incidence of 2.3 per 100,000 inhabitants. The age-specific incidence rate was highest between 50 and 70 years. In this series, there were 33 (11.6 %) PanNETs, and the overall annual incidence was 0.25 per 100,000 [56].

A Swedish study reported an annual incidence of 0.4 per 100,000 [45], and a study from Northern Ireland found an annual incidence of 0.18 per 100,000 [44]. The latter study was later updated reporting an incidence of 0.23 per 100,000 [46]. A Norwegian study on NETs of different sites made with data obtained from the Norwegian Registry of Cancer showed that the incidence of PanNETs was 0.23 per 100,000 with a male predominance (0.29 in males compared to 0.17 in females, per 100,000). However, the prognosis of PanNETs of this series was among the poorest of NET subtypes, probably reflecting the late diagnosis of malignant PanNETs and because well-differentiated G1 and G2 PanNETs were excluded from the two registries [57].

A French study using a population-based cancer registry found the overall annual crude incidence of malignant digestive endocrine tumors (MDETs) to be 2.16 per 100,000 inhabitants. PanNETs accounted for 20.5 % of all tumors in this cohort. The age-standardized incidence rate of PanNETs was 0.31 per 100,000, with a male-to-female ratio of 1.6 [48]. They observed that incidence rates were low in people under 40 years of age but increased with age, reaching a peak at the age of 75 for men and 65 for women. In England and Wales, a similar study on MDETs was done by using data from a National Cancer Registry. The 4,102 endocrine carcinomas collected in the period 1986–1999 represented 0.6 % of all the digestive cancers. They divided MDETs into well-differentiated tumors (78.8 %) and small cell carcinomas (21.2 %). Well-differentiated tumors included insulinomas, gastrinomas, VIPomas, glucagonomas, carcinoids, insular carcinomas, and neuroendocrine carcinomas. The mean age at diagnosis was 62.8 years for patients with well-differentiated tumors and 70.6 years for small cell carcinomas. The 240 cases of PanNETs represented the 5.8 % of MDETs and included 49 insulinomas, 31 gastrinomas, 17 glucagonomas, and 1 VIPoma [58].

In the USA, a study using SEER data between 1973 and 2003 found 1,310 islet cell carcinomas among 101,046 pancreatic cancers, representing 1.3 % of all pancreatic cancers. However, due to a better outcome of islet cell carcinoma, they represent almost 10 % of pancreatic cancers in prevalence analyses. Histologically, 1,117 cases were islet cell carcinomas, carcinoids, or NF-PanNETs, while of the F-PanNETs, 73 cases were gastrinoma, 49 insulinoma, 26 glucagonoma, and 16 VIPoma [31]. Obviously, this study underestimated the total number of patients with islet cell tumors because all cases from the SEER database are malignant. Over such a long time period, PETs had been classified in different ways, and in most cases there was more significant clinical presentation than histopathology. Many small islet cell tumors that may have been considered benign or of unclear malignant potential were not recorded in the SEER database. However, in the study from E. J. Kuo, using population-based data including patients diagnosed from 1988 (when SEER initiated the data collection of tumor size) to 2009, a total of 263 out of 1,371 NF-PanNETs were reported to be less than 2 cm in size. Over the 22-year study period, the incidence of PanNETs <2 cm increased, accounting for the 20.2 % in 2009 in contrast to the 12.3 % in 1988 [59].

In a SEER registry data from 1973 to 1987, the annual incidence of PanNETs was 0.6 per 100,000 for all age groups [47]. In the series of PanNETs from 1973 to 2000, the annual incidence was 0.2 per 100,000 with the highest incidence (0.7–0.8 per 100,000) in the sixth and seventh decades and with a slight male predominance [60]. In the same series that included 1,483 PanNETs, the majority were NF-PanNETs (90.8 %), while malignant F-PanNETs included gastrinomas (4.2 %), insulinomas (2.5 %), glucagonomas (1.6 %), and VIPomas (0.9 %) [60]. The annual incidence of insulinomas and gastrinomas in the SEER registry was 0.1/million, but this may be due to a substantial underestimation of F-PanNETs due to the fact that SEER registers only included malignant tumors and probably missed most of the insulinomas that frequently behave in a benign fashion [60]. The 5-year survival rate was 47.6 % in F-PanNETs versus 31.3 % in NF-PanNETs [60]. The SEER database was the source of 49,012 NETs recorded from 1973 to 2007. In these series, 29,664 cases were GEP-NETs and included 3,598 PanNETs which represented 7.34 % of all cases. PanNETs had the lowest 5-year survival rates (37.6 %), whereas rectal NETs showed the highest 5-year survival rates (88.5 %), reflecting the different behavior of NETs of different sites [32].

The frequency of the various subtypes of F-PanNETs has been described in several studies [49, 50, 58, 65–69]. Insulinomas (see Chap. 8) are the most frequently encountered F-PanNETs and are usually tumors with indolent behavior [54, 62, 63, 65–67]. Gastrinomas (see Chap. 12) are the second most commonly encountered F-PanNETs, but it is worth noting that gastrinomas can also arise outside of the pancreas [54, 64, 67, 70]. Pancreatic gastrinomas are generally more aggressive and frequently associated with liver metastases [71]. In a Japanese series, 30.2 % of gastrinomas had liver metastases at the time of the initial diagnosis, whereas insulinomas accounted for only 9.3 % of liver metastases [54]. Up to 30 % of gastrinomas are associated with MEN1 [68, 70]. In Denmark, the incidence of gastrinoma was estimated to be 0.5 per million per year [61]. A higher incidence of two to four per million has been found in Switzerland [68]. Other studies have reported an annual incidence of 0.5–1.2 cases per million [45, 46]. Epidemiological data on F-PanNETs other than insulinoma and gastrinoma are rare.

Functioning glucagon-secreting tumors (glucagonomas, see Chap. 9) represent <10 % of F-PanNETs and are almost exclusively found within the pancreas [72, 73]. Glucagonomas are very rare, and their annual incidence has been estimated to be around 0.1 per million [45, 46]. Functioning somatostatin-secreting PanNETs (somatostatinomas see Chap. 10) are extremely rare and account for <1 % of all F-PanNETs, and the true incidence of these tumors is not completely known. Somatostatinomas typically present in the fifth and sixth decades of life with a slight female preponderance. Up to 50 % of somatostatin-secreting tumors arise outside the pancreas, and these are not associated with a full-blown somatostatinoma syndrome [74–76].

PanNETs secreting vasoactive intestinal peptide (VIPomas, see Chap. 11) comprise <10 % of all F-PanNETs and appear to be slightly more common in females according to some but not all reports [72, 73, 77–79]. VIPomas are found in extrapancreatic locations in up to 25 % of cases [82].

Pancreatic tumors secreting other hormones are very rare. In the study by I. M. Modlin, a series of 13,715 carcinoid tumors were identified in the SEER database from January 1973 to December 1999. Seventy-nine cases were "pancreatic carcinoid" representing 0.73 % of all the carcinoids. However, the parameters utilized to distinguish pancreatic carcinoid tumors from PanNETs were not specified, and probably immunohistochemistry techniques were not applied to all the cases in these series because the antibodies were not available at the beginning of registry enrollment [80]. In the Netherlands Cancer Registry from 1989 to 1996, on a series of 2,391 patients harboring carcinoid tumor 68 (2.8 %), pancreatic carcinoids were found [81]. Fifteen cases of serotonin-producing PanNETs were reported in 2011 by La Rosa et al. who reviewed the medical literature and found 23 additional cases of nonfunctioning serotonin PanNETs and 17 cases of functional pancreatic carcinoids [82]. At present there are 71 nonfunctioning serotonin-producing PanNETs in the medical literature (see Chap. 14). There are 134 cases of adrenocorticotropin (ACTH)-secreting PanNETs (see Chap. 13) reported in the English medical literature [83] and 37 calcitonin-secreting PanNETs [84]. Growth hormone- and parathyroid hormone-related peptide F-PanNETs are extremely rare and are frequently associated with MEN1, but their incidence is unknown (see Chap. 15).

A European multicenter study collected 1,072 surgical PanNETs. There were 331 (30.9 %) F-PanNETs including 222 insulinomas (67.1 %), 37 gastrinomas (11.2 %), 22 glucagonomas

(6.5 %), and 19 VIPomas (5.7 %). There were 874 (94.6 %) sporadic PanNETs, while 36 (3.9 %) were associated with MEN1 and 14 (1.5 %) with VHL. According to the 2010 WHO classification, 488 (52.3 %) were PanNET G1, 382 (40.9 %) were PanNET G2, and lastly 63 (6.8 %) were PanNECs [65]. This study and the others that used the 2010 WHO classification show that there is good agreement in the diagnosis of PanNECs that is not always observed in NET G1 and G2.

In conclusion, there is evidence that PanNETs are a group of tumors with increasing incidence and prevalence. This is probably due to a longer life span, a widespread use of imagining, an increased awareness of physicians, and because more people benefit from a healthcare service. These tumors have a heterogeneous clinical presentation mostly with an advanced disease underscoring their malignant potential. However, F-PanNETs and incidentally discovered PanNETs have a better prognosis because of the small size and early detection. Nevertheless, to compare geographic or ethnic differences in incidence and survival, it is necessary that in the future pathologists should use the same diagnostic criteria and classification.

References

1. Fitzgerald PJ (1980) Medical anecdotes concerning some diseases of the pancreas. In: Fitzgerald PJ, Morrison AB (eds) The pancreas. Williams and Wilkins, Baltimore, pp 1–29
2. Singer C (1957) A short history of anatomy from the Greeks to Harvey. Dover Publications, New York, p 111
3. Garrison FH (1929) An introduction to the history of medicine. WB Saunders, Philadelphia, pp 554–690
4. Whipple AO (1960) A historical sketch of the pancreas. In: Howard JM, Jordan GH (eds) Surgical diseases of the pancreas. JB Lippincott, Philadelphia, pp 1–6
5. Langerhans P (1869) Beiträge zur mikroskopischen anatomie der bauchspeicheldrüse. Berlin Univ, Berlin
6. Laguesse E (1894) Sur la formation des ilots de Langerhans dans le pancréas. C R Soc Seances Soc Biol Fil Paris 46:819–820
7. Banting FG, Best CH, Collip JB et al (1922) Pancreatic extracts in the treatment of diabetes mellitus. Can Med Assoc J 12(3):141–146
8. Kimball CP, Murlin JR (1923) Aqueous extracts of pancreas: III. Some precipitation reactions of insulin. J Biol Chem 58:337–346
9. de Duve C (1951) Hyperglycemic principle of the pancreas (glucagon, H-G factor). Rev Med Liege 6(10):258–263
10. Diamare V (1899) Studi comparativi sulle isole di Langerhans del pancreas. Intern Monatschr für Anat und Physiol 16:155–209
11. Bensley RR (1911) Studies on the pancreas of the guinea pig. Am J Anat 12:297–388
12. Bloom W (1931) A new type of granular cell in the islet of Langerhans of man. Anat Rec 49:363–371
13. Deconinck JF, Potvliege PR, Gepts W (1971) The ultrastructure of the human pancreatic islets. I. The islets of adults. Diabetologia 7(4):266–282
14. Deconinck JF, Van Assche FA, Potvliege PR et al (1972) The ultrastructure of the human pancreatic islets. II. The islets of neonates. Diabetologia 8(5):326–333
15. Nicholls AG (1902) Simple adenoma of the pancreas arising from an island of Langerhans. J Med Res 8:385–395
16. Wilder RM, Allan FN, Power MH et al (1927) Carcinoma of islands of pancreas: hyperinsulinism and hypoglycemia. JAMA 89:348–355
17. Whipple AO (1938) The surgical therapy of hyperinsulinism. J Int Chir 3:237–276
18. Zollinger RM, Ellison EH (1955) Primary peptic ulcerations of the jejunum associated with islet cell tumors of the pancreas. Ann Surg 142:709–728
19. Gregory RA, Tracy HJ, French JM et al (1960) Extraction of a gastrin-like substance from a pancreatic tumour in a case of Zollinger-Ellison syndrome. Lancet I:1045–1048
20. Underdahl LO, Woolner LB, Black BM (1953) Multiple endocrine adenomas; report of 8 cases in which the parathyroids, pituitary and pancreatic islets were involved. J Clin Endocrinol Metab 13(1):20–47
21. Moldawer MP, Nardi GL, Raker JW (1954) Concomitance of multiple adenomas of the parathyroids and pancreatic islets with tumor of the pituitary: a syndrome with a familial incidence. Am J Med Sci 228(2):190–206
22. Laidlaw GF (1938) Nesidioblastoma, the islet tumor of the pancreas. Am J Pathol 14(2):125–134
23. Weichert RF, Roth LM, Krementz ET et al (1971) Carcinoid-islet cell tumors of the duodenum. Report of twenty-one cases. Am J Surg 121(2):195–205
24. Oberndorfer S (1907) Carcinoid tumors of the small intestine. Frankf Z Pathol 1:426–432
25. Szijj I, Csapó Z, László FA et al (1969) Medullary cancer of the thyroid gland associated with hypercorticism. Cancer 24(1):167–173
26. Solcia E, Klöppel G, Sobin SH (eds) (2000) Histological typing of endocrine tumours. Springer, Berlin
27. DeLellis R, Lloyd RV, Heitz PU et al (2004) WHO classification of tumours; pathology and genetics;

tumors of endocrine organs. IARC Press, Lyon, pp 177–208

28. Bosman FT, Carneiro F, Hruban RH et al (2010) WHO classification of tumors of the digestive system. IARC Press, Lyon, pp 13–14, 322–326

29. Jones S, Zhang X, Parsons DW et al (2008) Core signaling pathways in human pancreatic cancers revealed by global genomic analyses. Science 321(5897): 1801–1806

30. Jiao Y, Shi C, Edil BH et al (2011) DAXX/ATRX, MEN1, and mTOR pathway genes are frequently altered in pancreatic neuroendocrine tumors. Science 331:1199–1203

31. Yao JC, Hassan M, Phan A et al (2008) One hundred years after "carcinoid": epidemiology of and prognostic factors for neuroendocrine tumors in 35,825 cases in the United States. J Clin Oncol 26(18):3063–3072

32. Lawrence B, Gustafsson BI, Chan A et al (2011) The epidemiology of gastroenteropancreatic neuroendocrine tumors. Endocrinol Metab Clin North Am 40(1):1–18

33. Zhou J, Enewold L, Stojadinovic A et al (2010) Incidence rates of exocrine and endocrine pancreatic cancers in the United States. Cancer Causes Control 21(6):853–861

34. Lahat G, Ben Haim M, Nachmany I et al (2009) Pancreatic incidentalomas: high rate of potentially malignant tumors. J Am Coll Surg 209(3):313–319

35. Crippa S, Partelli S, Zamboni G et al (2014) Incidental diagnosis as prognostic factor in different tumor stages of nonfunctioning pancreatic endocrine tumors. Surgery 155(1):145–153

36. Korpàssy B (1939) Die Basalzellenmetaplasie des Ausfűhrungsgänge des Pankreas. Virchows Archiv A Pathol Pathol Anat 303:359–373

37. Frantz VK (1959) Tumors of the pancreas. In: Atlas of tumor pathology. Armed Forces Institute of Pathology, Washington, DC, pp 79–149

38. Warren S, Le Compte PM, Legg MA (1966) The pathology of diabetes mellitus. Lea & Febiger, Philadelphia

39. Becker V (1971) Pathologicoanatomical aspects of tumors with endocrine activity. Langenbecks Arch Surg 329:426–437

40. Grimelius L, Hultquist GT, Stenkvist B (1975) Cytological differentiation of asymptomatic pancreatic islet cell tumours in autopsy material. Virchows Arch Pathol Anat Physiol Klin Med 365:275–288

41. Kimura W, Kuroda A, Morioka Y (1991) Clinical pathology of endocrine tumors of the pancreas. Analysis of autopsy cases. Dig Dis Sci 36:933–942

42. Lam KY, Lo CY (1997) Pancreatic endocrine tumour: a 22-year clinico-pathological experience with morphological, immunohistochemical observation and a review of the literature. Eur J Surg Oncol 23:36–42

43. Kishi S, Sakamoto K, Mori M et al (2012) Asymptomatic insulinoma: a case report and autopsy series. Diabetes Res Clin Pract 98(3):445–451

44. Buchanan KD, Johnston CF, O'Hare MM et al (1986) Neuroendocrine tumors. A European view. Am J Med 81:14–22

45. Eriksson B, Öberg K, Skogseid B (1989) Neuroendocrine pancreatic tumors. Clinical findings in a prospective study of 84 patients. Acta Oncol 28:373–377

46. Watson RG, Johnston CF, O'Hare MM et al (1989) The frequency of gastrointestinal endocrine tumours in a well-defined population – Northern Ireland 1970–1985. Q J Med 72:647–657

47. Carriaga MT, Henson DE (1995) Liver, gallbladder, extrahepatic bile ducts, and pancreas. Cancer 75:171–190

48. Lepage C, Bouvier AM, Phelip JM et al (2004) Incidence and management of malignant digestive endocrine tumours in a well defined French population. Gut 53:549–553

49. Halfdanarson TR, Rubin J, Farnell MB et al (2008) Pancreatic endocrine neoplasms: epidemiology and prognosis of pancreatic endocrine tumors. Endocr Relat Cancer 15(2):409–427

50. Ito T, Sasano H, Tanaka M et al (2010) Epidemiological study of gastroenteropancreatic neuroendocrine tumors in Japan. J Gastroenterol 45(2):234–243

51. Garcia-Carbonero R, Capdevila J, Crespo-Herrero G (2010) Incidence, patterns of care and prognostic factors for outcome of gastroenteropancreatic neuroendocrine tumors (GEP-NETs): results from the National Cancer Registry of Spain (RGETNE). Ann Oncol 21(9):1794–1803

52. Scherübl H, Streller B, Stabenow R et al (2013) Clinically detected gastroenteropancreatic neuroendocrine tumors are on the rise: epidemiological changes in Germany. World J Gastroenterol 19(47): 9012–9019

53. O'Connor JM, Marmissolle F, Bestani C et al (2014) Observational study of patients with gastroenteropancreatic and bronchial neuroendocrine tumors in Argentina: results from the large database of a multidisciplinary group clinical multicenter study. Mol Clin Oncol 2(5):673–684

54. Ito T, Igarashi H, Nakamura K et al (2014) Epidemiological trends of pancreatic and gastrointestinal neuroendocrine tumors in Japan: a nationwide survey analysis. J Gastroenterol 50(1):58–64

55. Tsai HJ, Wu CC, Tsai CR et al (2013) The epidemiology of neuroendocrine tumors in Taiwan: a nationwide cancer registry-based study. PLoS One 8(4):e62487

56. Niederle MB, Hackl M, Kaserer K et al (2010) Gastroenteropancreatic neuroendocrine tumours: the current incidence and staging based on the WHO and European Neuroendocrine Tumour Society classification: an analysis based on prospectively collected parameters. Endocr Relat Cancer 17(4): 909–918

57. Hauso O, Gustafsson BI, Kidd M et al (2008) Neuroendocrine tumor epidemiology: contrasting

Norway and North America. Cancer 113(10): 2655–2664

58. Lepage C, Rachet B, Coleman MP (2007) Survival from malignant digestive endocrine tumors in England and Wales: a population-based study. Gastroenterology 132(3):899–904

59. Kuo EJ, Salem RR (2013) Population-level analysis of pancreatic neuroendocrine tumors 2 cm or less in size. Ann Surg Oncol 20(9):2815–2821

60. Halfdanarson TR, Rabe KG, Rubin J et al (2008) Pancreatic neuroendocrine tumors (PNETs): incidence, prognosis and recent trend toward improved survival. Ann Oncol 19(10):1727–1733

61. Jacobsen O, Bardram L, Rehfeld JF (1986) The requirement for gastrin measurements. Scand J Clin Lab Invest 46:423–426

62. Cullen RM, Ong CE (1987) Insulinoma in Auckland 1970–1985. N Z Med J 100:560–562

63. Service FJ, McMahon MM, O'Brien PC et al (1991) Functioning insulinoma – incidence, recurrence, and long-term survival of patients: a 60-year study. Mayo Clin Proc 66:711–719

64. Stamm B, Hacki WH, Klöppel et al (1991) Gastrin-producing tumors and the Zollinger-Ellison syndrome. In: Dayal EY (ed) Endocrine pathology of the gut and pancreas. CRC Press, Boca Raton, pp 155–194

65. Rindi G, Falconi M, Klersy C et al (2012) TNM staging of neoplasms of the endocrine pancreas: results from a large international cohort study. J Natl Cancer Inst 104(10):764–777

66. Soga J, Yakuwa Y (1994) Pancreatic endocrinomas: a statistical analysis of 1857 cases. J Hepatobiliary Pancreat Surg 1:522–529

67. Öberg K, Eriksson B (2005) Endocrine tumours of the pancreas. Best Pract Res Clin Gastroenterol 19:753–781

68. Soga J, Yakuwa Y (1998) The gastrinoma/Zollinger-Ellison syndrome: statistical evaluation of a Japanese series of 359 cases. J Hepatobiliary Pancreat Surg 5:77–85

69. Norton JA, Fraker DL, Alexander HR et al (1999) Surgery to cure the Zollinger-Ellison syndrome. N Engl J Med 341:635–644

70. Roy PK, Venzon DJ, Shojamanesh H et al (2000) Zollinger-Ellison syndrome. Clinical presentation in 261 patients. Medicine 79:379–411

71. Weber HC, Venzon DJ, Lin JT et al (1995) Determinants of metastatic rate and survival in patients with Zollinger-Ellison syndrome: a prospective long-term study. Gastroenterology 108(6):1637–1649

72. Kloppel G, Heitz PU (1988) Pancreatic endocrine tumors. Pathol Res Pract 183:155–168

73. Solcia E, Capella C, Klöppel G (1997) Tumors of the endocrine pancreas. In: Atlas of tumor pathology. Armed Forces Institute of Pathology, Washington, DC, pp 145–209

74. Harris GJ, Tio F, Cruz AB Jr (1987) Somatostatinoma: a case report and review of the literature. J Surg Oncol 36:8–16

75. Konomi K, Chijiiwa K, Katsuta T et al (1990) Pancreatic somatostatinoma: a case report and review of the literature. J Surg Oncol 43:259–265

76. Soga J, Yakuwa Y (1999) Somatostatinoma/inhibitory syndrome: a statistical evaluation of 173 reported cases as compared to other pancreatic endocrinomas. J Exp Clin Cancer Res 18:13–22

77. Smith SL, Branton SA, Avino AJ et al (1998) Vasoactive intestinal polypeptide secreting islet cell tumors: a 15-year experience and review of the literature. Surgery 124:1050–1055

78. Soga J, Yakuwa Y (1998) Vipoma/diarrheogenic syndrome: a statistical evaluation of 241 reported cases. J Exp Clin Cancer Res 17:389–400

79. Peng SY, Li JT, Liu YB et al (2004) Diagnosis and treatment of VIPoma in China: (case report and 31 cases review) diagnosis and treatment of VIPoma. Pancreas 28:93–97

80. Modlin IM, Lye KD, Kidd M (2003) A 5-decade analysis of 13,715 carcinoid tumors. Cancer 97(4): 934–959

81. Quaedvlieg PF, Visser O, Lamers CB et al (2001) Epidemiology and survival in patients with carcinoid disease in The Netherlands. An epidemiological study with 2391 patients. Ann Oncol 12(9):1295–1300

82. La Rosa S, Franzi F, Albarello L et al (2011) Serotonin-producing enterochromaffin cell tumors of the pancreas: clinicopathologic study of 15 cases and comparison with intestinal enterochromaffin cell tumors. Pancreas 40(6):883–895

83. Maragliano R, Vanoli A, Albarello L et al (2015) ACTH-secreting pancreatic neoplasms associated with cushing syndrome: clinicopathologic study of 11 cases and review of the literature. Am J Surg Pathol 39(3):374–382

84. Schneider R, Waldmann J, Swaid Z et al (2011) Calcitonin-secreting pancreatic endocrine tumors: systematic analysis of a rare tumor entity. Pancreas 40(2):213–221

85. Stringer MD, Ahmadj O (2009) Famous discoveries by medical students. ANZ J Surg 79:901–908

86. Lefèbvre PJ (2011) Early milestones in glucagon research. Diabetes Obes Metab 13(Suppl 1):1–4

Radiological Diagnosis of Pancreatic Neuroendocrine Neoplasms

2

Carlo Fugazzola, Maria Gloria Angeretti,
Natalie Lucchina, Ejona Duka, Valeria Molinelli,
and Fausto Sessa

2.1 Introduction

Neuroendocrine tumors (NETs) account for 1–2 % of all pancreatic neoplasms [1]; clinically they can be divided in functioning and nonfunctioning tumors. With the increased use of imaging and improved techniques, nonfunctioning NETs now account for approximately one-half of all NETs [1, 2].

In relation to their functional state, NETs can pose peculiar problems for imaging techniques. Indeed, in *functioning NETs* – in which the diagnosis is mainly based on clinical and laboratory findings – the primary imaging "goal" is the *localization* of the hormonal hypersecretion source/sources. On the contrary, in *nonfunctioning NETs* – which appear as symptomatic masses or as incidental findings – the priority questions for imaging are represented both by the *identification* and correct *histological typing*; in particular it is important to distinguish them from ductal pancreatic adenocarcinoma, because of a more

favorable prognosis of NETs. For all NETs – regardless of their functional state – an accurate *staging* and an appropriate *follow-up* are also required, as they are often malignant.

2.2 Pathologic Features

The gross appearance of NETs varies with size, ranging from smaller than 1 cm to larger than 20 cm, with most tumors being 1–5 cm in diameter [3]. Small NETs often present as solid, well-circumscribed masses with rounded appearance or lobulated borders; they are often richly vascular with a poor stromal component and tend to respect the adjacent anatomical structures, which are compressed rather than invaded [4]. More rarely, they present a highly abundant fibrotic stroma, which endows the tumor with an invasive behavior and indistinct margins: this type – albeit the small size – can obstruct the Wirsung duct, causing marked duct dilatation and onset of chronic obstructive pancreatitis [4]. Although cystic changes secondary to bleeding and/or necrosis are quite frequent in large solid NETs, true cystic NETs are rare [5].

Predicting biological behavior on the basis of the histological profile is difficult; moreover, unequivocal signs of malignancy include the invasion of surrounding organs and the presence

C. Fugazzola (✉) • M.G. Angeretti • N. Lucchina
E. Duka • V. Molinelli
Department of Radiology, University Hospital,
Varese, Italy
e-mail: carlo.fugazzola@uninsubria.it

F. Sessa
Department of Pathology, University Hospital,
Varese, Italy

S. La Rosa, F. Sessa (eds.), *Pancreatic Neuroendocrine Neoplasms: Practical Approach to Diagnosis,*
Classification, and Therapy, DOI 10.1007/978-3-319-17235-4_2,
© Springer International Publishing Switzerland 2015

of nodal, hepatic, and distant metastases [4]. Since the majority of these tumors – at the time of diagnosis – is locally confined and does not present with metastases, the World Health Organization (WHO) has proposed a classification more compliant with the prognosis, which considers three different categories [6, 7]: (1) grade 1 (G1) NET, (2) G2 NET, and (3) G3 neuroendocrine carcinoma (NEC).

2.3 Functioning Pancreatic Neuroendocrine Tumors (F-PanNETs)

The imaging modalities available for the detection of F-PanNETs are many and can be divided in four levels, depending on availability, cost, and invasiveness: first level (ultrasound, computed tomography), second level (magnetic resonance; nuclear medicine techniques), third level (echoendoscopy; stimulated venous sampling), and fourth level (intraoperative or laparoscopic ultrasound) [8].

The most common F-PanNETs (insulinoma and gastrinoma) are usually small (in particular insulinomas are smaller than 2 cm in diameter in 90 % of cases and in 40 % of cases smaller than 1 cm) [9]; the other histotypes (somatostatinoma, VIPoma, glucagonoma, carcinoid, etc.) are rarer and generally have larger size at diagnosis. Sporadic lesions are usually single, while multifocal lesions are more frequent in familial polyendocrine syndromes: indeed, gastrinomas are the most common F-PanNETs in patients with MEN-1 (20–25 % of all gastrinomas occur in these patients) [3].

Virtually all insulinomas are intrapancreatic and equally distributed throughout the gland; glucagonomas and VIPomas are mainly intrapancreatic (glucagonomas usually are located at the body or tail [3]; VIPomas most frequently are found in the tail [10]). On the contrary, gastrinomas and somatostatinomas have intrapancreatic or extrapancreatic location. Gastrinomas often arise in the "gastrinoma triangle" and in particular in the duodenum (about 80 % of sporadic lesions and 90 % of lesions associated

with MEN-1 [11]); somatostatinomas often occur in the duodenum, near the ampulla of Vater [12].

2.3.1 First-Level Methods: Ultrasound (US)

Small F-PanNETs appear as well-circumscribed round or oval hypoechoic masses with smooth margins (Fig. 2.1); rarely they may be hyperechoic or isoechoic with a hyperechoic peripheric rim [13]. The sensitivity of US is high (85–95 %) only for the detection of rare histotypes which usually are large, while for the most common histotypes, it is around 50 %, with a variable range from 19 to 40 % for gastrinomas and 25–64 % for insulinomas [8, 14–16].

Tumors may be heterogeneous or homogeneous, and when contrast material (CM) is administered, they demonstrate usually a hypervascular pattern [2, 17]. The advent of US contrast agents has not improved the detection of the F-PanNETs, so that it is used only for their characterization [18] (see paragraph on nonfunctioning PanNETs).

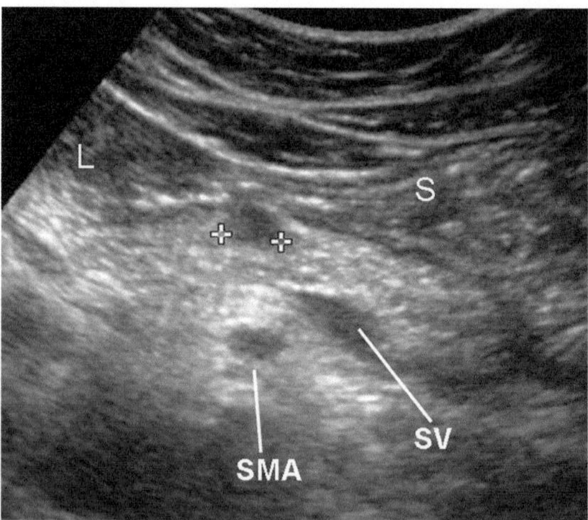

Fig. 2.1 Functioning PanNETs US. Small insulinoma of pancreatic body. Axial scan: hypoechoic mass (*calipers*) with smooth margins and about 1 cm in diameter, located at the anterior border of the pancreatic body. Liver (*L*); stomach (*S*); splenic vein (*SV*); superior mesenteric artery (*SMA*)

2.3.2 First-Level Methods: Multidetector Computed Tomography (MDCT)

MDCT, with and without IV injection of iodinated CM, is the most widely used imaging modality for diagnosing F-PanNETs [19]. Being usually hypervascular (see paragraph on pathologic features), F-PanNETs appear as round or oval masses with smooth margins, hyperattenuating in "pancreatic" parenchymal phase images (about 30 s after IV CM injection); the densitometric gradient between tumor and normal parenchyma is generally maximum in this phase, in which the tumor has the highest conspicuity [20]; in venous phase images (about 60–70 s after IV injection of CM), generally the attenuation of both the tumor and normal parenchyma decreases, so that the lesion is less visible [4] (Fig. 2.2a, b).

Tumors presenting a prevalent stromal component, with fibrohyaline structure and amyloid deposits, display iso-hypoattenuation in pancreatic phase and greater attenuation in venous phase [4] (Fig. 2.2c, d). Small cystic F-PanNETs appear hypoattenuating in pre-contrastographic and post-contrastographic phases; in venous portal phase cystic tumors are sometimes delimited by a hyperattenuating peripheral rim [21]. Large F-PanNETs

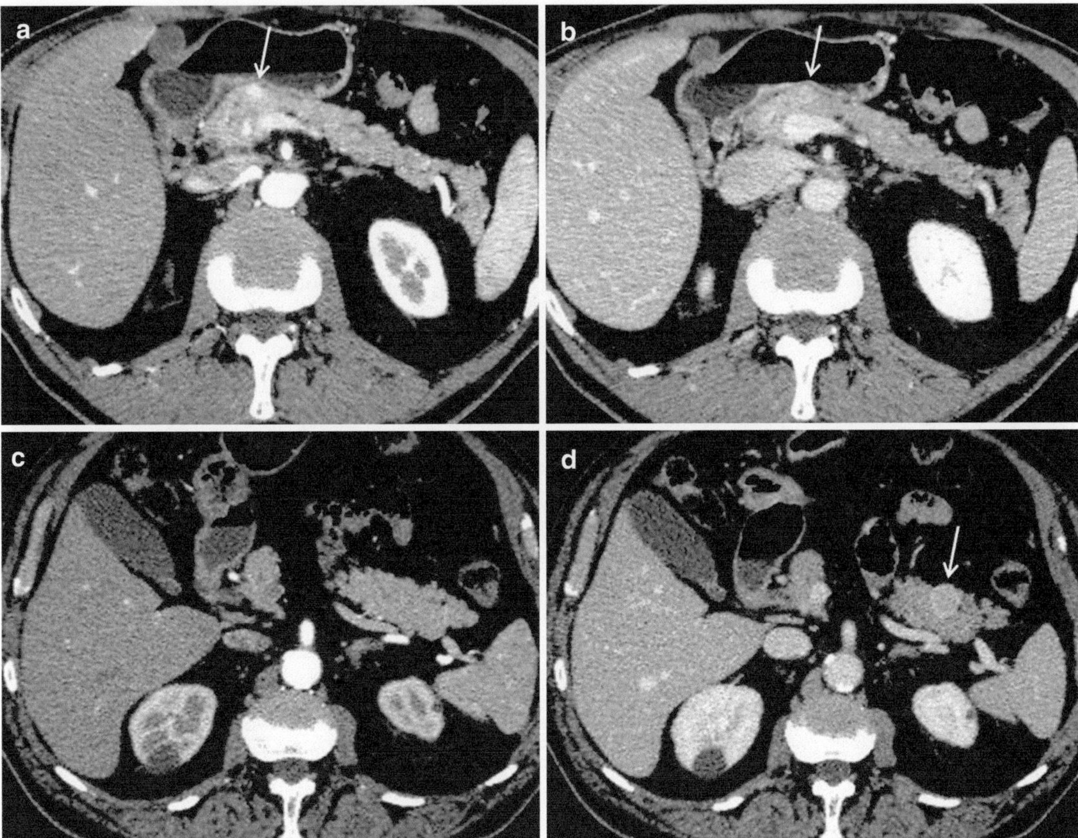

Fig. 2.2 Functioning PanNETs CT. (**a**, **b**) Small insulinoma of the pancreatic body (same case as Fig. 2.1). Round mass with smooth margins, located at the anterior border of the pancreatic body (*arrow*); the tumor, with a poor stromal component, is hyperattenuating both in pancreatic (**a**) and portal venous (**b**) phases; moreover, it presents the highest conspicuity in pancreatic phase. (**c**, **d**) Small glucagon-secretin tumor of the pancreatic tail. Round mass with smooth margins and about 1.5 cm in diameter, located at the anterior border of the pancreatic tail. The tumor, with a prevalent stromal component, is isodense in pancreatic phase (**c**) and hyperdense in portal venous phase (**d**), so it is visible only in the latter phase (*arrow*)

(diameter of more than 3 cm) usually demonstrate heterogeneous enhancement, due to cystic degeneration, necrosis, and hemorrhage; these tumors may present also fibrosis and calcifications [16].

At present it is well known that the pancreatic phase is the most sensitive for the detection of small F-PanNETs [14, 22] (Fig. 2.2a); it is equally known that the study of the pancreas should always be carried out also in the venous phase, because – as mentioned above – some lesions may be seen only on venous phase imaging [3] (Fig. 2.2d).

The CT detection rate of F-PanNETs has improved over time, together with the technological evolution (sequential CT, 28.6 %; helical CT, 57.1 %; MDCT, 94.4 % [20]); another study, carried on partially using MDCT, reports a prospective sensitivity of 63 % and a retrospective sensitivity of 83 % [14]. More recent studies, carried on using exclusively MDCT, report a detection rate of 77–89 % [23–26]. Even better results seem to be obtained with the most recent technological developments: in a study comparing MDCT and dual-energy spectral CT, the sensitivity of the former was 68.8 %, while that of the latter was 95.7 % [27].

With regard to the discrimination between benign and malignant tumors, malignant PanNETs are often larger, predominantly hypo-

vascular and with intratumoral calcifications (see paragraph on nonfunctioning PanNETs); in some cases peripancreatic vessels or bowel invasion, as well as lymph node or liver metastases, are observed [28].

2.3.3 Second-Level Methods: Magnetic Resonance Imaging (MRI)

The main indication of MRI is to localize a suspected lesion that has not been demonstrated by US and/or CT [19]. The tumors usually appear of low signal intensity on T_1-w sequences and high on T_2-w sequences relative to the normal pancreas; they are most conspicuous on fat-suppressed T_1-w and T_2-w sequences. Following IV injection of gadolinium, there is often a characteristic marked homogeneous enhancement, reflecting their highly vascular nature [19, 29]. Moreover, PanNETs have a quite broad spectrum of appearances [30]: as on CT, larger neoplasms tend to demonstrate more heterogeneous signal intensity and enhancement patterns [19]; rim enhancement may be seen in cystic lesions [31] (Fig. 2.3a, b); tumors which contain a high content of collagen or fibrous tissue may return a low signal on T_2-w images [32].

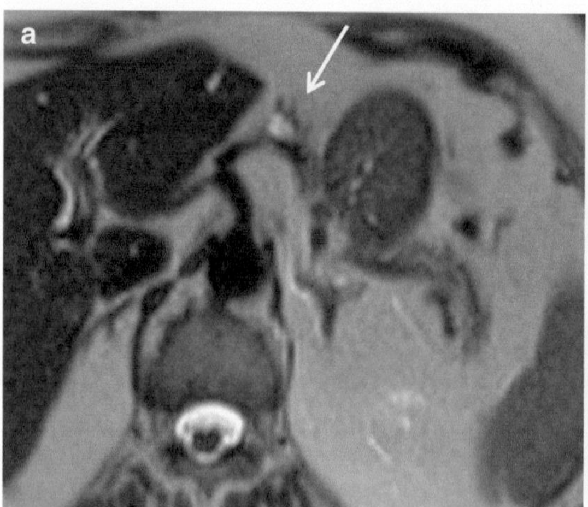
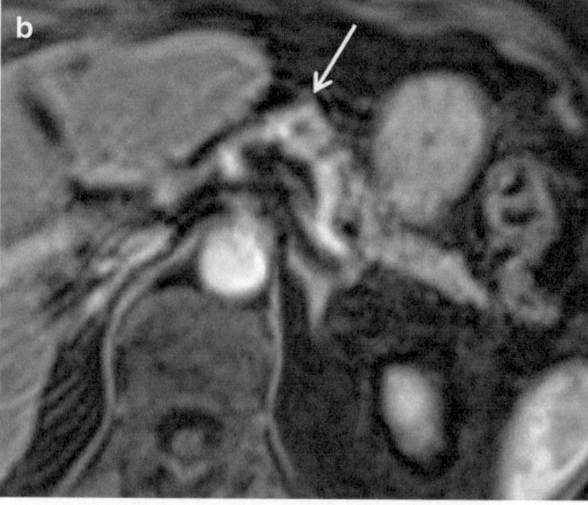
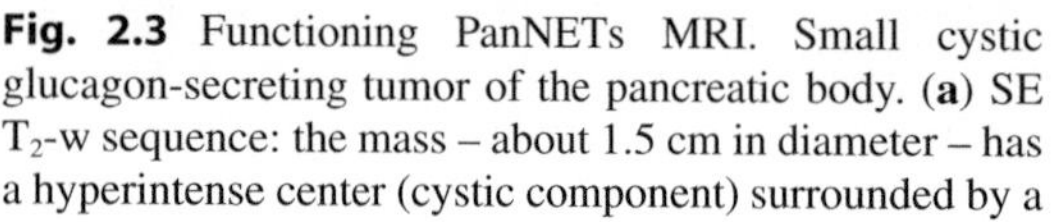

Fig. 2.3 Functioning PanNETs MRI. Small cystic glucagon-secreting tumor of the pancreatic body. (**a**) SE T_2-w sequence: the mass – about 1.5 cm in diameter – has a hyperintense center (cystic component) surrounded by a hypointense rim (*arrow*). (**b**) GRE T_1-w sequence after IV injection of gadolinium: the hypointense center (cystic component) is surrounded by an enhancing rim (*arrow*)

T_2-w sequences (Fig. 2.3a) and T_1-w in the arterial phase after CM (Fig. 2.3b) are the optimal pulse sequences: indeed hypervascular tumors are best depicted on the T_2-w, whereas hypovascular tumors are best depicted on the T_1-w sequence in the arterial phase [33].

The diagnostic performance of MRI has improved over time, showing now a sensitivity of up to 94–95 %, although sensitivity drops for extrapancreatic lesions [31, 33, 34]. As with CT, tumor detection increases with tumor size; moreover, multiple small tumors – as in patients with MEN-1 – are particularly difficult to identify [19].

Diffusion-weighted imaging (DWI) can be added to routine MRI protocol to detect the lesions in a limited number of patients with negative or doubtful imaging findings [35–38].

2.3.4 Second-Level Methods: Hybrid Techniques

As techniques of nuclear medicine are discussed in Chap. 3, we will only mention *hybrid techniques* and, in particular, PET-CT, since nowadays PET-CT scans routinely come with 8-, 16-, or even 64-slice capability, providing the same anatomic imaging capabilities of stand-alone CT scanners. In recent years, research has shown the value of contrast-enhanced CT examinations as part of PET-CT protocols, as multiphase CT and PET deliver highly synergistic information [39–41].

PET-CT with ^{68}Ga-labeled somatostatin analogues is not only more sensitive for the detection of well-differentiated PanNET lesions compared to SPECT-CT, due to its major spatial resolution [42, 43], but it is also more sensitive than morphological imaging of both first level and second level [37, 42, 43].

2.3.5 Third-Level Methods: Endoscopic Ultrasonography (EUS)

The high spatial resolution of this technique allows the detection of very small lesions and their precise anatomical localization [44]. The EUS characteristics of PanNETs are in most cases represented by a homogeneous echo pattern, often hypoechogenic, rarely nonhomogeneous with cystic or calcified areas, while margins are clear in the majority of cases, sometimes having a hyperechogenic border [45] (Fig. 2.4).

As concerns insulinoma, an overall detection rate of around 80 % (range between 57 and 94 %) is reported. Detection rate of lesions in the head and body is high (83–100 %), whereas detection of tumors in the tail ranges between 37 and 60 % [44]. As regards gastrinoma, duodenal lesions are more difficult to detect than pancreatic tumors: so, reported EUS detection rate varies between 40 and 100 %, with a mean of 67 % [44]. In particular, the sensitivity for the detection of pancreatic gastrinomas is between 75 and 94 %, and for peripancreatic lymph nodes it is between 58 and 82 %, while it drops to 11–50 % for tumors located in the duodenal wall [44, 45]. Finally, as concerns *MEN-1*, the identification of tumors is challenging, as many lesions are small and they are frequently multiple [46]; however, EUS is more sensitive than transabdominal US or CT in this respect [47].

Other works underscore the superior sensitivity of EUS for the detection of F-PanNETs compared to noninvasive morphological

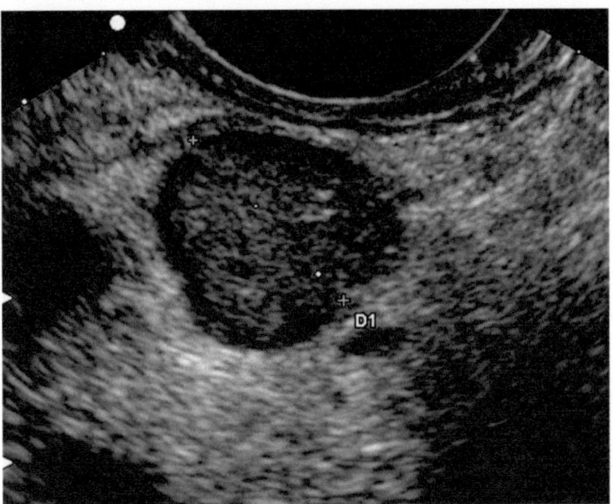

Fig. 2.4 Functioning PanNETs small EUS (Courtesy of Mario Montanari MD, Gastroenterology Unit, University Hospital of Varese) small insulinoma of the pancreatic body. Scan performed by probe located in the gastric body: hypoechoic mass (*calipers*) with smooth margins and about 1.9 cm in diameter

techniques [48–50]. These data are confirmed by a recent systematic review and meta-analysis, which, selecting 13 studies performed between 1992 and 2004, reported a pooled sensitivity of 87.2 % and a pooled specificity of 98 %. In particular, pooled sensitivity of EUS in detecting insulinomas was 87.5 % and pooled specificity 97.4 %, while pooled sensitivity in detecting gastrinomas was 84.5 % and pooled specificity 95.3 % [51]. Furthermore, EUS leads to the anatomically correct region of PanNETs and makes it possible to determine an appropriate excision range (enucleation vs resection), assessing the distance between the tumor and the main pancreatic duct [50].

2.3.6 Third-Level Methods: Arterial Stimulation Venous Sampling (ASVS)

Visceral angiography combined with ASVS is a highly sensitive investigation for the detection of small insulinomas and gastrinomas, which may prove difficult to localize by cross-sectional imaging modalities, despite the advances made in recent years [52]. When injected into the vessel supplying a functioning tumor, both calcium gluconate and secretin produce a release of insulin or gastrin into the portal venous system, resulting in a detectable rise in hormone level in venous samples obtained from the hepatic veins; the splenic, gastroduodenal, and superior mesenteric arteries are the vessels most commonly studied [52].

The large majority of reports on ASVS are limited to case studies or small series, which demonstrate a sensitivity of about 90 % for insulinomas and of 77–100 % for gastrinomas [52]. Moreover, in a recent paper encompassing 45 patients with insulinomas from 1996 to 2008, ASVS localized the tumors to the correct anatomical regions in 84 % of patients [53]; in the same institution, in the previous period 1989–1996, the method showed a sensitivity of 94 %, so that the overall sensitivity from 1989 to 2008 was 89 % [53].

2.3.7 Third-Level Methods: EUS vs ASVS

The published localization sensitivity of EUS for insulinoma is a little lower than that of ASVS. Furthermore, the ASVS detection rate was equal for head/neck (82 %) and body/tail lesions (88 %), while sensitivity of EUS for pancreatic tail tumors is lower; furthermore, EUS does not provide functional information, and pancreatic nodularities occasionally mistaken for insulinomas have been reported to affect the specificity of the test [54].

However, EUS is currently the localization test of choice in most Western centers [55], as it is less invasive than ASVS. It is also important to bear in mind that, although EUS is less successful in detecting tumors in the pancreatic tail, its sensitivity is excellent especially when used in combination with CT or MRI, whereby it has been reported to approach 100 % [20, 56].

2.3.8 Fourth-Level Methods: Intraoperative Ultrasonography (IOUS)

Currently, in view of the technological improvements of noninvasive methods and the availability of third-level invasive modalities, very few cases of occult F-PanNETs may still be encountered [56–58]. In fact, a diagnostic protocol providing a careful preoperative localization is usually applied, because it is known that some tumors – correctly located at the pancreatic tail by ASVS – may not be detected intraoperatively [55]. This approach may not be the most cost-effective, as it leads to an increase in the number of "unnecessary" tests. However, this may be a small price to pay for the patients in avoiding the need for a reoperation [55].

Moreover, ASVS has some limits in localizing tumors in the body of the pancreas [59]. Therefore, IOUS can still play a critical role in the identification of occult insulinomas [57], allowing detection in 95 % of the tumors [59]. In particular, IOUS is complementary to intraoperative exploration [60, 61], together with which – as shown in three recent studies – it has demonstrated a sensitivity of 88–92 % [55, 56, 62]. The method can detect small lesions in the pancreatic head parenchyma that are not palpable [61]; it is also able to provide an accurate assessment of the tumor's relationship with the adjacent structures (in particular the Wirsung duct), which can affect the choice of the best surgical technique [55, 62]. Furthermore, IOUS is helpful in patients with MEN-1 syndrome, because of the presence of multiple tumors of less than 1 cm that are not palpable [63].

Preoperative localization may become more important in the era of laparoscopic surgery [53], which is increasingly used to treat insulinomas [64], as the main disadvantage of this surgical technique is the loss of tactile sensation [65].

2.4 Nonfunctioning Pancreatic Neuroendocrine Tumors (NF-PanNETs)

Usually noninvasive imaging modalities easily identify the symptomatic NF-PanNETs, which often have significant size; moreover, as the use of high-quality cross-sectional imaging is becoming more widespread, incidental detection of small NF-PanNETs, real pancreatic "incidentalomas," is increasingly more frequent [6].

Regarding the histological characterization, the distinction from ductal adenocarcinoma is generally easy, because NF-PanNETs, as the functioning ones, are often hypervascular, and therefore they assume the CM. This justifies their hyperechogenicity in contrast-enhanced US [17, 18] and EUS [66] (Fig. 2.5a, b), their hyperdensity in contrast-enhanced CT [67] (Fig. 2.5c), and their high signal intensity on contrast-enhanced MRI [30] (Fig. 2.5d). Large tumors (diameter >3 cm) have inhomogeneous enhancement; it has to be emphasized that solid neoplasms measuring 3 cm or larger are commonly non-benign; however, about 30 % of tumors smaller than this size cutoff can be malignant [68].

Isovascular and hypovascular variants [69], as well as cystic lesions [70] (Fig. 2.5c, d), are more frequent than in F-PanNETs. In particular, cystic PanNETs were classically considered very rare [5]; however, recent published studies suggest that cystic PanNETs may be more common (17–17.8 %) than previously thought [70, 71].

A distinctive feature, reported in a recently published series [72], is the presence of venous tumor thrombus arising from malignant NF-PanNETs and growing into adjacent veins; another distinctive and unusual pattern of spread is intraductal growth: these findings are different from both the more common venous occlusion and ductal obstruction that can be seen in adenocarcinomas and NETs.

NF-PanNETs must be differentiated from multiple pancreatic and peripancreatic lesions [73–75]: in particular, hypervascular tumors should be distinguished from pancreatic metastases [76], acinar cell carcinoma [77], serous adenoma (solid type [78]), exophytic gastrointestinal stromal tumors [79], parapancreatic Castleman disease [80], and intrapancreatic accessory spleen [81, 82]. On the other hand, hypovascular NF-PanNETs should be distinguished from solid pseudopapillary tumors (SPTs) [74]; in particular, discrimination from small SPTs is difficult [83]. Finally, cystic tumors with a solid component that takes up intensively CM can be easily characterized (Fig. 2.5c, d); on the contrary almost completely cystic PanNETs are not specific in appearance and are impossible to differentiate from other cystic masses [70, 84].

Recent literature has tried to correlate some imaging findings (especially the post-contrast enhancement pattern) of both nonfunctioning and functioning PanNETs with the degree of cell differentiation, in particular by referring to the Ki-67 value. A recent paper reported that enhancement of tumors on CT decreases with higher tumor grading [85]. Other studies have shown an inverse correlation between the degree of enhancement on CT and value of Ki-67, with a qualitative [69, 86] or quantitative assessment [87]. At the same time a direct correlation between enhancement, "tumor blood flow"

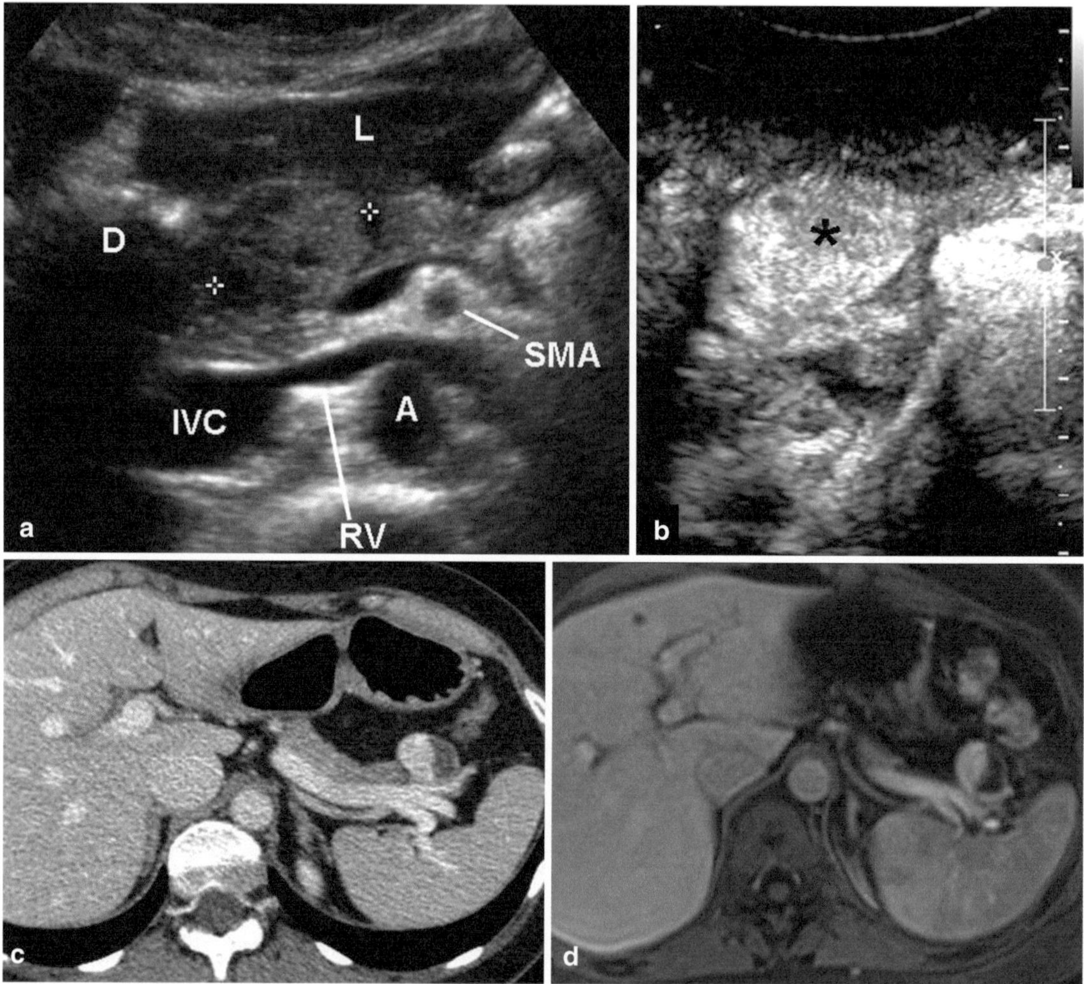

Fig. 2.5 Nonfunctioning PanNETs US, CT, MRI. (**a, b**) Solid tumor of the pancreatic head. US B-mode, axial scan (**a**): round mass, isoechoic vs normal parenchyma, about 2.5 cm in diameter. Liver (*L*); duodenum (*D*); superior mesenteric artery (*SMA*); aorta (*A*); renal vein (*RV*); inferior vena cava (*IVC*). The tumor, after IV injection of contrast medium (**b**), becomes hyperechoic (*asterisk*) because of its rich vascularization. (**c, d**) Cystic tumor of the pancreatic tail. CT, portal venous phase (**c**), shows a round mass, anterior to the splenic vein, about 3 cm in diameter; the medial solid component is hyperdense, while the lateral cystic one does not present contrast enhancement. MRI after IV injection of gadolinium, portal venous phase (**d**): similar enhancing pattern of the mass, which is partly hyperintense and partly hypointense

(evaluated by perfusion CT), and microvascular density (MVD) has been reported [87]. It is known that tumor angiogenesis – generally assessed by calculating MVD – is a prognostic indicator in several types of cancers: the presence of high intratumoral MVD has been correlated with local invasion and presence of metastases. Interestingly, angiogenesis is prominent in PanNETs, but the relationship between intratumoral MVD and tumor prognosis seems to be the opposite of that seen in other types of tumors [87]. Indeed, patients affected by hypovascular tumors showed a worse prognosis (5-year survival of 54 %) than those with isovascular or hypervascular tumors (survival, respectively, of 89 and 93 % at 5 years) [69].

Also intratumoral calcifications have a negative prognostic significance: this information – available preoperatively by MDCT – can support the routine dissection of regional lymph nodes through formal pancreatectomy rather than enucleation in calcified PanNETs [88].

As concerns MR-DWI, a recent contribution has demonstrated that PanNETs with different grade of differentiation have varying apparent diffusion coefficient (ADC) values. Tumor cellularity, ratio of nuclei and cytoplasm, and extracellular fibrosis may account for the variety of ADC values; ADCs correlate well with Ki-67 labeling index and may help to predict growth of PanNETs [89]. However, future studies allowing for larger patient populations are recommended to further evaluate the role of DWI in predicting the histopathology of NETs [89].

Therefore, NF-PanNETs often require *fine-needle aspiration biopsy* (*FNAB*) to establish a definitive diagnosis, because not only their appearance overlaps that of other pancreatic lesions [75], but also their imaging findings according to WHO classification are overlapped [90]. In particular, EUS-guided FNAB has a high accuracy for diagnosing PanNETs (71–91 %), as regards both cystic and solid tumors [48, 91, 92].

2.5 Staging of Pancreatic Neuroendocrine Tumors

The modified ENETS (European Neuroendocrine Tumor Society)-TNM system predicts survival based on the stage of the disease: the 5-year survival is almost 100 % for stage I (tumors <2 cm, restricted to the pancreas), 93 % for stage II (tumors >2 cm but still restricted to the pancreas), 65 % for stage III (tumors invading adjacent structures or with positive lymph nodes), and 35 % for stage IV (metastatic disease) [93]. Using the AJCC TNM classification, the 5-year overall survival rates for stage I, II, III, and IV tumors were 92 %, 84 %, 81 %, and 57 %, respectively [94].

Locoregional staging by CT or MRI should comprise a description of PanNET size, position within the pancreas, and its relation to the pancreatic duct and to the main bile duct. The relation of the PanNET to the superior mesenteric vessels, splenic vessels, and portal vein needs to be described, as should any vascular encasement [95] (Fig. 2.6a, b). In particular, MDCT seems to perform better than MRI in assessing vascular involvement [96].

As concerns *peripancreatic lymph node metastases*, they tend to resemble the primary tumor, with prominent enhancement typically seen [30] (Fig. 2.6c, d).

As regards *liver metastases*, they also are often hypervascular; however, hypovascular lesions are not infrequent [97]; sometimes a mixture of hypo- and hypervascular metastases may be seen in the same patient [95] (Fig. 2.7a, b). The sensitivity of CT to detect PanNET liver metastases is mean 82 % (range: 78–100 %), whereas the specificity is mean 92 % (range: 83–100 %) [98]. A comparison of CT, MRI, and somatostatin receptor scintigraphy (SRS) for detection of liver metastases showed 79 %, 95 %, and 49 % sensitivity for the respective methods [99]. In particular, MRI with hepatocyte-specific contrast agents is superior to CT [97], while the sensitivity of SRS with Octreoscan is low. However, PET-CT with a number of new tracers (^{68}Ga-labeled somatostatin analogues) has shown better detection rates than SRS with Octreoscan, because of the intrinsically better properties of PET tracers, which result in greater spatial resolution and less noise [97].

Contrast-enhanced ultrasonography (CEUS) also is sensitive for detection of metastases, and lesions less than 5 mm may be visualized [100]; therefore, for patients in whom liver metastases are difficult to depict at CT or in order to decrease the radiation dose in young patients, CEUS may be considered as an alternative to MRI [95].

As concerns *extrahepatic metastases*, contrast-enhanced MDCT of the thorax, abdomen, and pelvis can be used [101]; additional imaging with other modalities such as MRI of the spine may be necessary for characterization of nonspecific abnormalities identified on CT. Nevertheless, PET-CT with ^{68}Ga-labeled somatostatin analogues is the preferable modality, not only for its high sensitivity (see paragraph on hybrid techniques) but also for determining the likelihood that patients will respond to therapy with radiolabeled somatostatin analogues [97].

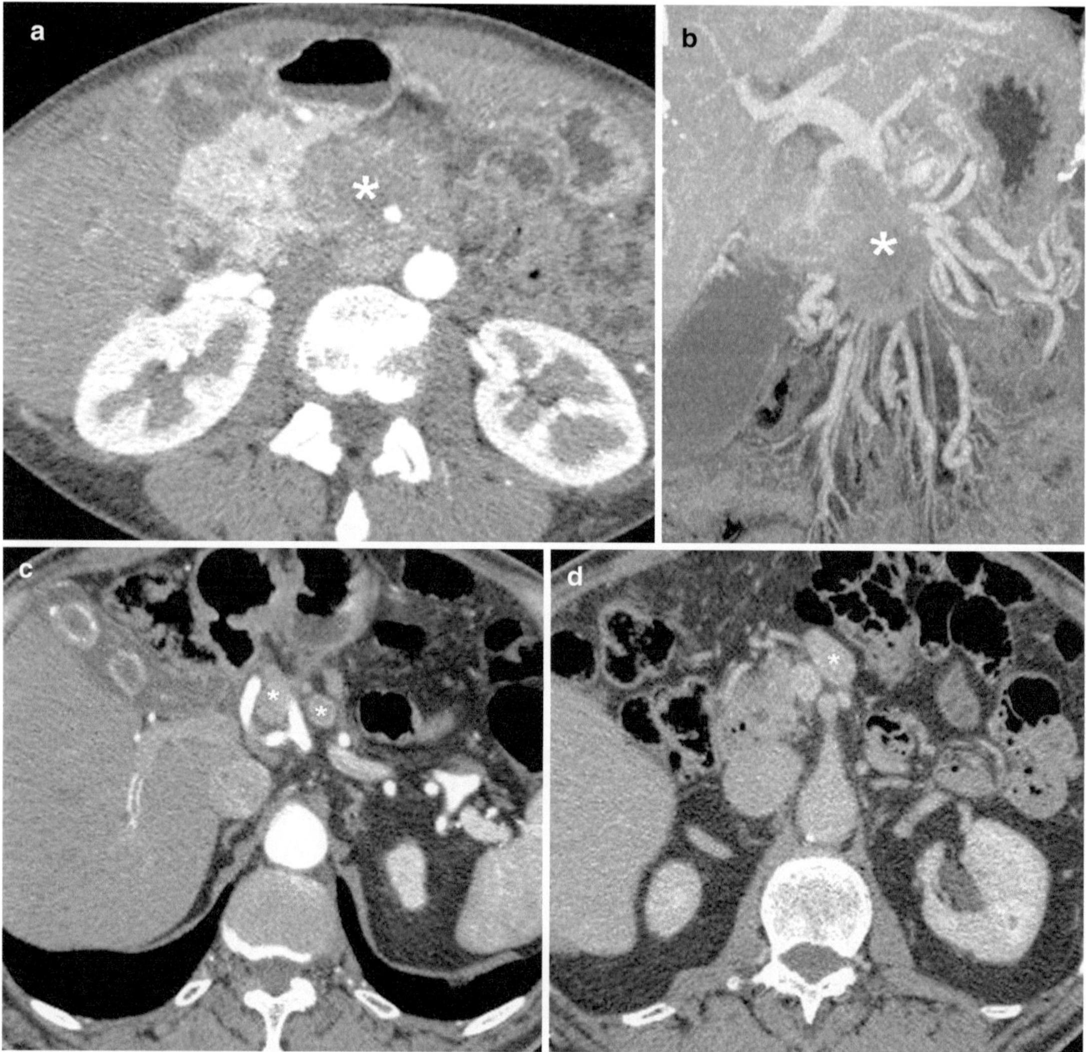

Fig. 2.6 Pancreatic NETs. Staging. (**a, b**) Involvement of peripancreatic vessels. CT (pancreatic phase), axial plan (**a**): a large hypovascular mass (*asterisk*) encases the superior mesenteric artery. CT (portal venous phase), coronal plane (**b**): the tumor (*asterisk*) obstructs the trunk of the superior mesenteric vein, involving also the portal carrefour. (**c, d**) Lymph node metastases. CT: hyperdense lesions (*asterisks*) in lymph nodes between celiac axis branches (**c**: pancreatic phase) and in lymph nodes located in front of the mesenteric vessels (**d** portal venous phase)

2.6   Monitoring of Therapy

After surgery with curative intent, surveillance of the patients is generally lifelong, because recurrences may be seen after many years. For monitoring PanNET therapy, CT or MRI every 3–6 months is generally appropriate in low-grade tumors and after the first year every 6 months. PET-CT is indicated after 1 or 2 years and when results of radiological modalities, biochemistry, and the patient's clinical status are conflicting [95].

Some of the characteristic features of PanNET disease make image monitoring of therapy problematic. In particular, detection and size measurement of hypervascular liver metastases require a constant CT/MRI protocol, because increase in lesion size and even appearance of new lesions or the reverse – a decrease in size and disappearance of lesions – may sometimes

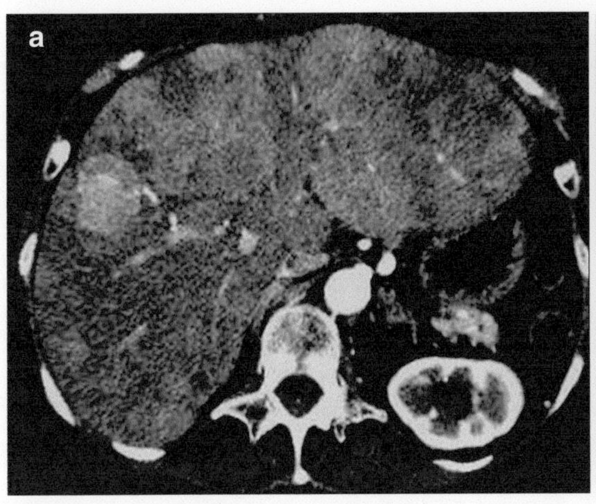
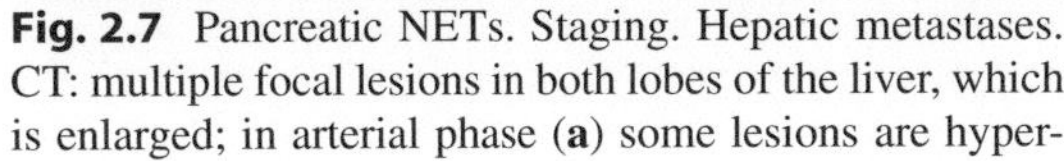
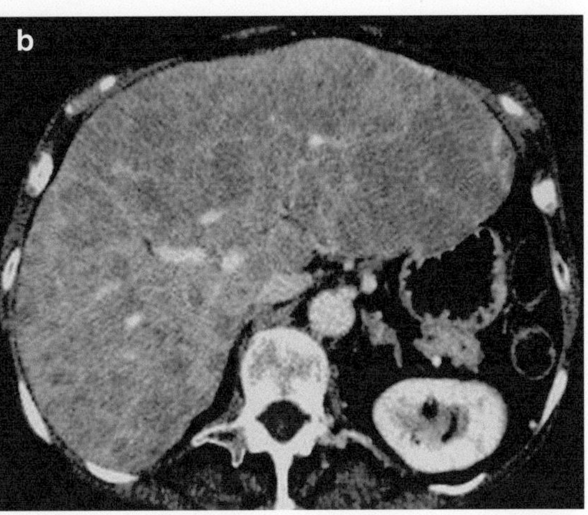

Fig. 2.7 Pancreatic NETs. Staging. Hepatic metastases. CT: multiple focal lesions in both lobes of the liver, which is enlarged; in arterial phase (**a**) some lesions are hyper- dense, while the majority are hypodense; the diffuse meta- static involvement is confirmed in portal venous phase (**b**)

only depend on differences in examination technique [95].

Furthermore, the response evaluation criteria in solid tumors (RECIST) – applied to common cancers, which are of generally high proliferative activity and have a measurable size response to chemotherapy – are not optimal for monitoring PanNETs, because the majority are low-grade and slow-growing tumors [95], so the patient outcome may not correlate with significant changes in tumor size [102].

Novel functional imaging techniques, which have the potential to measure changes in tumor physiology and metabolism, are now available; they include PET-CT with ^{68}Ga-labeled somatostatin analogues, molecular imaging with PET tracers that are not based on somatostatin receptor targeting, as well as dynamic contrast-enhanced CT/MRI and MR-DWI. However, the role of these techniques in monitoring treatment response requires further evaluation [102].

2.7 Conclusions

Actually, the basic modality for PanNET imaging is MDCT for both diagnosis and staging; although MRI is generally superior to CT for liver metastasis detection because of its high soft

tissue image contrast, the choice between the methods depends on the local availability and expertise.

Imaging techniques have an important role also in the follow-up of patients affected by PanNETs, for both diagnosis of recurrent disease and therapy monitoring. In this respect, it has to be stressed that the RECIST criteria, which were designed for general oncology, are less suited for PanNETs; so new criteria, which take the special characteristics of PanNETs into account, are currently under development.

Acknowledgment The authors wish to thank Miss Luisa Rinaldi (Department of Surgical and Morphological Sciences; University of Insubria, Varese) for her assistance in the preparation of this manuscript.

References

1. Hruban RH, Pitman MB, Klimstra DS (2007) Tumors of the pancreas. AFIP atlas of tumor pathology, 4th edn. American Registry of Pathology, Armed Forces Institute of Pathology, Washington, DC
2. Malagò R, D'Onofrio M, Zamboni GA et al (2009) Contrast-enhanced sonography of nonfunctioning pancreatic neuroendocrine tumors. AJR Am J Roentgenol 192(2):424–430
3. Lewis RB, Lattin GE Jr, Paal E (2010) Pancreatic endocrine tumors: radiologic-clinicopathologic correlation. Radiographics 30(6):1445–1464

4. Graziani R, Brandalise A, Bellotti M et al (2010) Imaging of neuroendocrine gastroenteropancreatic tumours. Radiol Med 115(7):1047–1064

5. Ligneau B, Lombard-Bohas C, Partensky C et al (2001) Cystic endocrine tumors of the pancreas: clinical, radiologic, and histopathologic features in 13 cases. Am J Surg Pathol 25(6):752–760

6. Zárate X, Williams N, Herrera MF (2012) Pancreatic incidentalomas. Best Pract Res Clin Endocrinol Metab 26(1):97–103

7. Rindi G, Arnold R, Bosman FT et al (2010) Nomenclature and classification of neuroendocrine neoplasms of the digestive system. In: Bosman FT, Carneiro F, Hruban RH, Theise ND (eds) WHO classification of tumours of the digestive system. IARC Press, Lyon, pp 13–14

8. Fugazzola C (2002) Ecotomografia pancreatica. In: Bazzocchi M (ed) Ecografia, vol 2. Idelson-Gnocchi, Napoli, pp 589–639

9. Mansour JC, Chen H (2004) Pancreatic endocrine tumors. J Surg Res 120(1):139–161

10. Soga J, Yakuwa Y (1998) Vipoma/diarrheogenic syndrome: a statistical evaluation of 241 reported cases. J Exp Clin Cancer Res 17(4):389–400

11. Klöppel G, Anlauf M (2006) Pancreatic endocrine tumors. Pathol Case Rev 11(6):256–267

12. Soga J, Yakuwa Y (1999) Somatostatinoma/inhibitory syndrome: a statistical evaluation of 173 reported cases as compared to other pancreatic endocrinomas. J Exp Clin Cancer Res 18(1):13–22

13. Gorman B, Charboneau JW, James EM et al (1986) Benign pancreatic insulinoma: preoperative and intraoperative sonographic localization. AJR Am J Roentgenol 147(5):929–934

14. Fidler JL, Fletcher JG, Reading CC et al (2003) Preoperative detection of pancreatic insulinomas on multiphasic helical CT. AJR Am J Roentgenol 181(3):775–780

15. Pitre J, Soubrane O, Palazzo L et al (1996) Endoscopic ultrasonography for the preoperative localization of insulinomas. Pancreas 13(1):55–60

16. Buetow PC, Miller DL, Parrino TV et al (1997) Islet cell tumors of the pancreas: clinical, radiologic, and pathologic correlation in diagnosis and localization. RadioGraphics 17(2):453–472

17. Recaldini C, Carrafiello G, Bertolotti E et al (2008) Contrast-enhanced ultrasonographic findings in pancreatic tumors. Int J Med Sci 5(4):203–208

18. D'Onofrio M, Mansueto G, Falconi M et al (2004) Neuroendocrine pancreatic tumor: value of contrast enhanced ultrasonography. Abdom Imaging 29(2):246–258

19. Rockall AG, Reznek RH (2007) Imaging of neuroendocrine tumours (CT/RM/US). Best Pract Res Clin Endocrinol Metab 21:43–68

20. Gouya H, Vignaux O, Augui J et al (2003) CT, endoscopic sonography, and a combined protocol for preoperative evaluation of pancreatic insulinomas. AJR Am J Roentgenol 181(4):987–992

21. Horton K, Hruban RH, Yeo C et al (2006) Multidetector row CT of pancreatic islet cell tumors. Radiographics 26:453–464

22. Gusmini S, Nicoletti R, Martinenghi C et al (2007) Arterial vs pancreatic phase: which is the best choice in the evaluation of pancreatic endocrine tumours with multidetector computed tomography (MDCT)? Radiol Med 112(7):999–1012

23. Alsohaibani F, Bigam D, Kneteman N et al (2008) The impact of preoperative endoscopic ultrasound on the surgical management of pancreatic neuroendocrine tumours. Can J Gastroenterol 22(10):817–820

24. Rappeport ED, Hansen CP, Kjaer A et al (2006) Multidetector computed tomography and neuroendocrine pancreaticoduodenal tumors. Acta Radiol 47(3):248–256

25. Liu Y, Song Q, Jin HT et al (2009) The value of multidetector-row CT in the preoperative detection of pancreatic insulinomas. Radiol Med 114(8):1232–1238

26. Khashab MA, Yong E, Lennon AM et al (2011) EUS is still superior to multidetector computerized tomography for detection of pancreatic neuroendocrine tumors. Gastrointest Endosc 73(4):691–696

27. Lin XZ, Wu ZY, Tao R et al (2012) Dual energy spectral CT imaging of insulinoma-Value in preoperative diagnosis compared with conventional multi-detector CT. Eur J Radiol 81(10):2487–2494

28. Xue HD, Liu W, Sun H et al (2008) Spectrum of functioning islet cell tumor on multislice computed tomography: experience on 70 patients. Chin Med Sci J 23(1):1–9

29. Semelka RC, Custodio CM, Cem Balci N et al (2000) Neuroendocrine tumors of the pancreas: spectrum of appearances on MRI. J Magn Reson Imaging 11(2):141–148

30. Herwick S, Miller FH, Keppke AL (2006) MRI of islet cell tumors of the pancreas. AJR Am J Roentgenol 187(5):W472–W480

31. Owen NJ, Sohaib SA, Peppercorn PD et al (2001) MRI of pancreatic neuroendocrine tumours. Br J Radiol 74(886):968–973

32. Ichikawa T, Peterson MS, Federle MP et al (2000) Islet cell tumor of the pancreas: biphasic CT versus MR imaging in tumor detection. Radiology 216(1):163–171

33. Caramella C, Dromain C, De Baere T et al (2010) Endocrine pancreatic tumours: which are the most useful MRI sequences? Eur Radiol 20(11):2618–2627

34. Thoeni RF, Mueller-Lisse UG, Chan R et al (2000) Detection of small, functional islet cell tumors in the pancreas: selection of MR imaging sequences for optimal sensitivity. Radiology 214(2):483–490

35. Anaye A, Mathieu A, Closset J et al (2009) Successful preoperative localization of a small pancreatic insulinoma by diffusion-weighted MRI. JOP 10(5):528–531

36. Bakir B, Salmaslioğlu A, Poyanli A et al (2010) Diffusion weighted MR imaging of pancreatic islet cell tumors. Eur J Radiol 74(1):214–220

37. Schmid-Tannwald C, Schmid-Tannwald CM, Morelli JN et al (2013) Comparison of abdominal MRI with diffusion-weighted imaging to 68Ga-DOTATATE PET/CT in detection of neuroendocrine tumors of the pancreas. Eur J Nucl Med Mol Imaging 40(6):897–907

38. Brenner R, Metens T, Bali M et al (2012) Pancreatic neuroendocrine tumor: added value of fusion of T2-weighted imaging and high b-value diffusion-weighted imaging for tumor detection. Eur J Radiol 81(5):e746–e749

39. Banks KP, Song WS (2013) Role of positron emission tomography-computed tomography in gastrointestinal malignancies. Radiol Clin N Am 51(5):799–831

40. Ruf J, Schiefer J, Furth C et al (2011) 68Ga-DOTATOC PET/CT of neuroendocrine tumors: spotlight on the CT phases of a triple-phase protocol. J Nucl Med 52(5):697–704

41. Ruf J, Heuck F, Schiefer J et al (2010) Impact of Multiphase 68Ga-DOTATOC-PET/CT on therapy management in patients with neuroendocrine tumors. Neuroendocrinology 91(1):101–109

42. Gabriel M, Decristoforo C, Kendler D et al (2007) 68Ga-DOTA-Tyr3-octreotide PET in neuroendocrine tumors: comparison with somatostatin receptor scintigraphy and CT. J Nucl Med 48(4):508–518

43. Etchebehere EC, de Oliveira SA, Gumz B et al (2014) 68Ga-DOTATATE PET/CT, 99mTc-HYNIC-Octreotide SPECT/CT, and whole-body MR imaging in detection of neuroendocrine tumors: a prospective trial. J Nucl Med 55(10):1598–1604

44. McLean AM, Fairclough PD (2005) Endoscopic ultrasound in the localisation of pancreatic islet cell tumours. Best Pract Res Clin Endocrinol Metab 19(2):177–193

45. De Angelis C, Brizzi RF, Pellicano R (2013) Endoscopic ultrasonography for pancreatic cancer: current and future perspectives. J Gastrointest Oncol 4(2):220–230

46. Gauger PG, Scheiman JM, Wamsteker EJ et al (2003) Role of endoscopic ultrasonography in screening and treatment of pancreatic endocrine tumours in asymptomatic patients with multiple endocrine neoplasia type 1. Br J Surg 90(6):748–754

47. Hellman P, Hennings J, Akerström G et al (2005) Endoscopic ultrasonography for evaluation of pancreatic tumours in multiple endocrine neoplasia type 1. Br J Surg 92(12):1508–1512

48. Pais SA, Al-Haddad M, Mohamadnejad M et al (2010) EUS for pancreatic neuroendocrine tumors: a single-center, 11-year experience. Gastrointest Endosc 71(7):1185–1193

49. Atiq M, Bhutani MS, Bektas M et al (2012) EUS-FNA for pancreatic neuroendocrine tumors: a tertiary cancer center experience. Dig Dis Sci 57(3):791–800

50. Ishikawa T, Itoh A, Kawashima H et al (2010) Usefulness of EUS combined with contrast-enhancement in the differential diagnosis of malignant versus benign and preoperative localization of pancreatic endocrine tumors. Gastrointest Endosc 71(6):951–959

51. Puli SR, Kalva N, Bechtold ML et al (2013) Diagnostic accuracy of endoscopic ultrasound in pancreatic neuroendocrine tumors: a systematic review and meta analysis. World J Gastroenterol 19(23):3678–3684

52. Jackson JE (2005) Angiography and arterial stimulation venous sampling in the localization of pancreatic neuroendocrine tumours. Best Pract Res Clin Endocrinol Metab 19(2):229–239

53. Guettier JM, Kam A, Chang R et al (2009) Localization of insulinomas to regions of the pancreas by intraarterial calcium stimulation: the NIH experience. J Clin Endocrinol Metab 94(4):1074–1080

54. Kann PH, Wirkus B, Keth A et al (2003) Pitfalls in endosonographic imaging of suspected insulinomas: pancreatic nodules of unknown dignity. Eur J Endocrinol 148(5):531–534

55. Goh BK, Ooi LL, Cheow PC et al (2009) Accurate preoperative localization of insulinomas avoids the need for blind resection and reoperation: analysis of a single institution experience with 17 surgically treated tumors over 19 years. J Gastrointest Surg 13(6):1071–1077

56. Nikfarjam M, Warshaw AL, Axelrod L et al (2008) Improved contemporary surgical management of insulinomas: a 25-year experience at the Massachusetts General Hospital. Ann Surg 247(1):165–172

57. Abboud B, Boujaoude J (2008) Occult sporadic insulinoma: localization and surgical strategy. World J Gastroenterol 14(5):657–665

58. Placzkowski KA, Vella A, Thompson GB et al (2009) Secular trends in the presentation and management of functioning insulinoma at the Mayo Clinic, 1987–2007. J Clin Endocrinol Metab 94(4):1069–1073

59. Hiramoto JS, Feldstein VA, LaBerge JM et al (2001) Intraoperative ultrasound and preoperative localization detects all occult insulinomas; discussion 1025–6. Arch Surg 136(9):1020–1025

60. Okabayashi T, Shima Y, Sumiyoshi T et al (2013) Diagnosis and management of insulinoma. World J Gastroenterol 19(6):829–837

61. Akerstrom G, Hellman P (2007) Surgery on neuroendocrine tumours. Best Pract Res Clin Endocrinol Metab 21:87–109

62. Wong M, Isa SH, Zahiah M et al (2007) Intraoperative ultrasound with palpation is still superior to intra-arterial calcium stimulation test in localising insulinoma. World J Surg 31(3):586–592

63. Shin LK, Brant-Zawadzki G, Kamaya A et al (2009) Intraoperative ultrasound of the pancreas. Ultrasound Q 25(1):39–48

64. Fernandez-Cruz L, Cesar-Borges G (2006) Laparoscopic strategies for resection of insulinomas. J Gastrointest Surg 10:752–760

65. Zhao YP, Zhan HX, Zhang TP et al (2011) Surgical management of patients with insulinomas: result of 292 cases in a single institution. J Surg Oncol 103(2):169–174

66. Matsubara H, Itoh A, Kawashima H et al (2011) Dynamic quantitative evaluation of contrast-enhanced endoscopic ultrasonography in the diagnosis of pancreatic diseases. Pancreas 40(7):1073–1079

67. Fugazzola C, Procacci C, Bergamo Andreis IA et al (1990) The contribution of ultrasonography and computed tomography in the diagnosis of nonfunctioning islet cell tumors of the pancreas. Gastrointest Radiol 15(2):139–144

68. Gallotti A, Perez Johnston R, Bonaffini P et al (2013) Incidental neuroendocrine tumors of the pancreas: MDCT findings and features of malignancy. AJR Am J Roentgenol 200:355–362

69. Worhunsky DJ, Krampitz GW, Poullos PD et al (2014) Pancreatic neuroendocrine tumours: hypoenhancement on arterial phase computed tomography predicts biological aggressiveness. HPB 16(4):304–311

70. Kawamoto S, Johnson PT, Shi C et al (2013) Pancreatic neuroendocrine tumor with cystlike changes: evaluation with MDCT. AJR Am J Roentgenol 200(3):W283–W290

71. Bordeianou L, Vagefi PA, Sahani D et al (2008) Cystic pancreatic endocrine neoplasms: a distinct tumor type? J Am Coll Surg 206:1154–1158

72. Balachandran A, Tamm EP, Bhosale PR et al (2012) Venous tumor thrombus in nonfunctional pancreatic neuroendocrine tumors. AJR Am J Roentgenol 199(3):602–608

73. Procacci C, Carbognin G, Accordini S et al (2001) Nonfunctioning endocrine tumors of the pancreas: possibilities of spiral CT characterization. Eur Radiol 11(7):1175–1183

74. Xue HD, Liu W, Xiao Y et al (2011) Pancreatic and peri-pancreatic lesions mimic pancreatic islet cell tumor in multidetector computed tomography. Chin Med J 124(11):1720–1725

75. Bhosale PR, Menias CO, Balachandran A et al (2013) Vascular pancreatic lesions: spectrum of imaging findings of malignant masses and mimics with pathologic correlation. Abdom Imaging 38(4):802–817

76. Raman SP, Hruban RH, Cameron JL et al (2012) Pancreatic imaging mimics: part 2, pancreatic neuroendocrine tumors and their mimics. AJR Am J Roentgenol 199(2):309–318

77. Raman SP, Hruban RH, Cameron JL et al (2013) Acinar cell carcinoma of the pancreas: computed tomography features – a study of 15 patients. Abdom Imaging 38(1):137–143

78. Hayashi K, Fujimitsu R, Ida M et al (2012) CT differentiation of solid serous cystadenoma vs endocrine tumor of the pancreas. Eur J Radiol 81(3):e203–e208

79. Uchida H, Sasaki A, Iwaki K et al (2005) An extramural gastrointestinal stromal tumor of the duodenum mimicking a pancreatic head tumor. J Hepatobiliary Pancreat Surg 12(4):324–327

80. Mangini M, Aiani L, Bertolotti E et al (2007) Parapancreatic Castleman disease: contrast-enhanced sonography and CT features. J Clin Ultrasound 35(4):207–211

81. Coquia SF, Kawamoto S, Zaheer A et al (2014) Intrapancreatic accessory spleen: possibilities of computed tomography in differentiation from nonfunctioning pancreatic neuroendocrine tumor. J Comput Assist Tomogr 38(6):874–878

82. Jang KM, Kim SH, Lee SJ et al (2013) Differentiation of an intrapancreatic accessory spleen from a small (<3-cm) solid pancreatic tumor: value of diffusion-weighted MR imaging. Radiology 266(1):159–167

83. Yu MH, Lee JY, Kim MA et al (2010) MR imaging features of small solid pseudopapillary tumors: retrospective differentiation from other small solid pancreatic tumors. AJR Am J Roentgenol 195(6):1324–1332

84. Barral M, Soyer P, Dohan A et al (2014) Magnetic resonance imaging of cystic pancreatic lesions in adults: an update in current diagnostic features and management. Abdom Imaging 39(1):48–65

85. Luo Y, Dong Z, Chen J et al (2014) Pancreatic neuroendocrine tumours: correlation between MSCT features and pathological classification. Eur Radiol 24:2945–2952

86. Rodallec M, Vilgrain V, Couvelard A et al (2006) Endocrine pancreatic tumours and helical CT: contrast enhancement is correlated with microvascular density, histoprognostic factors and survival. Pancreatology 6(1–2):77–85

87. D'Assignies G, Couvelard A, Bahrami S et al (2009) Pancreatic endocrine tumors: tumor blood flow assessed with perfusion CT reflects angiogenesis and correlates with prognostic factors. Radiology 250(2):407–416

88. Poultsides GA, Huang LC, Chen Y et al (2012) Pancreatic neuroendocrine tumors: radiographic calcifications correlate with grade and metastasis. Ann Surg Oncol 19(7):2295–2303

89. Yi W, Chen ZE, Yaghmai V et al (2011) Diffusion-weighted MR imaging in pancreatic endocrine tumors correlated with histopathologic characteristics. J Magn Reson Imaging 33:1071–1079

90. Rha SE, Jung SE, Lee KH et al (2007) CT and MR imaging findings of endocrine tumor of the pancreas according to WHO classification. Eur Radiol 62:371–377

91. Morales-Oyarvide V, Yoon WJ, Ingkakul T et al (2014) Cystic pancreatic neuroendocrine tumors: the value of cytology in preoperative diagnosis. Cancer Cytopathol 122(6):435–444

92. Figueiredo FA, Giovannini M, Monges G et al (2009) Pancreatic endocrine tumors: a large single-center experience. Pancreas 38(8):936–940

93. Scarpa A, Mantovani W, Capelli P et al (2010) Pancreatic endocrine tumors: improved TNM staging and histopathological grading permit a clinically efficient prognostic stratification of patients. Mod Pathol 23(6):824–833

94. Muniraj T, Vignesh S, Shetty S et al (2013) Pancreatic neuroendocrine tumors. Dis Mon 59(1):5–19
95. Sundin A (2012) Radiological and nuclear medicine imaging of gastroenteropancreatic neuroendocrine tumours. Best Pract Res Clin Gastroenterol 26(6):803–818
96. Foti G, Boninsegna L, Falconi M et al (2013) Preoperative assessment of nonfunctioning pancreatic endocrine tumours: role of MDCT and MRI. Radiol Med 118:1082–1101
97. McDermott S, O'Neill AC, Skehan SJ (2013) Staging of gastroenteropancreatic neuroendocrine tumors: how we do it based on an evidence-based approach. Clin Imaging 37:194–200
98. Sundin A, Vullierme MP, Kaltsas G et al (2009) ENETS consensus guidelines for the standards of care in neuroendocrine tumors: radiological examinations. Neuroendocrinology 90:167–183
99. Dromain C, de Baere T, Lumbroso J et al (2005) Detection of liver metastases from endocrine tumors: a prospective comparison of somatostatin receptor scintigraphy, computed tomography, and magnetic resonance imaging. J Clin Oncol 23:70–78
100. Hoeffel C, Job L, Ladam-Marcus V et al (2009) Detection of hepatic metastases from carcinoid tumor: prospective evaluation of contrast-enhanced ultrasonography. Dig Dis Sci 54:2040–2046
101. Kumbasar B, Kamel IR, Tekes A et al (2004) Imaging of neuroendocrine tumors: accuracy of helical CT versus SRS. Abdom Imaging 29(6):696–702
102. Sundin A, Rockall A (2012) Therapeutic monitoring of gastroenteropancreatic neuroendocrine tumors: the challenges ahead. Neuroendocrinology 96(4):261–271

The Role of Nuclear Medicine in the Diagnosis of Pancreatic Neuroendocrine Neoplasms

Vittoria Rufini, Paola Castaldi, and Valerio Lanni

Pancreatic neuroendocrine neoplasms are a heterogeneous group of tumors with variable clinical behavior and prognosis. Imaging modalities play an essential role in identifying the tumor lesion, defining the regional and distant involvement, planning the most appropriate treatment, assessing the therapeutic efficacy, and periodically monitoring the disease. Usually, a combination of morphologic and functional techniques is required to optimize diagnostic accuracy and obtain clinically relevant information [1]. Based on the biological properties of neuroendocrine neoplasms (NENs), specific radiopharmaceuticals for NEN imaging have been developed, thus assigning to nuclear medicine imaging an important role in the functional characterization of these neoplasms [2]. Nuclear medicine imaging consists of conventional scintigraphy and positron emission tomography (PET), which differ for the physical properties of the radionuclides employed, i.e., gamma-emitters for conventional scintigraphy and positron emitters for PET. Somatostatin receptor scintigraphy (SRS) including single-photon emission computed tomography (SPECT) with ^{111}In-DTPA-octreotide has been considered for a long time the first choice imaging modality for NENs, due to the specific binding to somatostatin receptors, which are expressed by the majority of NENs [2]. In the last 10-year period, great progress has been made with the development and clinical application of highly specific radiopharmaceuticals for PET, which reflect different metabolic pathways of NENs, such as the expression of receptors (^{68}Ga-labeled somatostatin analogs), the uptake of hormone precursors (^{11}C-5-hydroxytryptophan, ^{18}F-dihydroxyphenylalanine), and glucose metabolism (^{18}F-fluorodeoxyglucose). Among these radiopharmaceuticals, ^{68}Ga-labeled somatostatin analogs are increasingly used for PET imaging. Moreover, the standard use of image fusion by hybrid machines such as PET/computed tomography (CT) allows to correlate anatomic detail with function, with great benefit on diagnostic accuracy [2].

This chapter will focus on the functional imaging of pancreatic NENs by means of radiolabeled peptides, mainly stressing the use of ^{111}In-DTPA-octreotide for SPECT or SPECT/CT and ^{68}Ga-peptides for PET/CT, with special emphasis to the advantages and limitations of their use in the clinical practice. Other SPECT and PET radiopharmaceuticals exploiting different molecular properties of these neoplasms will be described.

V. Rufini (✉) • P. Castaldi • V. Lanni
Institute of Nuclear Medicine,
Università Cattolica del Sacro Cuore,
Largo Agostino Gemelli, 8, Rome 00168, Italy
e-mail: v.rufini@rm.unicatt.it; pcastaldi80@yahoo.it;
valerio.lanni@gmail.com

S. La Rosa, F. Sessa (eds.), *Pancreatic Neuroendocrine Neoplasms: Practical Approach to Diagnosis, Classification, and Therapy*, DOI 10.1007/978-3-319-17235-4_3,
© Springer International Publishing Switzerland 2015

3.1 Radiopharmaceuticals for SPECT Imaging

^{111}In-DTPA-octreotide. The cyclic octapeptide octreotide conjugated with diethylenetriamine pentaacetic acid (DTPA) and labeled with indium-111 is the only worldwide-approved and commercially available radiopharmaceutical for NEN imaging (OctreoScan®). This tracer is a somatostatin analog that specifically binds to somatostatin receptors, preferentially subtypes 2 and 5. To ensure good imaging quality and obtain adequate clinical information, an optimal imaging protocol should be adopted, also including SPECT imaging and possibly high-resolution CT co-registration. Procedure guidelines for tumor imaging with ^{111}In-DTPA-octreotide have been published in Europe and in the USA [3–5]. Normal scintigraphic pattern includes visualization of organs that express somatostatin receptors, including the pituitary, spleen (and accessory spleen, when present), liver, renal parenchyma, and thyroid; the gallbladder, bowel, and urinary collecting system are seen as a result of ^{111}In-DTPA-octreotide clearance. Any uptake in nonphysiologic areas or any focal accumulation of the tracer higher than the surrounding physiologic uptake reflects the presence of lesions with overexpression of somatostatin receptors. Sensitivity of SRS is related to various factors such as type and density of somatostatin receptors expressed by the tumor, target-to-background ratio, tumor size and site, and tumor histology. As somatostatin receptors are also expressed in peritumoral vessels and inflammatory and immune cells, uptake can be seen in tumors other than NENs as well as in infections and granulomatous or autoimmune diseases [2].

[99m]Tc-labeled Somatostatin Analogs. Various somatostatin analogs for ^{99m}Tc labeling have been developed. Among these, ^{99m}Tc-hydrazino-nicotinamide (HYNIC)-octreotide(TOC) is commercially available in some European countries and is registered in Poland [6, 7]. The corresponding ^{99m}Tc-HYNIC-TATE has also been used for NEN imaging, giving high-quality images at low cost and low patient dose [7, 8].

3.2 Radiopharmaceuticals for PET Imaging

Radiolabeled Somatostatin Analogs. In the last 10-year period, many different somatostatin analogs labeled with gallium-68 has been introduced for the diagnostic workup of gastroenteropancreatic NENs with PET/CT. The most used in clinical practice are DOTANOC, DOTATATE, and DOTATOC. DOTA stands for 1,4,7,10-tetraazacyclododecane-1,4,7,10-tetraacetic acid, and it is the macrocyclic chelator that enables stable labeling with various metal ions (indium, gallium, yttrium, lutetium, copper, and others). The three somatostatin analogs (TOC, TATE, and NOC) differ in their individual binding affinity to the different somatostatin receptor subtypes. Among the three peptides, ^{68}Ga-DOTANOC shows the widest receptor binding profile with good affinity for subtypes 2, 3, and 5; ^{68}Ga-DOTATOC has a high affinity for subtype 2 and 5, while ^{68}Ga-DOTATATE binds to subtype 2 only, but with the highest affinity [9]. Even though rare mismatches have been reported when comparing different ^{68}Ga-labeled peptides in the same patient, at present there is no evidence that such differences are associated with major advantages in the clinical practice [10–13]. The synthesis of ^{68}Ga-peptides does not require an on-site cyclotron as the radionuclide is eluted from a commercially available Ge-68/Ga-68 generator. A European Pharmacopoeia monograph is currently available for DOTATOC only; neither of the ^{68}Ga-DOTA-peptides is registered, with consequent logistic difficulties and regulatory implications. Procedure guidelines for PET/CT tumor imaging with ^{68}Ga-DOTA-peptides have been published in Europe [14]. Some differences exist between ^{68}Ga-DOTA-peptides and ^{111}In-DTPA-octreotide regarding physiologic uptake areas, as more evident physiologic uptake of ^{68}Ga-DOTA-peptides is usually seen in the adrenal glands and the head/uncinate process of the pancreas [15–18]. When studying the pancreas, apart from the focal physiologic uptake in the head/uncinate process, which can mimic a pancreatic NEN, potential pitfalls in image interpretation derive from the presence of pancreatitis or intrapancreatic accessory spleen, both characterized by high tracer uptake [19, 20] (Fig. 3.1). The mean effective dose equivalent in adults is 0.025 ± 0.004 mSv/MBq, less than one-half of the effective dose with ^{111}In-DTPA-octreotide [21]. Recently, somatostatin analogs labeled with copper-64 (12.5 h half-life) have

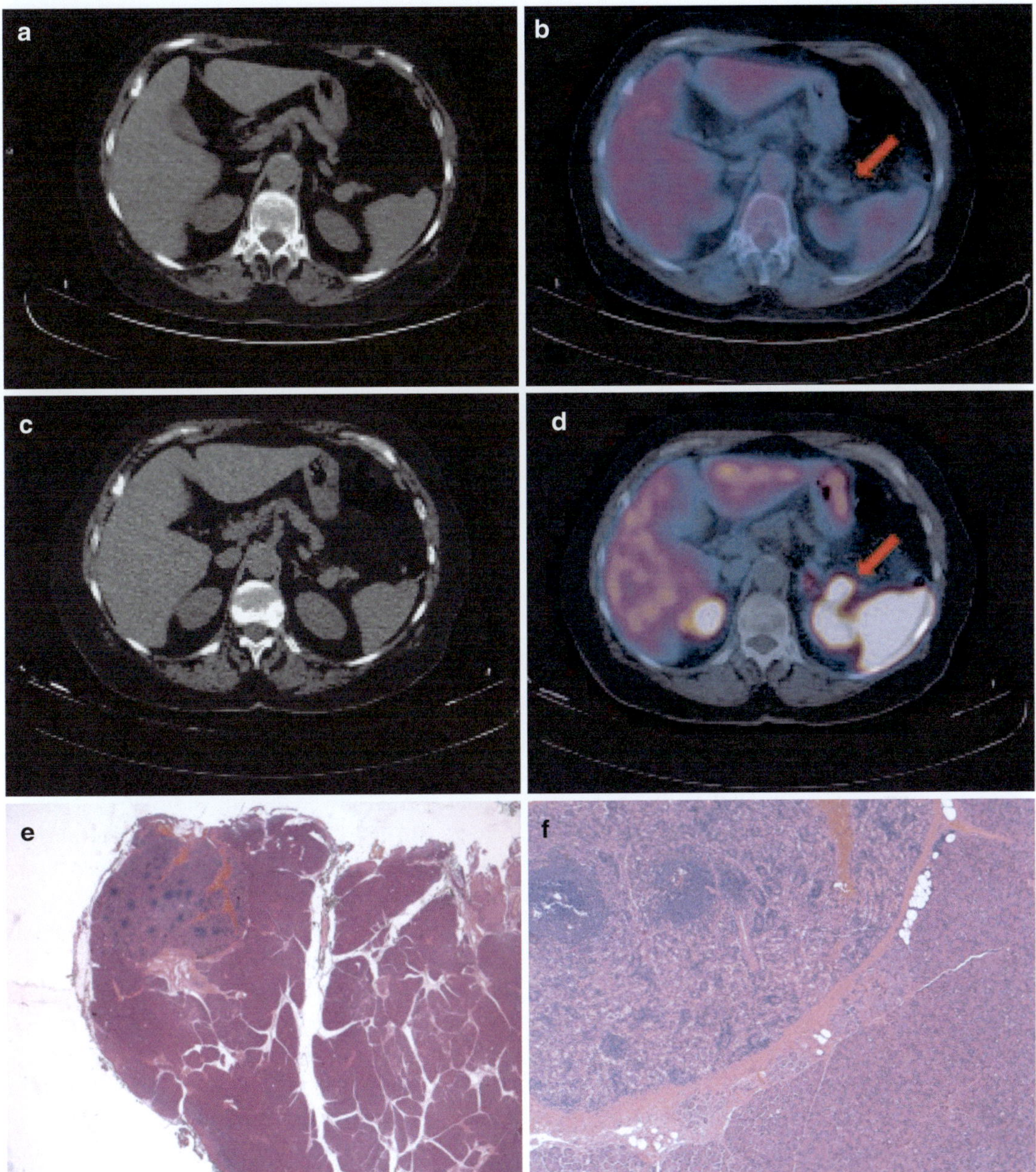

Fig. 3.1 Comparison between ^{18}F-FDG PET/CT and ^{68}Ga-DOTANOC PET/CT in a patient with a nodule in the pancreatic tail incidentally detected at CT. ^{18}F-FDG PET/CT showed no ^{18}F-FDG uptake in the pancreatic lesion (**a, b**) (*arrow*), while ^{68}Ga-DOTANOC PET/CT showed intense focal tracer uptake (**c, d**) (*arrow*), thus suggesting the presence of a pancreatic NEN. The patient underwent distal pancreasectomy; surprisingly histology showed the presence of an intrapancreatic spleen. (**e**) Pancreatic tissue showing a peripheral (left upper corner) well-demarcated nodule approximately 1 cm in size corresponding to a benign intrapancreatic accessory spleen (**f**). H&E (**e, f**) (Courtesy of Dr. Frediano Inzani, Institute of Pathology, Università Cattolica del Sacro Cuore, Rome, Italy)

been developed for PET/CT studies and tested in NENs [22].

18F-DOPA. Dihydroxyphenylalanine (DOPA) is an amino acid intermediate in the catecholamine synthesis pathway, which is taken up into the cells via the large neutral amino acid transporter and converted to dopamine by aromatic amino acid decarboxylase (AADC) [23]; via the vesicular monoamine transporters, DOPA is stored in the secretory granules where enzymatic degradation is prevented [24]. AADC is usually upregulated in neuroendocrine tumor cells, especially pheochromocytomas/paragangliomas and gastroenteric NENs with the exception of pancreatic islet cell tumors, where lower AADC levels have been reported [24]. For imaging purposes, DOPA can be labeled with both ^{11}C and ^{18}F; however, ^{11}C-DOPA is not widely used because of limited availability of ^{11}C (physical half-life of 20 min with need of an on-site cyclotron for production) and high costs. ^{18}F-DOPA has been registered in France in 2006 and is commercially available in Europe but not in the USA. A potential limitation of ^{18}F-DOPA is the physiologic uptake in the abdomen (liver, gallbladder, biliary tract, pancreas, and duodenum), which might mask tumors in this site [2]. Premedication with carbidopa, an inhibitor of the peripheral AADC, can improve image quality by decreasing background activity [23]. ^{18}F-DOPA PET/CT performs well in patients with functioning carcinoid tumors, with lower sensitivity for pancreatic islet cell tumors due to the physiologic pancreatic uptake [25].

11C-5-HTP. ^{11}C-5-hydroxytryptophan (^{11}C-5-HTP) is a serotonin precursor and DOPA decarboxylase substrate, which is specifically and irreversibly trapped by serotonin-producing tumors. Unfortunately, ^{11}C-5-HTP is produced only in centers with a cyclotron on site and at high costs; so, its use is essentially limited to clinical trials in specialized centers [26]. As for ^{18}F-DOPA PET, carbidopa premedication increases tumor-to-background ratio so improving image interpretation [27]. ^{11}C-5-HTP PET seems to be useful in many tumor entities of the heterogeneous NEN group, especially in detecting small pancreatic neoplasms [28].

18F-FDG. ^{18}F-Fluorodeoxyglucose (FDG) is a glucose analog and the most used PET tracer in oncology with very high sensitivity in many types of tumors, especially the rapid-growing and aggressive ones. FDG uptake in neoplastic cells reflects the highest glucose metabolism which is linked to the cellular proliferative activity [2]. Procedure guidelines for PET and PET/CT tumor imaging with ^{18}F-FDG have been published in Europe, the USA, and Japan [29–31]. Pitfalls in the interpretation of FDG images may be caused by the physiologic activity in the brain, vocal cords, esophagus, heart, stomach, bowel, bladder, and brown fat. An increased FDG uptake can be seen also in infections and other inflammatory processes [2, 30]. The usefulness of FGD PET/CT in the diagnosis of NEN is strictly related to the grade of differentiation, as high ^{18}F-FDG uptake is usually associated with more aggressive GEP-NENs and a less favorable prognosis [28].

3.3 New Tracers for SPECT and PET

Besides radiolabeled somatostatin analogs, the use of radiolabeled somatostatin antagonists represents a highly promising strategy for both SPECT and PET imaging [1, 32]. Preliminary experiences showed that the radiolabeled antagonist ^{111}In-DOTA-BASS may be preferable to agonists because of a higher and longer retention in tumors and better imaging results [33]; so, a greater benefit on radioreceptor therapy is expected [34]. Among new SPECT tracers, specific radioligands for glucagon-like peptide-1 (GLP-1) receptors have been recently developed and evaluated in animal models and in humans [35, 36]. GLP-1 is an intestinal hormone that stimulates insulin secretion through receptors expressed in islet cells. GLP-1 receptors are greatly expressed in insulinomas, and recent studies demonstrated that an ^{111}In-labeled GLP-1 analog (^{111}In-exendin-4) can detect occult insulinomas, which were not localized by other imaging modalities [35, 36]. ^{68}Ga-exendin-4 has been recently applied for PET/CT imaging [37].

3.4　Clinical Applications

Many different radiopharmaceuticals are available for imaging of pancreatic neuroendocrine neoplasms (as other GEP-NENs) based on their physiopathology, which is characterized by different metabolic pathways and different receptor expression.

SRS with ^{111}In-octreotide still today is a widely used functional imaging modality for GEP tumors, due to its worldwide availability together with good diagnostic sensitivity, which is ≥80 % in various studies with the only exception of insulinomas due to the low density of sstr2 in these tumors and its ability in changing patient management in approximately 30 % of cases [2]. [99mTc]-labeled somatostatin analogs ([99mTc]-HYNIC-TOC and [99mTc]-HYNIC-TATE) have been proposed as promising candidates for an alternative to ^{111}In-DTPA-octreotide for SRS [6]. The main limitations of SRS are its relatively low spatial resolution (about 1 cm) and the lack of a precise localization of the neoplastic lesions when a SPECT/CT device is not available.

The initial clinical applications of ^{68}Ga-DOTA-peptides have shown several advantages over ^{111}In-DTPA-octreotide [38–40]: higher diagnostic sensitivity (>90 %), especially in detecting small primary tumors and metastatic lesions, due to the higher spatial resolution (4–6 mm) and higher count rate sensitivity of PET devices; quantification of the uptake by the standardized uptake value (SUV); lower radiation exposure; single-day procedure (versus 2–3 days for SRS if a hybrid machine is not available), with better patient comfort and faster reporting; and lower costs [40, 41]. Also the superiority of ^{68}Ga-DOTATATE over [99mTc]-HYNIC-TOC has been recently demonstrated [42]. ^{68}Ga-DOTA-peptide PET/CT has shown to be the most sensitive procedure for the detection of unknown primary NENs; among the detected primary tumors, a significant number is located in the pancreas (46 % in the experience by Prasad et al.) [43]. In the presence of a pancreatic mass, a positive scan suggests the presence of a well-differentiated NEN (Fig. 3.2). On the contrary, a negative scan suggests an adenocarcinoma or a poorly differentiated neuroendocrine neoplasm; in these cases, an intense ^{18}F-FDG uptake is frequently observed. In any case, preoperative cytologic/histologic confirmation is needed. In addition, ^{68}Ga-DOTA-peptide PET/CT can affect either stage or therapy in approximately 50 % of patients with NEN [44] and plays a distinctive role in guiding the selection of therapy with cold or radiolabeled somatostatin analogs.

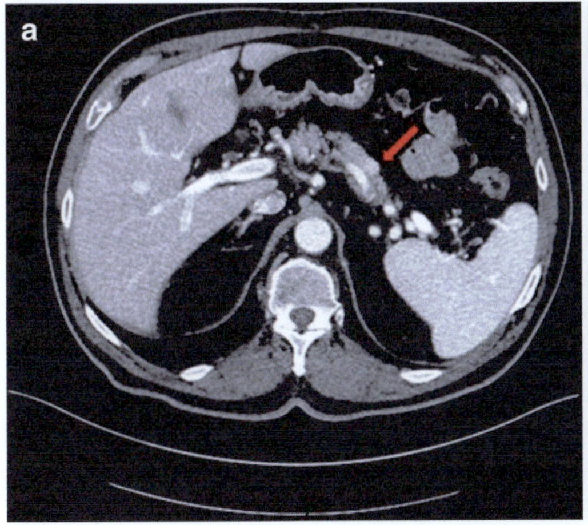
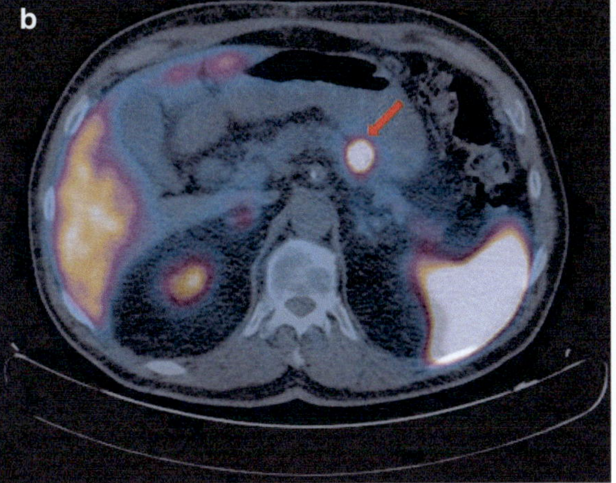

Fig. 3.2 (**a**) Axial contrast-enhanced CT image obtained in the arterial phase showing a 1 cm homogeneous hyperenhancing mass at the junction of the pancreatic body and tail (*arrow*). (**b**) Axial fused ^{68}Ga-DOTANOC PET/CT images demonstrating intense and focal tracer uptake in the same pancreatic nodule, leading to the diagnosis of neoplastic disease characterized by elevated expression of somatostatin receptors (*arrow*)

^{18}F-DOPA is particularly suited to visualize carcinoid tumors with elevated serotonin levels [2, 45] and is the imaging technique of choice in children with congenital hyperinsulinism to distinguish focal from diffuse forms [46, 47]. On the contrary, controversial results have been reported in localizing neuroendocrine pancreatic tumors in adults [48–50]. Due to the physiologic pancreatic uptake, false-negative findings with ^{18}F-DOPA PET have been reported both in functioning and nonfunctioning neuroendocrine pancreatic tumors in adults as well as in patients with pancreatic islet cell tumors who had been pretreated with carbidopa, suggesting that carbidopa premedication should be avoided when such tumors are suspected [48]. Recent observations seem to reassess the value of ^{18}F-DOPA PET/CT after carbidopa premedication in insulin-secreting tumors in adults [51]. Abnormal ^{18}F-DOPA uptake in a pancreatic tumor not of neuroendocrine origin (i.e., solid pseudopapillary tumor) has been recently reported, doubting the specificity of this tracer [52].

The uptake of ^{11}C-5-HTP in NENs is based on the same mechanism as for ^{18}F-DOPA; however, few data are available about the use of ^{11}C-5-HTP due to its complex production and limited availability. ^{11}C-5-HTP can be used both in patients with increased serotonin synthesis, i.e., with carcinoid tumors, and patients without elevation of urinary 5-HIAA, i.e., with neuroendocrine pancreatic neoplasms [53]. In comparative studies, ^{11}C-5-HTP PET showed the highest sensitivity (96 %) for the detection of pancreatic NENs as compared with CT, SRS, and ^{18}F-DOPA PET [28]. False-negative results may occur in poorly differentiated neoplasms [48, 53].

^{18}F-FDG frequently fails to visualize tumors with a low proliferation rate, i.e., well-differentiated NENs (G1), whereas it is recommended for identification and assessment of poorly differentiated (G3) neuroendocrine carcinomas [54, 55]. In patients with NEN, the so-called "flip flop" pattern of uptake may be observed, i.e., ^{68}Ga-peptide positive and ^{18}F-FDG negative in well-differentiated tumors and vice versa in poorly differentiated carcinomas [2] (Fig. 3.3). However, ^{18}F-FDG positivity has been reported also in a substantial percentage of G1 and G2 NENs, where it offers important prognostic information, predicting early progression and influencing the therapeutic management [56]. Recently, a metabolic grading system based on the tumor-to-liver ratio of ^{18}F-FDG uptake has been assessed in patients with inoperable multifocal gastroenteropancreatic NEN [57].

Considering the wide availability of radiopharmaceuticals that target endocrine tumor cells, how to choose the most appropriate one in the clinical practice for imaging endocrine pancreatic neoplasms? The choice depends on several factors including:

- The biologic characteristics of the tumor, i.e., the metabolic activity as well as receptor subtype and specific amine profile, the functional activity, and the histologic grading (Ki-67)
- The clinical information needed, i.e., diagnostic or prognostic
- The diagnostic efficacy of each tracer in the various clinical situations, as well as the impact on patient management and on therapeutic decision
- Practical issues, such as availability and costs as well as local expertise

Therefore, the preferential use of a given tracer should be defined in the specific clinical context (Table 3.1). When the diagnostic information is needed, i.e., for lesion identification and localization (including unknown primary) and disease staging and restaging after therapy, the choice should be primarily guided by tumor differentiation and grading. In well-differentiated pancreatic neuroendocrine tumors (G1 and low G2), functional imaging with radiolabeled peptides should be performed. In this context, ^{68}Ga-DOTA-peptide PET/CT is currently regarded as the nuclear medicine technique of choice; where available, it has replaced OctreoScan®, which maintains a role just for evaluating the receptor status prior to therapy with cold or radiolabeled somatostatin analogs ([90]Y- or ^{177}Lu-DOTA-peptides) [58]. In fact, PET/CT with ^{68}Ga-DOTA-peptides provides the same information of SRS with a higher diagnostic accuracy and a lower patient discomfort.

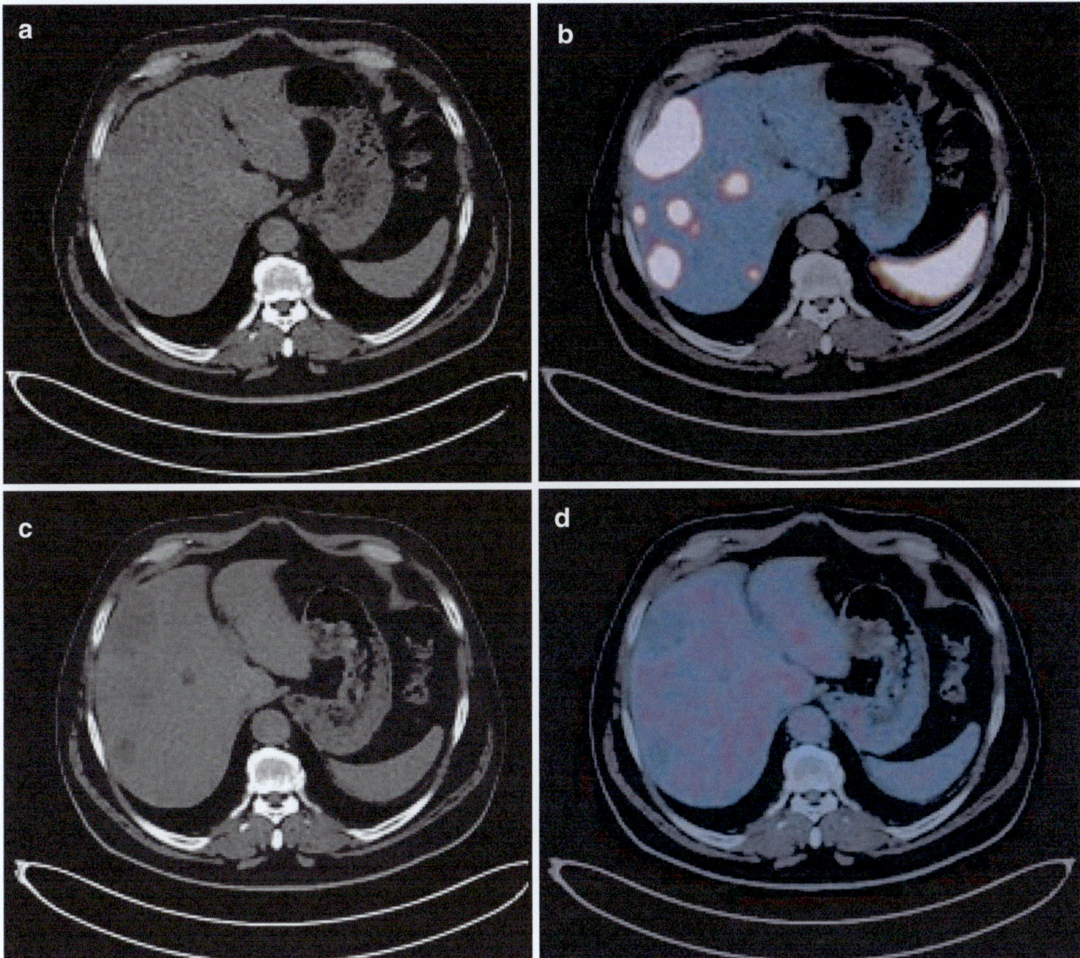

Fig. 3.3 Comparison between ⁶⁸Ga-DOTANOC PET/CT and ¹⁸F-FDG PET/CT in a patient with liver metastases from previously removed well-differentiated pancreatic neuroendocrine tumor (G1). The images show multiple liver metastatic lesions characterized by intense ⁶⁸Ga-DOTANOC uptake (**a**, **b**); the same lesions showed no FDG uptake (**c**, **d**), confirming the biological behavior of a G1 NEN

For diagnostic purposes, ¹⁸F-FDG is the tracer of choice in poorly differentiated neoplasms with high proliferative activity (high G2 and G3), where a loss of NEN features and increased glucose metabolism are expected [48, 55, 59]. The presence of ¹⁸F-FDG-positive lesions correlates with a poor prognosis, independently from tumor grading; in well/moderately differentiated tumors, this prognostic information is complimentary to the diagnostic one provided by ⁶⁸Ga-DOTA-peptides and very useful to plan the most appropriate treatment [60].

In the clinical practice, the use of other PET tracers in well/moderately differentiated pancreatic NENs is currently restricted to particular situations. ¹⁸F-DOPA is considered of poor utility both in functioning and nonfunctioning tumors, even though recent observations seem to reassess its value in insulin-secreting tumors in adults [51]. The use of ¹⁸F-DOPA should be considered when ⁶⁸Ga-DOTA-peptides are not available or provide doubtful information. ¹¹C-5-HTP seems to perform better than ¹⁸F-DOPA, but its use is limited to specialized centers [26, 61].

Table 3.1 Choice of the radiopharmaceutical for imaging pancreatic neuroendocrine neoplasms

	^{111}In-DTPA-octreotide	^{68}Ga-DOTA-peptides	^{18}F-FDG	^{18}F-DOPA
Tumor biologic features	SMS receptor status	SMS receptor status	Glucose metabolism	Amine metabolism
Diagnostic information needed (unknown primary, staging and restaging after therapy)	Obsolete	In well/moderately differentiated NENs (G1, low G2)	In poorly differentiated NENs (high G2, G3)	In well/moderately differentiated NENs (G1, low G2)
Prognostic information needed	–	–	In G1, G2, G3 NENs	–
Corresponding therapeutic information	Receptor status prior to therapy with cold or radiolabeled SMS analogs	Receptor status prior to therapy with cold or radiolabeled SMS analogs	–	–
Practical issues	Registered, commercially available	Not registered on-site production	Registered, commercially available on-site production	Registered, commercially available

SMS somatostatin, *NEN* neuroendocrine neoplasm

References

1. Bodei L, Sundin A, Kidd M et al (2015) The status of neuroendocrine tumor imaging: from darkness to light? Neuroendocrinology 101:1–17
2. Rufini V, Calcagni ML, Baum RP (2006) Imaging of neuroendocrine tumors. Semin Nucl Med 36:228–247
3. Kwekkeboom DJ, Krenning EP, Scheidhauer K et al (2009) ENETS consensus guidelines for the standards of care in neuroendocrine tumors: somatostatin receptor imaging with (111)In-pentetreotide. Neuroendocrinology 90:184–189
4. Bombardieri E, Ambrosini V, Aktolun C et al (2010) ^{111}In-pentetreotide scintigraphy: procedure guidelines for tumour imaging. Eur J Nucl Med Mol Imaging 37:1441–1448
5. Balon HR, Brown TL, Goldsmith SJ et al (2011) The SNM practice guideline for somatostatin receptor scintigraphy 2.0. J Nucl Med Technol 39:317–324
6. Decristoforo C, Melendez-Alafort L, Sosabowski JK et al (2000) ^{99m}Tc-HYNIC-[Tyr3]-octreotide for imaging somatostatin-receptor-positive tumors: preclinical evaluation and comparison with ^{111}In-octreotide. J Nucl Med 41:1114–1119
7. Ambrosini V, Fani M, Fanti S et al (2011) Radiopeptide imaging and therapy in Europe. J Nucl Med 52(Suppl 2):42S–55S
8. Hubalewska-Dydejczyk A, Fross-Baron K, Mikolajczak R et al (2006) ^{99m}Tc-EDDA/HYNIC-octreotate scintigraphy, an efficient method for the detection and staging of carcinoid tumours: results of 3 years' experience. Eur J Nucl Med Mol Imaging 33:1123–1133
9. Ambrosini V, Campana D, Tomassetti P et al (2012) ^{68}Ga-labelled peptides for diagnosis of gastroentero-pancreatic NET. Eur J Nucl Med Mol Imaging 39(Suppl 1):S52–S60
10. Kabasakal L, Demirci E, Ocak M et al (2012) Comparison of ^{68}Ga-DOTATATE and ^{68}Ga-DOTANOC PET/CT imaging in the same patient group with neuroendocrine tumours. Eur J Nucl Med Mol Imaging 39:1271–1277
11. Poeppel TD, Binse I, Petersenn S et al (2013) Differential uptake of (68)Ga-DOTATOC and (68)Ga-DOTATATE in PET/CT of gastroenteropancreatic neuroendocrine tumors. Recent Results Cancer Res 194:353–371
12. Wild D, Bomanji JB, Benkert P et al (2013) Comparison of ^{68}Ga-DOTANOC and ^{68}Ga-DOTATATE PET/CT within patients with gastroenteropancreatic neuroendocrine tumors. J Nucl Med 54:364–372
13. Velikyan I, Sundin A, Sörensen J et al (2014) Quantitative and qualitative intrapatient comparison of ^{68}Ga-DOTATOC and ^{68}Ga-DOTATATE: net uptake rate for accurate quantification. J Nucl Med 55:204–210
14. Virgolini I, Ambrosini V, Bomanji JB et al (2010) Procedure guidelines for PET/CT tumour imaging with ^{68}Ga-DOTA-conjugated peptides: ^{68}Ga-DOTA-TOC, ^{68}Ga-DOTA-NOC, ^{68}Ga-DOTA-TATE. Eur J Nucl Med Mol Imaging 37:2004–2010
15. Castellucci P, Pou Ucha J, Fuccio C et al (2011) Incidence of increased ^{68}Ga-DOTANOC uptake in the pancreatic head in a large series of extrapancreatic NET patients studied with sequential PET/CT. J Nucl Med 52:886–890
16. Al-Ibraheem A, Bundschuh RA, Notni J et al (2011) Focal uptake of ^{68}Ga-DOTATOC in the pancreas: pathological or physiological correlate in patients with neuroendocrine tumours? Eur J Nucl Med Mol Imaging 38:2005–2013

17. Krausz Y, Rubinstein R, Appelbaum L et al (2012) Ga-68 DOTA-NOC uptake in the pancreas: pathological and physiological patterns. Clin Nucl Med 37:57–62
18. Jacobsson H, Larsson P, Jonsson C et al (2012) Normal uptake of ^{68}Ga-DOTA-TOC by the pancreas uncinate process mimicking malignancy at somatostatin receptor PET. Clin Nucl Med 37:362–365
19. Treglia G, Farchione A, Stefanelli A et al (2013) Masking effect of chronic pancreatitis in the interpretation of somatostatin receptor positron emission tomography in pancreatic neuroendocrine tumors. Pancreas 42:726–728
20. Collarino A, Del Ciello A, Perotti G et al (2015) Intrapancreatic accessory spleen detected by ^{68}Ga-DOTANOC PET/CT and ^{99m}Tc-colloid SPECT/CT scintigraphy. Clin Nucl Med 40:415–418
21. Pettinato C, Sarnelli A, Di Donna M et al (2008) ^{68}Ga-DOTANOC: biodistribution and dosimetry in patients affected by neuroendocrine tumors. Eur J Nucl Med Mol Imaging 35:72–79
22. Pfeifer A, Knigge U, Mortensen J et al (2012) Clinical PET of neuroendocrine tumors using ^{64}Cu-DOTATATE: first-in-humans study. J Nucl Med 53:1207–1215
23. Jager PL, Chirakal R, Marriott CJ et al (2008) 6-L-18F-fluorodihydroxyphenilalanine PET in neuroendocrine tumors: basic aspects and emerging clinical applications. J Nucl Med 49:573–586
24. Dudczak R, Traub-Weidinger T (2010) PET and PET/CT in endocrine tumours. Eur J Radiol 73:481–493
25. Wong KK, Waterfield RT, Marzola MC et al (2012) Contemporary nuclear medicine imaging of neurodocrine tumours. Clin Radiol 67:1035–1050
26. Koopmans KP, Neels OC, Kema IP et al (2008) Improved staging of patients with carcinoid and islet cell tumors with ^{18}F-fluorodihydroxyphenilalanine and ^{11}C-5-hydroxytryptophan positron emission tomography. J Clin Oncol 26:1489–1495
27. Orlefors H, Sundin A, Lu L et al (2006) Carbidopa pretreatment improves image interpretation and visualisation of carcinoid tumours with ^{11}C-5-hydroxytryptophan positron emission tomography. Eur J Nucl Med Mol Imaging 33:60–65
28. de Herder WW (2014) Functional localisation and scintigraphy in neuroendocrine tumours of the gastrointestinal tract and pancreas (GEP-NETs). Eur J Endocrinol 170:173–183
29. Delbeke D, Coleman RE, Guiberteau MJ et al (2006) Procedure guideline for tumor imaging with 18F-FDG PET/CT 1.0. J Nucl Med 47:885–895, Erratum (2006) in J Nucl Med 47:903
30. Boellaard R, O'Doherty MJ, Weber WA et al (2010) FDG PET and PET/CT: EANM procedure guidelines for tumour PET imaging: version 1.0. Eur J Nucl Med Mol Imaging 37:181–200
31. Fukukita H, Senda M, Terauchi T et al (2010) Japanese guideline for the oncology FDG-PET/CT data acquisition protocol: synopsis of version 1.0. Ann Nucl Med 24:325–334
32. Ginj M, Zhang H, Waser B et al (2006) Radiolabeled somatostatin receptor antagonists are preferable to agonists for in vivo peptide receptor targeting of tumors. Proc Natl Acad Sci 103:16436–16441
33. Wild D, Fani M, Behe M et al (2011) First clinical evidence that imaging with somatostatin receptor antagonists is feasible. J Nucl Med 52:1412–1417
34. Cescato R, Waser B, Fani M et al (2011) Evaluation of ^{177}Lu-DOTA-sst2 antagonist versus ^{177}Lu-DOTA-sst2 agonist binding in human cancers in vitro. J Nucl Med 52:1886–1890
35. Wild D, Macke H, Christ E et al (2008) Glucagon-like peptide-1 receptor scans to localize occult insulinomas. N Engl J Med 359:766–768
36. Christ E, Wild D, Forrer F et al (2009) Glucagon-like peptide-1 receptor imaging for localization of insulinomas. J Clin Endocrinol Metab 94:4398–4405
37. Eriksson O, Velikyan I, Selvaraju RK et al (2014) Detection of metastatic insulinoma by positron emission tomography with [^{68}Ga]exendin-4-a case report. J Clin Endocrinol Metab 99:1519–1524
38. Gabriel M, Decristoforo C, Kendler D et al (2007) ^{68}Ga-DOTATyr3-Octreotide PET in neuroendocrine tumors: comparison with somatostatin receptor scintigraphy and CT. J Nucl Med 48:508–518
39. Krausz Y, Freedman N, Rubinstein R et al (2011) ^{68}Ga-DOTANOC PET/CT imaging of neuroendocrine tumors: comparison with ^{111}In-DTPA-octreotide (octreoscan). Mol Imaging Biol 13:583–593
40. Schreiter NF, Brenner W, Nogami M et al (2012) Cost comparison of ^{111}In-DTPA-octreotide scintigraphy and ^{68}Ga-DOTATOC PET-CT for staging enteropancreatic neuroendocrine tumours. Eur J Nucl Med 39:72–82
41. Mansi L, Cuccurullo V (2014) Diagnostic imaging in neuroendocrine tumors. J Nucl Med 55:1576–1577
42. Etchebehere EC, de Oliveira SA, Gumz B et al (2014) ^{68}Ga-DOTATATE PET/CT, ^{99m}Tc-HYNIC-octreotide SPECT/CT, and whole-body MR imaging in detection of neuroendocrine tumors: a prospective trial. J Nucl Med 55:1598–1604
43. Prasad V, Ambrosini V, Hommann M et al (2010) Detection of unknown primary neuroendocrine tumours (CUP-NET) using (68)Ga-DOTA-NOC receptor PET/CT. Eur J Nucl Med Mol Imaging 37:67–77
44. Ambrosini V, Campana D, Bodei L et al (2010) ^{68}Ga-DOTANOC PET/CT clinical impact in patients with neuroendocrine tumors. J Nucl Med 51:669–673
45. Koopmans KP, de Vries EG, Kema IP et al (2006) Staging of carcinoid tumours with ^{18}F-DOPA PET: a prospective, diagnostic accuracy study. Lancet Oncol 7:728–734
46. Treglia G, Mirk P, Giordano A et al (2012) Diagnostic performance of fluorine-18-dihydroxyphenylalanine positron emission tomography in diagnosing and localizing the focal form of congenital hyperinsulinism: a meta-analysis. Pediatr Radiol 42:1372–1379

47. Yang J, Hao R, Zhu X (2013) Diagnostic role of ^{18}F-dihydroxyphenylalanine positron emission tomography in patients with congenital hyperinsulinism: a meta-analysis. Nucl Med Commun 34:347–353

48. Rufini V, Baum RP, Castaldi P et al (2012) Role of PET/CT in the functional imaging of endocrine pancreatic tumors. Abdom Imaging 37:1004–1020

49. Treglia G, Inzani F, Campanini N et al (2013) A case of insulinoma detected by (68)Ga-DOTANOC PET/CT and missed by (18)F-dihydroxyphenylalanine PET/CT. Clin Nucl Med 38:e267–e270

50. Santhanam P, Taieb D (2014) Role of ^{18}F-FDOPA PET/CT imaging in endocrinology. Clin Endocrinol 81:789–798

51. Imperiale A, Sebag F, Vix M et al (2014) ^{18}F-FDOPA PET/CT imaging of insulinoma revisited. Eur J Nucl Med Mol Imaging 42:409–418

52. Imperiale A, Addeo P, Averous G (2013) Solid pseudopapillary pancreatic tumor mimicking a neuroendocrine neoplasm on ^{18}F-FDOPA PET/CT. J Clin Endocrinol Metab 98:2643–2644

53. Eriksson B, Orlefors H, Oberg K et al (2005) Developments in PET for the detection of endocrine tumors. Best Pract Res Clin Endocrinol Metab 19:311–324

54. Garin E, Le Jeune F, Devillers A et al (2009) Predictive value of ^{18}F-FDG PET and somatostatin receptor scintigraphy in patients with metastatic endocrine tumors. J Nucl Med 50:858–864

55. Binderup T, Knigge U, Loft A et al (2010) 18F-fluorodeoxyglucose positron emission tomography predicts survival of patients with neuroendocrine tumors. Clin Cancer Res 16:978–985

56. Severi S, Nanni O, Bodei L et al (2013) Role of ^{18}F-FDG PET/CT in patients treated with ^{177}Lu-DOTATATE for advanced differentiated neuroendocrine tumours. Eur J Nucl Med Mol Imaging 40:881–888

57. Ezziddin S, Adler L, Sabet A et al (2014) Prognostic stratification of metastatic gastroenteropancreatic neuroendocrine neoplasms by ^{18}F-FDG PET: feasibility of a metabolic grading system. J Nucl Med 55:1260–1266

58. Bodei L, Kidd M, Prasad V et al (2014 Jul 22) The future of nuclear medicine imaging of neuroendocrine tumors: on a clear day one might see forever…. Eur J Nucl Med Mol Imaging 41:2189–2193

59. Toumpanakis C, Kim MK, Rinke A et al (2014) Combination of cross-sectional and molecular imaging studies in the localization of gastroenteropancreatic neuroendocrine tumors. Neuroendocrinology 99:63–74

60. Naswa N, Sharma P, Gupta SK et al (2014) Dual tracer functional imaging of gastroenteropancreatic neuroendocrine tumors using ^{68}Ga-DOTA-NOC PET-CT and ^{18}F-FDG PET-CT: competitive or complimentary? Clin Nucl Med 39:27–34

61. Koopmans KP, Glaudemans AW (2014) Other PET tracers for neuroendocrine tumors. PET Clin 9:57–62

Endocrinological Approach to the Diagnosis of Pancreatic Neuroendocrine Neoplasms

4

Wouter W. de Herder

4.1 Introduction

Pancreatic neuroendocrine tumors (PanNETs) may produce specific hypersecretory symptoms and hormones. The diagnosis of PanNETs is based on their clinical presentation, hormone assays, radiological and nuclear medicine imaging, and pathology. In patients with so-called functioning, or syndromic PanNETs, specific biochemical tests should be requested in blood or 24-h urine samples obtained with or without provocative testing. Levels of circulating markers or urinary excreted products can be monitored and used for tumor follow-up.

Gastrinomas and insulinomas are the more frequent functioning or syndromic PanNETs [1, 2]. VIPoma (secreting vasoactive intestinal polypeptide [VIP]), glucagonoma (secreting glucagon), GHRHoma (secreting growth hormone-releasing hormone [GHRH]), ACTHoma (secreting adrenocorticotropin [ACTH]), PTHrPoma (secreting parathyroid hormone-related peptide [PTHrP]), somatostatinoma (secreting somatostatin), and PanNETs causing the carcinoid syndrome are relatively rare [1–5]. PanNETs secreting cholecystokinin (CCK), insulinlike growth factor II (IGF-II), renin, luteinizing hormone (LH), and erythropoietin are extremely rare [1, 2, 6]. Some experts also suggest to include those PanNETs secreting calcitonin, neurotensin, pancreatic polypeptide (PP), and ghrelin in the group of functioning PanNETs [1, 2, 7, 8].

4.2 Gastrinoma: Zollinger-Ellison Syndrome

The diagnosis of gastrinoma – Zollinger-Ellison syndrome (ZES) – requires the demonstration of an inappropriately elevated fasting serum gastrin (FSG) in the presence of gastric acid (hyper) secretion (gastric pH <2) [1, 9–13]. The assessment of the gastric pH is obligatory since conditions which present with fasting, or stimulated (see below) hypergastrinemia, such as atrophic gastritis, pernicious anemia, *Helicobacter pylori* infections, or the use of proton pump inhibitors (PPIs), are much more prevalent in the general population and, therefore, should be excluded first [2, 14–16].

In 40 % of ZES patients, the FSG is >10-fold elevated and the gastric pH <2, thus establishing the diagnosis. However, in the remaining 60 % of ZES patients, the FSG is <10-fold elevated with a gastric pH <2 [9, 10], and an additional secretin test is needed [1, 9]. Many commercial laboratories also use poorly characterized

W.W. de Herder, MD, PhD
Department of Internal Medicine,
Section of Endocrinology, Erasmus MC,
's Gravendijkwal 230, 3015 CE Rotterdam,
The Netherlands
e-mail: w.w.deherder@erasmusmc.nl

S. La Rosa, F. Sessa (eds.), *Pancreatic Neuroendocrine Neoplasms: Practical Approach to Diagnosis,
Classification, and Therapy*, DOI 10.1007/978-3-319-17235-4_4,
© Springer International Publishing Switzerland 2015

antibodies for the assessment of serum gastrin levels, and test results may, therefore, be unreliable [17, 18].

In patients taking PPIs in which ZES is suspected, it should be remembered that diagnostic procedures should only be initiated when the patient is stable and free of active acid-peptic disease and PPIs should not be abruptly stopped [2, 11, 15, 18, 19]. Abrupt stopping of PPIs may result in the development or recurrence of life-threatening acid-peptic complications [20]. Either the patient should be referred to a center experienced in the diagnosis, or if this is not possible, an attempt can be made to reduce the PPI dose and/or frequency of the PPI while monitoring the gastric pH. Alternatively, the PPIs can be slowly withdrawn with adequate coverage by high doses of H2 blockers and careful patient monitoring [2, 11, 15].

The criterion for a positive secretin test (using a rapid infusion of 2 U/kg secretin) is a >120 pg/mL increase in FSG over basal. This test has a sensitivity of 94 % and a specificity of 100 % [9]. A small percentage of patients with gastric acid hypersecretion and clinical features of ZES demonstrates normal fasting serum gastrin levels and negative secretin tests [9–11]. In light of the clinical and biochemical features described with CCKoma [6], these patients should have plasma CCK levels assessed. A secretin test cannot be used while a patient is taking PPIs because this can lead to a false-positive test [21]. Another problem is that secretin is increasingly becoming unavailable in many countries [16, 22]. This issue might be circumvented by substituting the secretin test by a glucagon stimulation test, but the experience with this test is still very limited, and its sensitivity and specificity are yet unclear [22].

The assessment of chromogranin A (CgA) is not reliable in the diagnosis of ZES, because up to 30 % of patients will have normal plasma CgA levels, whereas on the other hand the use of PPIs cause false-positive elevations of this nonspecific tumor marker [23–25].

4.3 Insulinoma

The exact criteria for the diagnosis of insulinoma continue to evolve and vary in different consensus documents and reviews [26–32]. In the most recent consensus report from the US Endocrine Society, the following diagnostic criteria were proposed: endogenous hyperinsulinism documented by the finding of symptoms, signs, or both with plasma concentrations of glucose <3.0 mmol/l (<55 mg/dl), insulin ≥3.0 mU/ml (18 pmol/l), C peptide ≥0.6 ng/ml (0.2 nmol/l), and proinsulin ≥5.0 pmol/l [27]. The presence of a plasma β-hydroxybutyrate levels of ≤2.7 mmol/l and an increase in plasma glucose 1.4 mmol/l (≥25 mg/dl) after IV glucagon indicates mediation of the hypoglycemia by insulin (or by an insulinlike growth factor). The use of an insulin cutoff value of ≥3 mU/ml instead of the older recommended value ≥5 mU/ml is supported by a recent study showing that 9 % of patients with insulinoma would be missed using the insulin cutoff value of ≥5 mU/ml [30].

The evaluation of serum CgA levels is generally not helpful for diagnosing patients with insulinoma, with an elevated CgA value having only a low specificity (73 %) [33].

4.4 VIPoma: Verner-Morrison or WDHA Syndrome

The most prevalent biochemical abnormalities in VIPoma patients are hypokalemia (virtually all patients), hypophosphatemia, acidosis, hypomagnesemia, hypo- or achlorhydria (75 % of patients), and hypercalcemia (25–75 % of patients). Glucose intolerance occurs in 50 % of patients, and elevated plasma glucose levels can be found in 18 % of cases. The diagnosis can be confirmed by demonstrating elevated fasting plasma VIP and peptide histidine-methionine (PHM) concentrations. Plasma CgA levels are generally elevated [24, 25].

4.5 Somatostatinoma

The most prevalent biochemical abnormalities in somatostatinoma patients are elevated plasma glucose levels and elevated fasting plasma somatostatin levels. Plasma CgA levels are generally elevated [24, 25].

4.6 Glucagonoma

The most prevalent biochemical abnormalities in glucagonoma patients are diabetes mellitus (>50 % of patients), normochromic normocytic anemia (33 % of patients), and elevated fasting plasma glucagon levels. Plasma CgA levels are generally elevated [24, 25].

References

1. Jensen RT, Cadiot G, Brandi ML et al (2012) ENETS consensus guidelines for the management of patients with digestive neuroendocrine neoplasms: functional pancreatic endocrine tumor syndromes. Neuroendocrinology 95(2):98–119
2. Ito T, Igarashi H, Jensen RT (2012) Pancreatic neuroendocrine tumors: clinical features, diagnosis and medical treatment: advances. Best Pract Res Clin Gastroenterol 26(6):737–753
3. Kamp K, Feelders RA, van Adrichem RC et al (2014) Parathyroid hormone-related peptide (PTHrP) secretion by gastroenteropancreatic neuroendocrine tumors (GEP-NETs): clinical features, diagnosis, management, and follow-up. J Clin Endocrinol Metab 99(9):3060–3069
4. Garby L, Caron P, Claustrat F et al (2012) Clinical characteristics and outcome of acromegaly induced by ectopic secretion of growth hormone-releasing hormone (GHRH): a French nationwide series of 21 cases. J Clin Endocrinol Metab 97(6):2093–2104
5. Borson-Chazot F, Garby L, Raverot G, Claustrat F, Raverot V, Sassolas G (2012) Acromegaly induced by ectopic secretion of GHRH: a review 30 years after GHRH discovery. Ann Endocrinol (Paris) 73(6): 497–502
6. Rehfeld JF, Federspiel B, Bardram L (2013) A neuroendocrine tumor syndrome from cholecystokinin secretion. N Engl J Med 368(12):1165–1166
7. Schneider R, Waldmann J, Swaid Z et al (2011) Calcitonin-secreting pancreatic endocrine tumors: systematic analysis of a rare tumor entity. Pancreas 40(2):213–221
8. Wang HS, Oh DS, Ohning GV, Pisegna JR (2007) Elevated serum ghrelin exerts an orexigenic effect that may maintain body mass index in patients with metastatic neuroendocrine tumors. J Mol Neurosci 33(3):225–231
9. Berna MJ, Hoffmann KM, Long SH, Serrano J, Gibril F, Jensen RT (2006) Serum gastrin in Zollinger-Ellison syndrome: II. Prospective study of gastrin provocative testing in 293 patients from the National Institutes of Health and comparison with 537 cases from the literature. Evaluation of diagnostic criteria, proposal of new criteria, and correlations with clinical and tumoral features. Medicine (Baltimore) 85(6): 331–364
10. Berna MJ, Hoffmann KM, Serrano J, Gibril F, Jensen RT (2006) Serum gastrin in Zollinger-Ellison syndrome: I. Prospective study of fasting serum gastrin in 309 patients from the National Institutes of Health and comparison with 2229 cases from the literature. Medicine (Baltimore) 85(6):295–330
11. Ito T, Cadiot G, Jensen RT (2012) Diagnosis of Zollinger-Ellison syndrome: increasingly difficult. World J Gastroenterol 18(39):5495–5503
12. Jensen RT, Niederle B, Mitry E et al (2006) Gastrinoma (duodenal and pancreatic). Neuroendocrinology 84(3):173–182
13. Roy PK, Venzon DJ, Feigenbaum KM et al (2001) Gastric secretion in Zollinger-Ellison syndrome. Correlation with clinical expression, tumor extent and role in diagnosis–a prospective NIH study of 235 patients and a review of 984 cases in the literature. Medicine (Baltimore) 80(3):189–222
14. Ito T, Igarashi H, Jensen RT (2013) Zollinger-Ellison syndrome: recent advances and controversies. Curr Opin Gastroenterol 29(6):650–661
15. Metz DC (2012) Diagnosis of the Zollinger-Ellison syndrome. Clin Gastroenterol Hepatol 10(2): 126–130
16. Poitras P, Gingras MH, Rehfeld JF (2013) Secretin stimulation test for gastrin release in Zollinger-Ellison syndrome: to do or not to do? Pancreas 42(6):903–904
17. Rehfeld JF, Gingras MH, Bardram L, Hilsted L, Goetze JP, Poitras P (2011) The Zollinger-Ellison syndrome and mismeasurement of gastrin. Gastroenterology 140(5):1444–1453
18. Rehfeld JF, Bardram L, Hilsted L, Poitras P, Goetze JP (2012) Pitfalls in diagnostic gastrin measurements. Clin Chem 58(5):831–836
19. O'Toole D, Salazar R, Falconi M et al (2006) Rare functioning pancreatic endocrine tumors. Neuroendocrinology 84(3):189–195
20. Poitras P, Gingras MH, Rehfeld JF (2012) The Zollinger-Ellison syndrome: dangers and conse-

quences of interrupting antisecretory treatment. Clin Gastroenterol Hepatol 10(2):199–202

21. Shah P, Singh MH, Yang YX, Metz DC (2013) Hypochlorhydria and achlorhydria are associated with false-positive secretin stimulation testing for Zollinger-Ellison syndrome. Pancreas 42(6):932–936

22. Shibata C, Kakyo M, Kinouchi M et al (2013) Criteria for the glucagon provocative test in the diagnosis of gastrinoma. Surg Today 43(11):1281–1285

23. Rehfeld JF, Bardram L, Hilsted L, Goetze JP (2014) An evaluation of chromogranin A versus gastrin and progastrin in gastrinoma diagnosis and control. Biomark Med 8(4):571–580

24. de Herder WW (2007) Biochemistry of neuroendocrine tumours. Best Pract Res Clin Endocrinol Metab 21(1):33–41

25. Kanakis G, Kaltsas G (2012) Biochemical markers for gastroenteropancreatic neuroendocrine tumours (GEP-NETs). Best Pract Res Clin Gastroenterol 26(6):791–802

26. Agin A, Charrie A, Chikh K, Tabarin A, Vezzosi D (2013) Fast test: clinical practice and interpretation. Ann Endocrinol (Paris) 74(3):174–184

27. Cryer PE, Axelrod L, Grossman AB et al (2009) Evaluation and management of adult hypoglycemic disorders: an endocrine society clinical practice guideline. J Clin Endocrinol Metab 94(3):709–728

28. Cryer PE, Axelrod L, Grossman AB, Heller SR, Seaquist ER, Service FJ (2013) Diagnostic accuracy of an "amended" insulin-glucose ratio for the biochemical diagnosis of insulinomas. Ann Intern Med 158(6):500–501

29. Buffet A, Vezzosi D, Maiza JC, Grunenwald S, Bennet A, Caron P (2013) Increased plasma beta-hydroxybutyrate levels during the fasting test in patients with endogenous hyperinsulinaemic hypoglycaemia. Eur J Endocrinol 169(1):91–97

30. Guettier JM, Lungu A, Goodling A, Cochran C, Gorden P (2013) The role of proinsulin and insulin in the diagnosis of insulinoma: a critical evaluation of the endocrine society clinical practice guideline. J Clin Endocrinol Metab 98(12):4752–4758

31. De Leon DD, Stanley CA (2013) Determination of insulin for the diagnosis of hyperinsulinemic hypoglycemia. Best Pract Res Clin Endocrinol Metab 27(6):763–769

32. Nauck MA, Meier JJ (2012) Diagnostic accuracy of an "amended" insulin-glucose ratio for the biochemical diagnosis of insulinomas. Ann Intern Med 157(11):767–775

33. Qiao XW, Qiu L, Chen YJ et al (2014) Chromogranin A is a reliable serum diagnostic biomarker for pancreatic neuroendocrine tumors but not for insulinomas. BMC Endocr Disord 14:64. doi:10.1186/1472-6823-14-64.:64-14

Cytological Diagnosis of Pancreatic Neuroendocrine Neoplasms

5

Massimo Bongiovanni, Christine Sempoux, and Antoine Nobile

5.1 Introduction

With the development of ultrasound endoscopic procedures to investigate pancreatic masses, *fine-needle aspiration* (FNA) has become an essential technique in the initial management of patients diagnosed with pancreatic lesions.

Pancreatic neuroendocrine tumors (PanNETs) are rare, accounting for approximately 2 % of all pancreatic neoplasia [1–5]. They can be functioning or nonfunctioning. Functioning tumors synthesize and secrete various hormones including, among many others, insulin and glucagon. This uncontrolled activity can sometimes lead to clinically obvious symptoms that are of great help to locate and diagnose these tumors in their early stage. By contrast, nonfunctioning tumors are discovered incidentally ("incidentaloma") in case of abdominal scanning for other conditions, compressive pancreatic mass with or without jaundice, or liver metastasis. Because of the absence of secretion, they are usually found later and are thus larger.

When a pancreatic mass is discovered in the setting of multiple endocrine neoplasia type 1 (MEN1), von Hippel-Lindau or von Recklinghausen diseases, and tuberous sclerosis, the diagnosis can be suspected clinically and eventually helps the cytopathologist to narrow his or her differential diagnosis. Different approaches are possible for pancreatic masses (and/or liver metastasis):

1. *Endoscopic ultrasound-guided (EUS) FNA* [6]
2. Percutaneous ultrasound-guided or *CT-guided FNA*

EUS-FNA of pancreatic masses is gaining importance, an increasing number of PanNETs being diagnosed with this procedure [7]. Among young people (<35 years old), PanNET has been reported as the most frequent diagnosis done by EUS-FNA [8]. In one of the largest series evaluating the performance of EUS-FNA in diagnosing PanNET preoperatively as compared to histological final diagnosis, PanNETs were recognized in 38 of 48 cases (79 %) based on cytomorphological analysis and immunocytochemical studies [6]. As to cystic PanNET, cytology has been shown to be the most accurate test for preoperative diagnoses compared with imaging and fluid analysis [9]. In particular, EUS-FNA can be used to diagnose very small lesions, as compared with computed tomography (CT) and magnetic resonance imaging, where such small lesions cannot be seen [10, 11]. Moreover, EUS-FNA seems to have a higher yield of neoplastic cells and

M. Bongiovanni, MD (✉) • C. Sempoux, MD
A. Nobile, MD
Department of Laboratory,
Institute of Pathology, CHUV, Rue du Bugnon, 25,
Lausanne CH-1011, Switzerland
e-mail: massimo.bongiovanni@chuv.ch

S. La Rosa, F. Sessa (eds.), *Pancreatic Neuroendocrine Neoplasms: Practical Approach to Diagnosis,*
Classification, and Therapy, DOI 10.1007/978-3-319-17235-4_5,

consequently a lower rate of nondiagnostic cases, as compared to CT-guided biopsies [12].

EUS-FNA has a relatively high sensitivity for diagnosing neuroendocrine pancreatic lesions, with rates ranging from 83 to 94 % and specificity rates up to 95 % [6, 13].

5.2 Techniques

Several articles have shown that EUS-guided FNA is now established as an accurate and cost-effective procedure not only to detect PanNETs but also for their staging. Actually, peripancreatic lymph nodes and other peripancreatic tissues are well visualized during pancreatic EUS and can be aspirated in the same session [6, 14].

Working with a skilled endoscopist is of prime importance to obtain good-quality material. Briefly, a linear endosonographic device is used along with a 22- or 25-gauge needle. Under US guidance, the lesion is visualized with the best possible angle, followed by insertion of the needle and eventually aspiration of material [15].

Usually 2–3 passes are performed: the first and second passes are useful for quantitative evaluation of the material by the on-site cytopathologist (*rapid on-site evaluation (ROSE)*) after performing a rapid toluidine blue staining or a modified Papanicolaou (Pap) staining. The third pass is kept exclusively to enrich the material for cell block preparation. The rapid toluidine blue staining is then washed out and replaced in the cytology lab by a usual PAP staining.

The on-site presence of a cytopathologist is preferred in order to reduce the number of unsatisfactory specimens, by asking the gastroenterologist additional passes into the lesion if necessary [16]. Actually, a material quantitatively insufficient to produce paraffin-embedded cell blocks and to perform ancillary techniques represents a limiting factor to ascertain the diagnosis [10, 14, 17]. Thus, nondiagnostic or false-negative FNA diagnosis can be seen in a limited number of cases, especially with small-sized tumors [6]. For cystic PanNETs, additional passes in solid areas are usually required to reduce the possibility of acellular specimens (Fig. 5.1a–f).

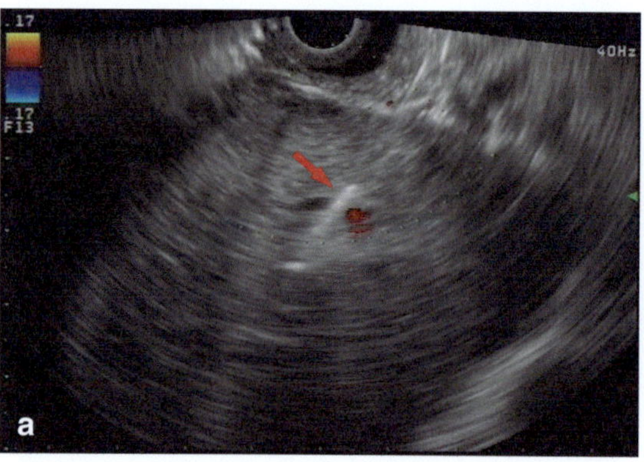

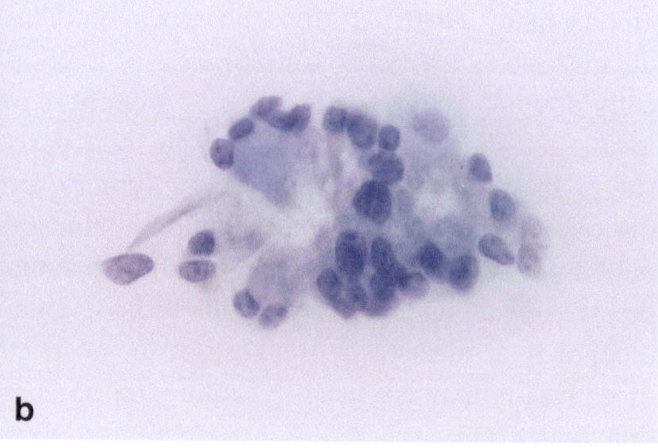

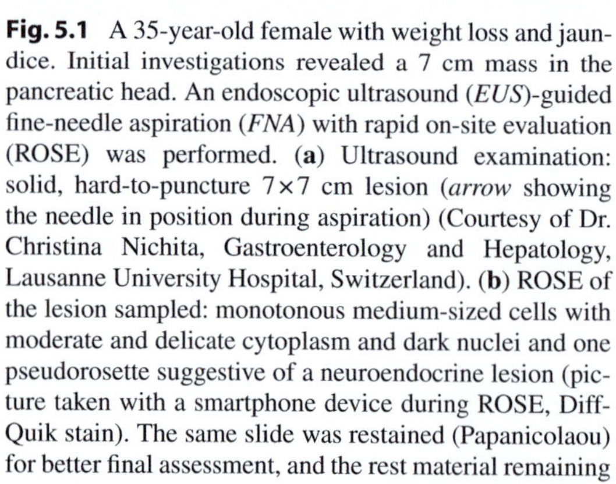

Fig. 5.1 A 35-year-old female with weight loss and jaundice. Initial investigations revealed a 7 cm mass in the pancreatic head. An endoscopic ultrasound (*EUS*)-guided fine-needle aspiration (*FNA*) with rapid on-site evaluation (ROSE) was performed. (**a**) Ultrasound examination: solid, hard-to-puncture 7×7 cm lesion (*arrow* showing the needle in position during aspiration) (Courtesy of Dr. Christina Nichita, Gastroenterology and Hepatology, Lausanne University Hospital, Switzerland). (**b**) ROSE of the lesion sampled: monotonous medium-sized cells with moderate and delicate cytoplasm and dark nuclei and one pseudorosette suggestive of a neuroendocrine lesion (picture taken with a smartphone device during ROSE, Diff-Quik stain). The same slide was restained (Papanicolaou) for better final assessment, and the rest material remaining

in the needle was rinsed in preservative solution for liquid-based preparations (*LB*). (**c**) LB-Papanicolaou-stained slide: bland appearing group of cells, some with larger salt and pepper nuclei, others with small amount of cytoplasm. (**d**) Following the initial ROSE diagnosis, two dedicated passes were performed for cell block preparation (hematoxylin and eosin stain) and immunocytochemical stains (*inset*, chromogranin A immunostain). The final diagnosis was neoplastic lesion, consistent with a low-grade neuroendocrine tumor. (**e**) Tumor resection specimen: a 4×5 cm mass, corresponding to the ultrasonographic image (**a**). (**f**) The histological examination confirmed the diagnosis of a neuroendocrine pancreatic tumor, NET G2

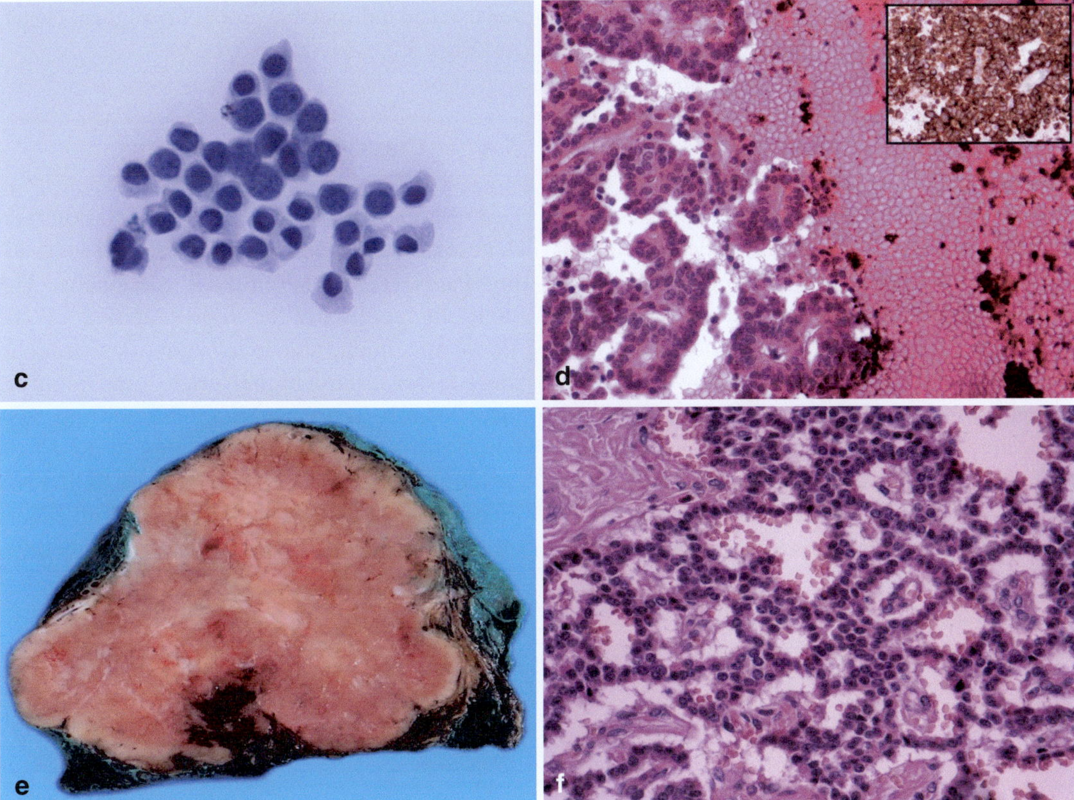

Fig. 5.1 (continued)

5.3 Cytomorphological Features of PanNETs

At low-power view, one can observe a clean or hemorrhagic background. In the wide spectrum of tumors with neuroendocrine differentiation, clear-cut tumor necrosis is always associated with malignant behavior. FNA material is highly cellular and contains predominantly isolated cells. Sometimes, cohesive groups show some hints of neuroendocrine architecture (ribbons and rosettes). PanNETs are highly vascular; it is thus not uncommon to find palisaded tumor cells polarized toward a capillary lumen (Table 5.1).

Around 15 % of PanNETs are partly or entirely cystic and can be confused with other cystic neoplasms. However, cytomorphology is specific of PanNETs and remains identical in cystic and solid forms. Cyst fluid can be misleading because of important variations of macro- and microscopic aspects and should be interpreted carefully. As expected, CEA and amylase levels are usually low in these lesions.

At high-power view, cells are of variable size (usually not large) and show an eccentric nucleus and enough typically granular cytoplasm to exhibit a plasmacytoid appearance. High nucleocytoplasmic

Table 5.1 Main cytomorphological features of PanNETs

Clean or hemorrhagic background
Highly cellular smear with a predominance of isolated cells
Some cohesive groups sometimes with a typical neuroendocrine architecture (rosettes, ribbons)
Small- to medium-sized cells with plasmacytoid appearance
Nuclei round to oval with "salt and pepper" chromatin
Cytoplasmic changes (e.g., clearing) not to be confused with primary or metastatic carcinoma
A cystic lesion does not rule out a PanNET!

ratio and nuclear molding are not characteristic of PanNETs: if found, they should prompt alternate diagnoses in the category of small-blue-round-cell tumors, small cell carcinoma being at the top of the differential. Nuclei are round to oval and regular in size. Nuclear pleomorphism, if any, does not correlate with biological behavior. Chromatin is usually described as salt and pepper, and nucleoli of various sizes can be appreciated. Cytoplasmic changes define uncommon morphological variants of PanNETs (lipid rich, clear cell, oncocytic, etc.) that should be kept in mind to avoid a wrong diagnosis of primary or metastatic carcinoma [9, 18, 19].

Features associated with malignancy include spindling or multinucleation of tumor cells, high mitotic count, and necrotic background. Histo-/cytologically proven metastasis remains the most reliable and indisputable proof of malignant behavior (Figs. 5.2, 5.3a–d, and 5.4a, b).

5.4 Classification/Grading

Grading PanNET is based on proliferation rate. A note of caution should be addressed on grading PanNETs on cytological specimens. The sampling could not be representative of the whole specimen, and local variations occur in these lesions; thus, higher-grade zone could be insufficiently represented in the scoring system. Proliferation index evaluated by Ki-67 on cytological material obtained from EUS-FNA procedures has shown good results, and this is either with alcohol-fixed or paraffin-embedded

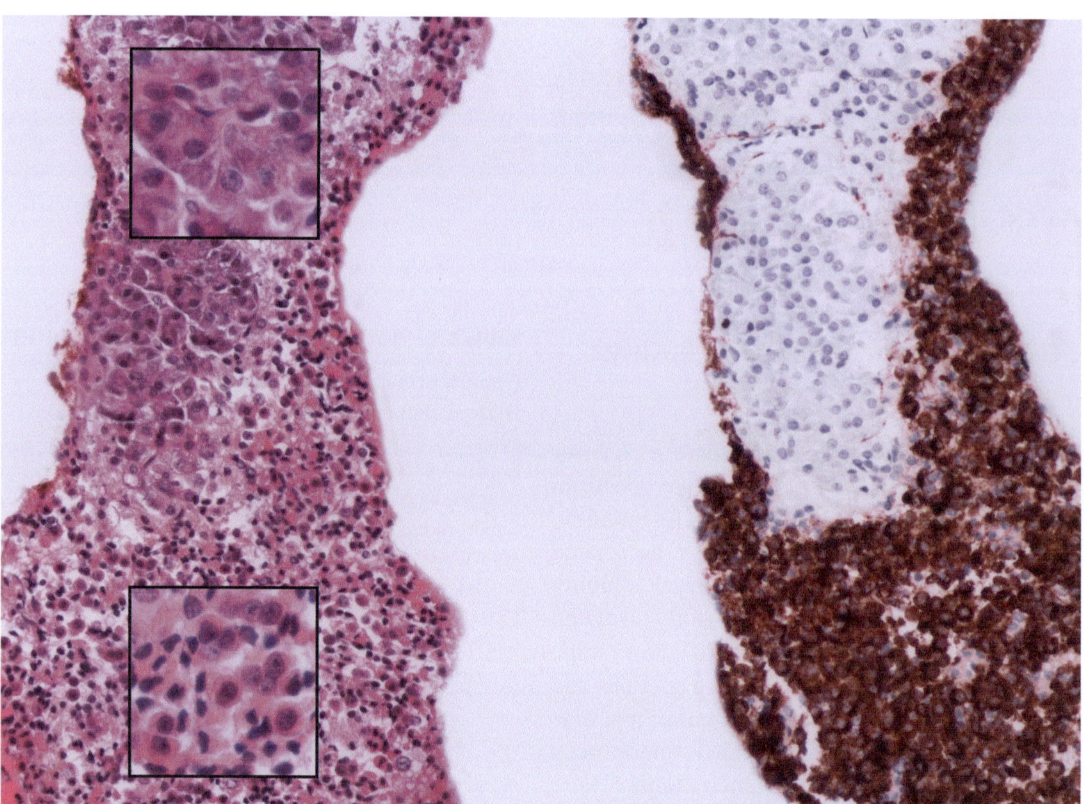

Fig. 5.2 The cell block preparation is a fundamental complement to assist in the final diagnosis as it allows to perform immunohistochemistry. In this case normal exocrine acinar cells (*upper part* of the picture) were intimately admixed with neoplastic cells (*lower part* of the picture) that stained positive for chromogranin A. The insets show at higher magnification the morphological aspect of medium-sized acinar cells (*upper inset*), with abundant eosinophilic cytoplasm, and small- to medium-sized neuroendocrine-looking cells (*lower inset*) with obvious nucleoli (*left picture*, hematoxylin and eosin stain; *right picture*, chromogranin A stain)

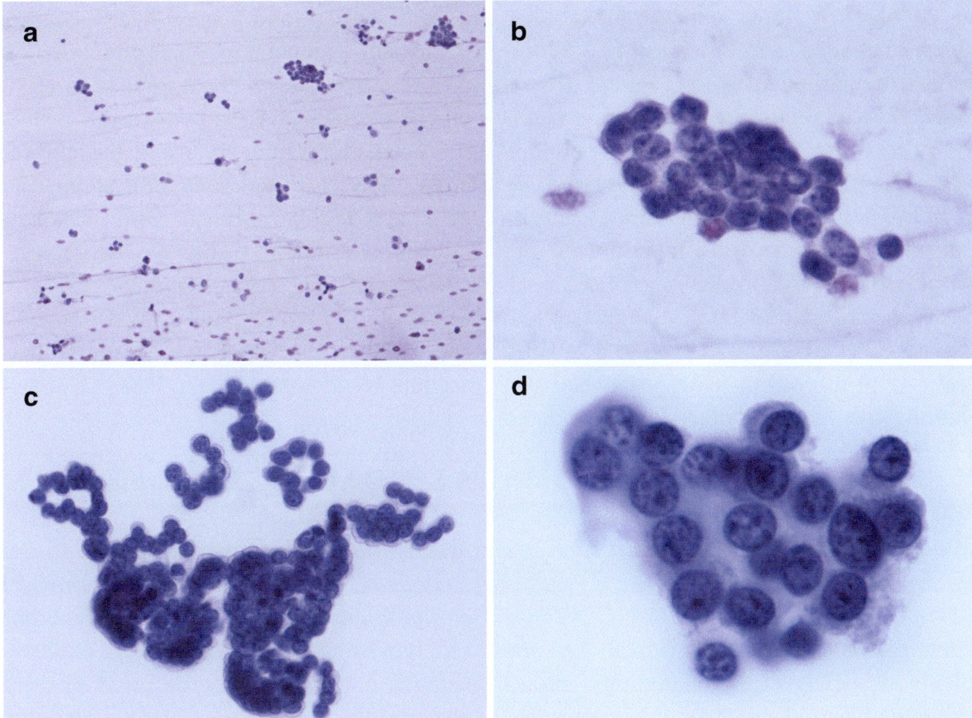

Fig. 5.3 Morphological aspects of well-differentiated neuroendocrine neoplasms (smear, Papanicolaou stains). (**a**) At low magnification the background is slightly hemorrhagic, without necrosis or inflammation. Moderate cellularity is seen with a predominantly discohesive pattern. (**b**) Higher magnification shows a group of cohesive cells with crowded nuclei and dark chromatin, without particular differentiation. (**c**) Other regions of the same slide show trabecular and rosette-like structures. This architecture, a plasmacytoid aspect of some cells, the high nucleocytoplasmic ratio, and the finely granular chromatin suggest a neuroendocrine differentiation. (**d**) Nuclear details: round- to oval-shaped nuclei with regular nuclear membrane contour and nucleoli

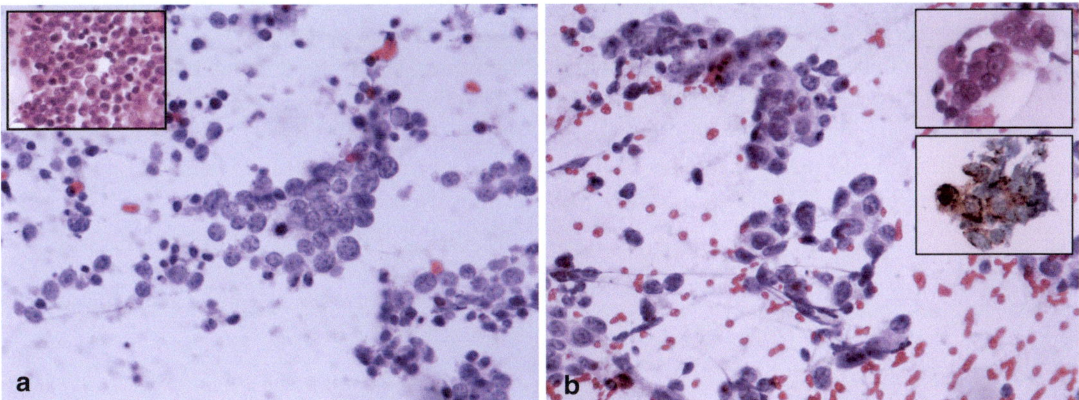

Fig. 5.4 Morphological aspects of poorly differentiated neuroendocrine carcinomas (smear, Papanicolaou stains). Crowded smears with high cellularity and background cell debris (necrosis). (**a**) Small-sized and loosely cohesive cells showing obvious nuclear molding, with salt and pepper chromatin and apoptotic debris. The cell block preparation (*inset*, hematoxylin and eosin stain) shows the same aspect. The final diagnosis was consistent with a small cell neuroendocrine carcinoma, NEC G3. (**b**) Larger cells with salt and pepper chromatin and macronucleoli. The cell block preparation showed only a small group of neoplastic cells (*inset, upper part*) that were intensely and diffusely positive for chromogranin A (*inset, lower part*). The final diagnosis was consistent with large cell neuroendocrine carcinoma, NEC G3

tumors. Moreover, high concordances have been found between cytological and histological grading to distinguish G1-G2 PanNET from G3 PanNEC (pancreatic neuroendocrine carcinoma), by counting a minimum of 100 neoplastic cells [20–22]. The grading obtained by Ki-67 on cytological material is more accurate than mitotic count, as mitotic count is not always possible on cytological samples. As an alternative to Ki-67 proliferative index, phosphohistone-H3 (PHH3) has proved to be a valid surrogate of proliferation assessment and can be paired with a computer for automated count [23].

5.5　Cytological Reporting Systems

The new *nomenclature* established by the Papanicolaou Society of Cytopathology applies also for PanNET, and we strongly recommend its use [4]. Briefly, the new terminology is based on a six-tiered diagnostic category system (Table 5.2).

PanNET usually falls in the neoplastic category, under the specification "other" if they are of low grade (well differentiated), as it happens in the majority of cases. This decision has been justified by the fact that placing neuroendocrine lesions in this neoplastic category allows broader management options in comparison to placing neuroendocrine lesions in the malignant category (where the only possible management decision is surgery). Final management decision is then done in accordance with clinical-pathological

Table 5.2 The new proposed classification systems for reporting pancreatobiliary cytology

Nondiagnostic
Negative
Atypical
Neoplastic (benign or other)
Suspicious
Positive/malignant

Modified by Pitman et al. [4]
Most of the well-differentiated PanNETs fall into the neoplastic category (see text)

conditions (age and general health condition of the patient, clinical hormonal symptoms, size and proliferation rate of the lesion, compression of other structures).

When the architectural and the nuclear features show neuroendocrine differentiation, but cells are highly atypical with anisokaryosis, mitosis, and necrosis, then the cytological diagnosis fall under the "suspicious" or "positive" category. These are poorly differentiated small and large cell neuroendocrine carcinomas that account for less than 5 % of PanNET.

5.6　Ancillary Techniques

Ancillary techniques are fundamental to establish a correct diagnosis and can be performed either on cytological smears or on paraffin-embedded cell blocks. Almost all PanNETs express cytokeratins and neuroendocrine markers (synaptophysin, chromogranin, CD56). Positivity has been shown also for CD57 and CA 19-9. Ki-67 is used for grading purposes and has excellent performance on cytological material.

Hormones detected in the serum in cases of functioning PanNET can also be used on cytological material (i.e., insulin, glucagon, somatostatin, etc.), but not all labs have established the correct protocols, and sometimes, even in case of clinical symptoms, the presence of such hormones cannot be demonstrated at the immunocytochemical level. New markers, such as Islet 1, Pax8, and CDX-2, are useful to demonstrate a primary pancreatic versus a small bowel origin especially in metastatic location with unknown primary [24]. Moreover, somatostatin receptor type 2A can be detected in cytological specimens for therapeutic and monitoring approach [25, 26].

5.7　Molecular Testing

Molecular genetic tests (in case of confirmed or suspected MEN1 or von Hippel-Lindau disease) and *fluorescent in situ hybridization* (FISH) analysis can be easily performed on cytological material, either from smears, liquid-based cytology, and/or cell block preparation. The quality of DNA/RNA is excellent [25].

5.8 Differential Diagnosis

Apart from neuroendocrine carcinomas (e.g., originating from the digestive tract or the lungs) metastatic to the pancreas, the *differential diagnosis* typically includes "stroma-poor and parenchyma-rich" tumors, such as acinar cell carcinoma (ACC), solid pseudopapillary tumor (SPT), and pancreatoblastoma or plasmacytoma.

ACC is a tough differential diagnosis. Among other patterns, it presents with acinar structures that can be easily confused with rosettes. Luminal space outline is usually sharply demarcated, a feature not seen in neuroendocrine tumors. A minor expression of neuroendocrine markers can be found in up to 50 % of ACC. However, pancreatic enzymes (especially trypsin) and BCL10 immunoreactivities help to confirm this diagnosis.

SPT typically arise in young women and display pseudopapillae with hyalinized fibrovascular cores. These pseudopapillae are lined by cells with granular chromatin and sometimes a PAS-positive intracytoplasmic hyaline body. These structures can be misinterpreted as perivascular palisades or rosettes. Cytokeratins are usually patchy or negative, but positivity for β-catenin (nuclear and cytoplasmic expression), CD10, and vimentin is usually found. Focally, expression of synaptophysin and CD56 can be noted. Enzymes such as trypsin may be produced.

In case of tumors with plasmacytoid appearance (i.e., plasmacytoma, some melanomas, and some lymphomas), a panel of antibodies comprising CD45, CD138, Melan-A, and S-100 besides cytokeratins and neuroendocrine markers is indicated.

A variety of metastatic tumors can involve the pancreas and thus widen the differential diagnosis. Appropriate clinical information about the patient history is crucial, as usual. To note, metastatic clear cell renal carcinoma to the pancreas is not infrequent and can be considered in the differential diagnosis with benign or malignant serous tumors (e.g., pancreatic microcystic cystadenoma), as well as the rare lipid-rich or clear cell PanNETs.

References

1. Chatzipantelis P, Salla C, Konstantinou P, Karoumpalis I, Sakellariou S, Doumani I (2008) Endoscopic ultrasound-guided fine-needle aspiration cytology of pancreatic neuroendocrine tumors: a study of 48 cases. Cancer 114:255–262
2. Frankel WL (2006) Update on pancreatic endocrine tumors. Arch Pathol Lab Med 130:963–966
3. Fesinmeyer MD, Austin MA, Li CI, De Roos AJ, Bowen DJ (2005) Differences in survival by histologic type of pancreatic cancer. Cancer Epidemiol Biomark Prev Publ Am Assoc Cancer Res Cosponsored Am Soc Prev Oncol 14:1766–1773
4. Pitman MB, Centeno BA, Ali SZ et al (2014) Standardized terminology and nomenclature for pancreatobiliary cytology: the papanicolaou society of cytopathology guidelines. Diagn Cytopathol 42: 338–350
5. Klimstra DS, Capella C, Hruban RH, Arnold R, Kloppel G (2010) Neuroendocrine neoplasms of the pancreas. In: Carneiro F, Bosman C, Hruban RH, Theise ND (eds) WHO classification of tumours of the digestive system, 4th edn. WHO PRESS, Lyon, pp 322–326
6. Bernstein J, Ustun B, Alomari A et al (2013) Performance of endoscopic ultrasound-guided fine needle aspiration in diagnosing pancreatic neuroendocrine tumors. Cyto J 10:10
7. Fernandez-del Castillo C (2014) Standardized cytopathology reporting for the pancreas: the time is right. Cancer Cytopathol 122:397–398
8. Redelman M, Cramer HM, Wu HH (2014) Pancreatic fine-needle aspiration cytology in patients < 35-years of age: a retrospective review of 174 cases spanning a 17-year period. Diagn Cytopathol 42:297–301
9. Morales-Oyarvide V, Yoon WJ, Ingkakul T et al (2014) Cystic pancreatic neuroendocrine tumors: the value of cytology in preoperative diagnosis. Cancer Cytopathol 122:435–444
10. Patel KK, Kim MK (2008) Neuroendocrine tumors of the pancreas: endoscopic diagnosis. Curr Opin Gastroenterol 24:638–642
11. Rosch T, Lightdale CJ, Botet JF et al (1992) Localization of pancreatic endocrine tumors by endoscopic ultrasonography. N Engl J Med 326:1721–1726
12. Jhala D, Eloubeidi M, Chhieng DC et al (2002) Fine needle aspiration biopsy of the islet cell tumor of pancreas: a comparison between computerized axial tomography and endoscopic ultrasound-guided fine needle aspiration biopsy. Ann Diagn Pathol 6:106–112

13. Lee LS (2010) Diagnosis of pancreatic neuroendocrine tumors and the role of endoscopic ultrasound. Gastroenterol Hepatol 6:520–522

14. Chang F, Chandra A, Culora G, Mahadeva U, Meenan J, Herbert A (2006) Cytologic diagnosis of pancreatic endocrine tumors by endoscopic ultrasound-guided fine-needle aspiration: a review. Diagn Cytopathol 34:649–658

15. Brugge W, Dewitt J, Klapman JB et al (2014) Techniques for cytologic sampling of pancreatic and bile duct lesions. Diagn Cytopathol 42:333–337

16. Klapman JB, Logrono R, Dye CE, Waxman I (2003) Clinical impact of on-site cytopathology interpretation on endoscopic ultrasound-guided fine needle aspiration. Am J Gastroenterol 98:1289–1294

17. Gu M, Ghafari S, Lin F, Ramzy I (2005) Cytological diagnosis of endocrine tumors of the pancreas by endoscopic ultrasound-guided fine-needle aspiration biopsy. Diagn Cytopathol 32:204–210

18. Zhang Z, Lee JG, Gu M (2014) Cytologic features of lipid-rich variant of pancreatic endocrine tumor – report of two cases with literature review. Diagn Cytopathol 42:308–313

19. Chen S, Lin J, Wang X, Wu HH, Cramer H (2014) EUS-guided FNA cytology of pancreatic neuroendocrine tumour (PanNET): a retrospective study of 132 cases over an 18-year period in a single institution. Cytopathology 25:396–403 doi:10.1111/cyt.12137 [Epub ahead of print]

20. Carlinfante G, Baccarini P, Berretti D et al (2014) Ki-67 cytological index can distinguish well-differentiated from poorly differentiated pancreatic neuroendocrine tumors: a comparative cytohistological study of 53 cases. Virchows Arch 465:49–55

21. Farrell JM, Pang JC, Kim GE, Tabatabai ZL (2014) Pancreatic neuroendocrine tumors: accurate grading with Ki-67 index on fine-needle aspiration specimens using the WHO 2010/ENETS criteria. Cancer Cytopathol 122:770–778

22. Weynand B, Borbath I, Bernard V et al (2013) Pancreatic neuroendocrine tumour grading on endoscopic ultrasound-guided fine needle aspiration: high reproducibility and inter-observer agreement of the Ki-67 labelling index. Cytopathology 25:389–395 doi:10.1111/cyt.12111 [Epub ahead of print]

23. Draganova-Tacheva R, Bibbo M, Birbe R, Daskalakis C, Solomides C (2013) The potential value of phosphohistone-h3 mitotic index determined by digital image analysis in the assessment of pancreatic endocrine tumors in fine-needle aspiration cytology specimens. Acta Cytol 57:291–295

24. Koo J, Mertens RB, Mirocha JM, Wang HL, Dhall D (2012) Value of islet 1 and PAX8 in identifying metastatic neuroendocrine tumors of pancreatic origin. Mod Pathol 25:893–901

25. Layfield LJ, Ehya H, Filie AC et al (2014) Utilization of ancillary studies in the cytologic diagnosis of biliary and pancreatic lesions: the papanicolaou society of cytopathology guidelines for pancreatobiliary cytology. Diagn Cytopathol 42:351–362

26. Volante M, Brizzi MP, Faggiano A et al (2007) Somatostatin receptor type 2A immunohistochemistry in neuroendocrine tumors: a proposal of scoring system correlated with somatostatin receptor scintigraphy. Mod Pathol 20:1172–1182

Classification and Staging of Pancreatic Neuroendocrine Neoplasms

6

Frediano Inzani, Gianluigi Petrone, and Guido Rindi

6.1 The Significance of Classification

The classification of cancer relies on multiple information, and the pathology classification mainly derives from morphology, i.e., the morphological study of the surgical specimen. The technological expansion in pathology practice is reflected in current pathological cancer classifications, now containing not only morphological but also molecular descriptors. An ideal pathological classification conveys information that uniquely describes a cancer disease or a cancer subset. Most importantly, the pathological classification is a clinical tool intended to direct to the best possible management of the patient, associating cancer definitions to prognosis appraisal. The continuous growth in cancer knowledge and the constant technological development in pathology practice have been widely expanding the pathological classification concept, not any more an algid taxonomic list of cancer disease but an evolving clinical instrument. Needless to say, the limits of a pathological classification do reflect the limits of the current knowledge on each specific cancer disease. In any case, the major property requested for an effective pathological classification is its robustness and reproducibility in clinical practice as proven from published evidence. The present chapter reports the current classification of pancreatic neuroendocrine neoplasms as developed in the last years and reflects the current status of knowledge on this cancer disease.

6.2 Terminology

Carcinoid, apudoma, insulinoma, glucagonoma, tumors of the diffuse endocrine system, endocrine tumor, endocrine carcinoma, well-differentiated endocrine tumor, well-differentiated endocrine carcinoma, poorly differentiated endocrine carcinoma, neuroendocrine carcinoma, small cell carcinoma, and large cell neuroendocrine carcinoma are all terms that have been used to describe the neuroendocrine neoplasms of the pancreas [1–9]. These are indeed the terms used in the classifications developed since 1980 by the World Health Organization (WHO) [5, 7, 8]. The WHO represents the ideal place for a world-shared and updated vision of cancer classification meant to provide a worldwide guide for pathologist. The present chapter will adopt the current WHO classification principles and standard definitions from now on defined as WHO 2010 [10–12].

F. Inzani • G. Petrone • G. Rindi (✉)
Institute of Pathology,
Università Cattolica-Policlinico A. Gemelli,
Rome, Italy
e-mail: guido.rindi@rm.unicatt.it

S. La Rosa, F. Sessa (eds.), *Pancreatic Neuroendocrine Neoplasms: Practical Approach to Diagnosis, Classification, and Therapy*, DOI 10.1007/978-3-319-17235-4_6,
© Springer International Publishing Switzerland 2015

6.3 Principles of WHO 2010 Classification

All previous WHO classifications were centered either on basic morphofunctional descriptors only, as embedded in terms like carcinoid, insulinoma, and glucagonoma or, more recently, on differentiation as defined by morphology and staging parameters like tumor size, gross local invasion, and presence of metastasis. The current WHO classification is based on grading and staging as separate tools [11]. The reasons for such choice derived from the need for standard cancer measure in patients with neuroendocrine neoplasm, alike all other types of cancer disease. Aligning neuroendocrine cancer with type-specific cancer measure tools was felt as one major requirement for a better understanding of such rare cancer disease. It is implied that neuroendocrine neoplasms all bear a potential for malignancy that is further defined by grade and stage. The term "neoplasm" was adopted to embrace all grades of neuroendocrine cancer given its broad though specific significance of new, independent growth. The adjective "neuroendocrine" was adopted to describe the presence of shared neural antigens as observed in both normal epithelial cells of the diffuse neuroendocrine system and cancer cells [13]. No embryological derivative implication is considered for this connotative adjective. The term "neuroendocrine tumor" (NET) was adopted for low to intermediate grade neoplasms and embeds the prognostic significance of relatively good survival as measurable in years. A NET definition gives clinician time for managing a malignant though relatively torpid cancer disease. By converse, the term "neuroendocrine carcinoma" (NEC) was adopted since associating with manifest malignancy and implying a prognostic significance of poor survival as measurable in months. NECs are further subdivided in small cell and large cell types according to morphology. A NEC definition gives the message to the clinician that the patient needs immediate attention for management and cure.

6.4 Clinical Classification

The neuroendocrine neoplasm of the pancreas is differently defined according to the presence/absence of overt hyperfunctional syndromes [6, 9, 12]. If this is the case, the lesion may be defined using the peptide-oma appropriate description, like insulinoma when a hypoglycemic/hyperinsulinemic condition is present. Functioning pancreatic neuroendocrine neoplasms account for about one third of cases in current literature and are mostly low- to intermediate-grade neoplasms. They comprise the most frequent insulinoma accounting for about 67 % of functioning NETs, the less frequent gastrinoma (11 %), glucagonoma (6 %), VIPoma (5.7 %), serotonin-producing "carcinoid" NET (4.5 %), and PPoma (4 %) [9, 14–17]. Other rare NETs associated with the unregulated production of various hormones (ACTH, calcitonin, GHRH, ghrelin, PTH, and somatostatin) account altogether for about 4.8 % of functioning NETs.

The majority of neuroendocrine neoplasms of the pancreas are nonfunctioning and account for about 70 % of recently reported series [9, 14–17]. This probably reflects the increased incidence of neuroendocrine neoplasms as recently observed worldwide [18–21]. This phenomenon likely is the result of increased diffusion and sensitivity of diagnostic procedures, the adoption of cancer screening programs, and increased awareness of neuroendocrine cancer disease. The vast majority of nonfunctioning neuroendocrine neoplasms of the pancreas are low- to intermediate-grade NETs and account for about 93 % of cases, while only about 7 % are high-grade NECs [15, 17]. Nonfunctioning neuroendocrine neoplasms present with local mass symptoms or, more frequently, are discovered by chance during diagnostic procedures established for other clinical reasons including the presence of distant metastasis. The unspecific presentation of nonfunctioning pancreatic neuroendocrine neoplasms demands a complex protocol of diagnostic tests and procedures culminating with the definitive histological diagnosis, most frequently on small samples obtained at endoscopic ultrasound (EUS), fine-needle aspiration (FNA), or fine-needle tissue acquisition (FNTA) procedures [22]. Such complex diagnostic voyage needs to be tailored for each patient after multidisciplinary clinical discussion to minimize duplications, costs, and errors and should be performed in expert referral centers, as suggested and practiced for rare cancer management [23, 24].

6.5 Pathological Classification: Grading

The well-known limits of morphology for neuroendocrine neoplasm definition and prognostication required a more effective tool. Differentiation, the basis of the previous WHO classification [7, 8], is a robust and familiar method for the practicing pathologist; however, it is experience-dependent and carries a significant load of subjectivity. In addition, it proved somehow ineffective in predicting prognosis for the "uncertain behavior" category, probably the largest fraction of pancreatic neuroendocrine neoplasms [25]. The grading of neuroendocrine neoplasms is based only on proliferation measured by both mitotic count and Ki67 indexes (Table 6.1). The proliferation measure was chosen as an effective method for cancer prognostication similar to what was experienced in other types of cancer even of neuroepithelial type [26]. A three-tier system was adopted as originally proposed by the European Neuroendocrine Tumor Society (ENETS) [27, 28]. Mitoses are counted in areas of higher frequency (the so-called hot spots) and expressed per 10 high power fields (HPF, considered as 2 mm^2) after counting at least 50 HPFs. Mitotic count was chosen since it is robust and reproducible in the higher-grade cancer range. It is also a more familiar method for practicing pathologist based on routine hematoxylin and eosin (H&E) preparations. The limits of mitotic counting are also well known and acknowledged as experienced, for instance, in other cancer types like the gastrointestinal stromal tumors

Table 6.1 Grading of pancreatic neuroendocrine neoplasms as proposed by ENETS and endorsed by WHO 2010

WHO class	Definition	Grade	Mitosis	Ki67%
I	NET	G1	<2	≤2
II	NET	G2	2–20	3–20
III	NEC	G3	>20	>20
IV	MANEC	nd	nd	nd
V	Hyperplasia/dysplasia	na	na	na

Modified from Rindi et al. [11, 27]

ENETS European Neuroendocrine Tumor Society, *WHO* World Health Organization, *NET* neuroendocrine tumor, *NEC* neuroendocrine carcinoma, *MANEC* mixed adeno-neuroendocrine carcinoma, *nd* not determined, *na* not available

(GIST) [29]. Ki67 index definition has a shorter track of application in pathology compared to mitotic count. Nonetheless, it is proven effective in diverse cancer areas including neuroendocrine neoplasms [30]. Ki67 is measured in area of highest nuclear labeling by counting 400–2,000 cells [11]. The efficacy of these grading rules was demonstrated effective in spite of cancer heterogeneity, sampling, and methodology limits [31–36]. It is understood that grading as such only in part overlaps the information derived by morphology, which in any instance is the first driver for diagnostic pathology (Fig. 6.1). The advantage deriving from adopting a grading system is that it gives relatively simple and reproducible parameters for cancer categorization. The major drawback is that baptizing specific cases according to strict cutoffs for specific variables does elicit interpretative problems for cases at grade borders and for which morphology is necessarily and equivocally similar. This aspect, though largely expected, may generate discomfort for the practicing pathologist. This issue is particularly evident for G3 NECs, which, by definition, contain neuroendocrine cancers of high grade as for proliferation but cases with classical morphology of poor differentiation, and cases that do not, and thus variably considered as "well" or, more likely, "moderately" differentiated. Given that mitotic count and Ki67 index are both continuous variables, the prognostic significance is reflected in increased death risk which proceeds stepwise only by arbitrary definition. Therefore, it is largely expected that cases belonging to the same category within large variable intervals may display different prognosis. This is particularly evident in the G3 NEC category comprising cases embracing Ki67 >20–100 % and mitotic count >20–100 per 10 HPF [37–40].

Despite such limits, the current grading proved essentially effective for death prediction in multiple independent studies [15, 17, 25, 41, 42]. For pancreas, it was demonstrated that Ki67 5 % is the value above which the death risk increases in a statistically significant fashion as previously suggested [15, 25]. This value needs to be taken into adequate account for any specific decision for NET G2 patients.

G1-G2 NETs may display most types of the structures described originally by Soga and Tazawa in 1971 for carcinoids [43], namely, solid islet (type A), trabecular (type B), and glandular (type C) (Figs. 6.2 and 6.3). Usually, a pancreatic NET may display a mixture of types. The margins are usually expansive, with a delicate stroma rich in vessels, a feature typical of neuroendocrine cancer. Often, the stroma may become more solid with desmoplastic, parenchyma-substituting aspects reminiscent of the more aggressive adenocarcinoma. This latter feature may associate with deposits of amorphous eosinophilic material defined as amyloid and displaying metachromasia at Congo red stain. Amyloid deposits have been classically described in insulinomas and are composed by fragments of the hormonal peptide islet amyloid polypeptide (IAPP) as produced by the tumor beta cells [44]. NET cells are usually rather monomorphic, with abundant eosinophilic cytoplasm, round,

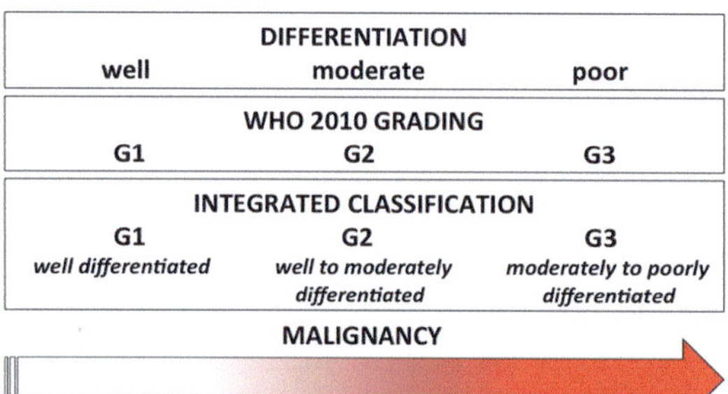

Fig. 6.1 Diagram illustrating the theoretical relationship existing between morphological differentiation, grading, and malignancy for neuroendocrine neoplasms. It is understood and accepted that the lower the degree of differentiation, the higher the malignancy is expected in a biological continuum. Grading, since based on unique and fixed descriptors, lies in between, and for G2 and G3, classes may well incorporate cases with different degree of differentiation along the very same continuum (see text)

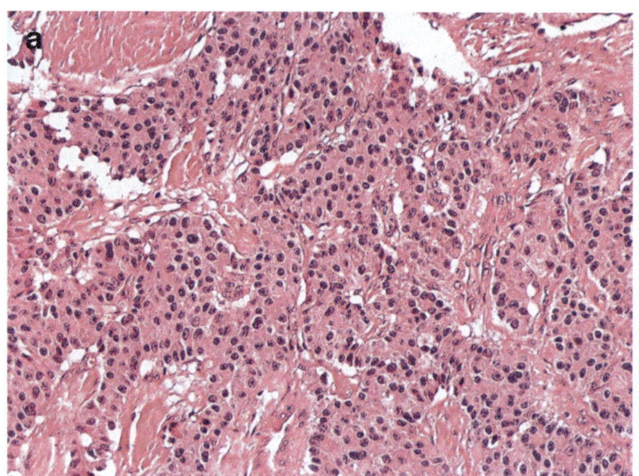

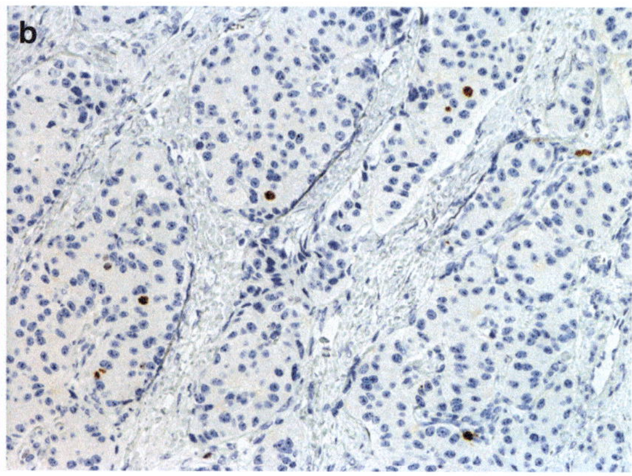

Fig. 6.2 Morphology of a PanNET G1 (WHO 2010) showing a mixed structure with trabeculae and solid islets, evident hyalinized stroma, mild atypia in absence of necrosis (**a**), and very few cells labeled for Ki67 corresponding to about 1 % (**b**); this case was a functioning, insulin-producing PanNET (insulinoma; see also Figs. 6.5 and 6.6) of 2 cm in size void of local lymph nodes and distant metastases (pT1 pN0 pM0, AJCC 2010; pT2 pN0 pM0 ENETS staging). (**a**) H & E (**b**) immunoperoxidase

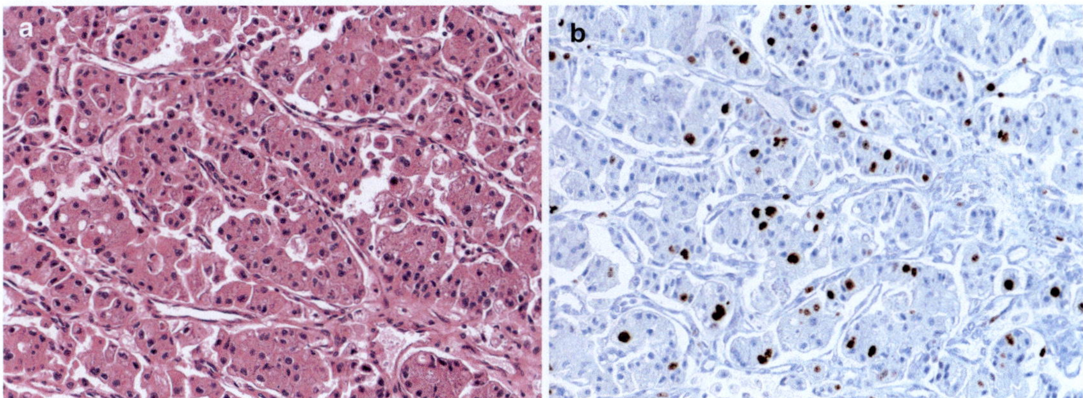

Fig. 6.3 Morphology of a PanNET G2 (WHO 2010) showing a relatively more compact, trabecular structure with highly vascularized stroma, mild to moderate atypia with irregularly shaped nuclei (**a**) several of which are labeled for Ki67 and accounting for about 16 % (**b**); occasional foci of necrosis were also observed as well as 5 mitoses per 10 HPF (not shown); the case was a nonfunctioning PanNET of 2.7 cm in size, void of local lymph nodes and distant metastases (pT2 pN0 pM0, AJCC 2010, and ENETS staging). (**a**) H & E (**b**) immunoperoxidase

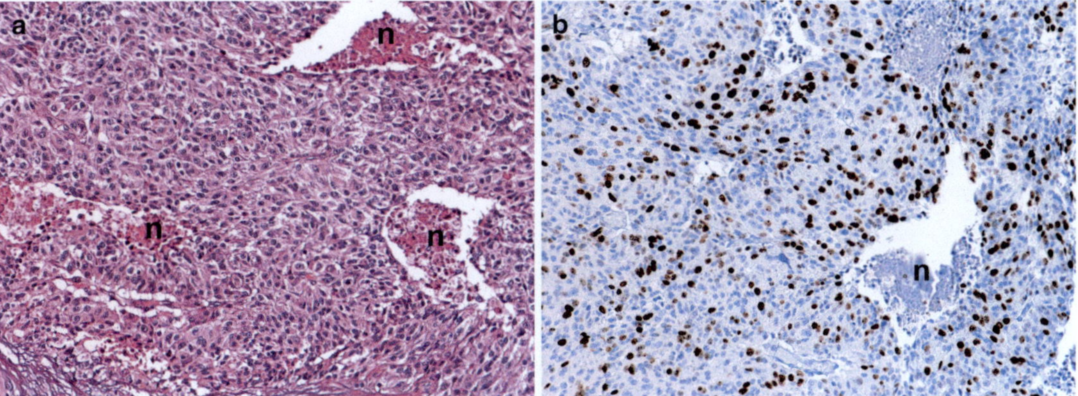

Fig. 6.4 Morphology of a high-grade neuroendocrine carcinoma, G3 NEC (WHO 2010) showing a packed trabecular-solid structure with multiple foci of necrosis (*n*), moderate atypia with irregular though monomorphic nuclei (**a**), and high Ki67 index accounting for about 40 % (**b**); the case was 2.5 cm in size with synchronous liver metastases in the absence of local lymph node deposits (pT2 pN0 pM1 AJCC 2010 and ENETS staging). (**a**) H & E (**b**) immunoperoxidase

monomorphic nuclei with spotted chromatin and rather rare mitoses, only exceptionally atypical. The degree of atypia does however increase in G2 cases, with prevalent solid structure, polymorphic cytological features including irregular cell size, pronounced atypia with increased nuclear/cytoplasmic ratio, evident nucleoli, and mitoses, sometimes atypical. Necrosis is absent and when present usually heralds the more severe cytological-histological features of NEC (Fig. 6.4). Angioinvasion and perineural space invasion may also be observed and, though of potential prognostic significance,

are not included in the current classification criteria.

G1-G2 NETs stain positive for all markers of neuroendocrine differentiation, including chromogranin A and synaptophysin, the two minimum stains recommended for diagnosis by ENETS (Fig. 6.5) [16]. It is usually considered good practice that at least two neuroendocrine-specific stains should be positive in the large majority of tumor cells to set the diagnosis of NET. The degree of specificity of neuroendocrine stains is the highest for chromogranin A and

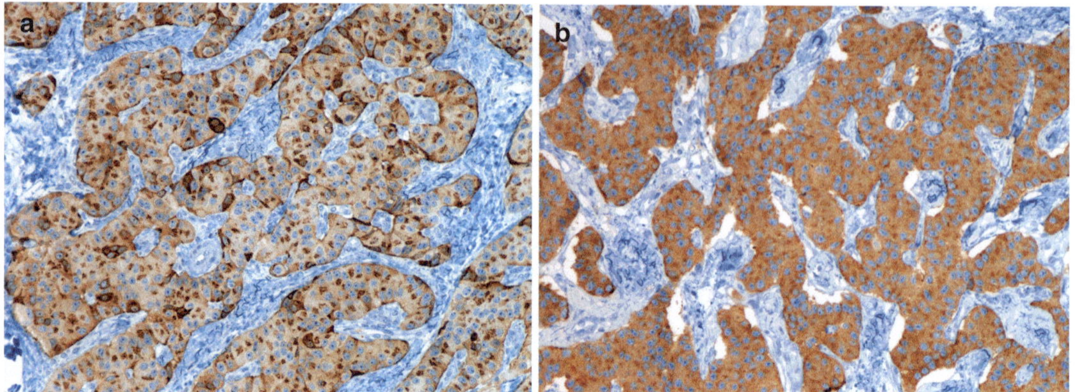

Fig. 6.5 Diffuse and intense expression of chromogranin A (**a**) and synaptophysin (**b**) in a functioning, insulin-producing PanNET G1 (insulinoma, same case of Figs. 6.2 and 6.6); note the irregular distribution of chromogranin A staining likely reflecting the chromogranin A-containing large dense-core vesicles (LDCV) as compared to the more uniform staining of synaptophysin (**b**). A and B immunoperoxidase

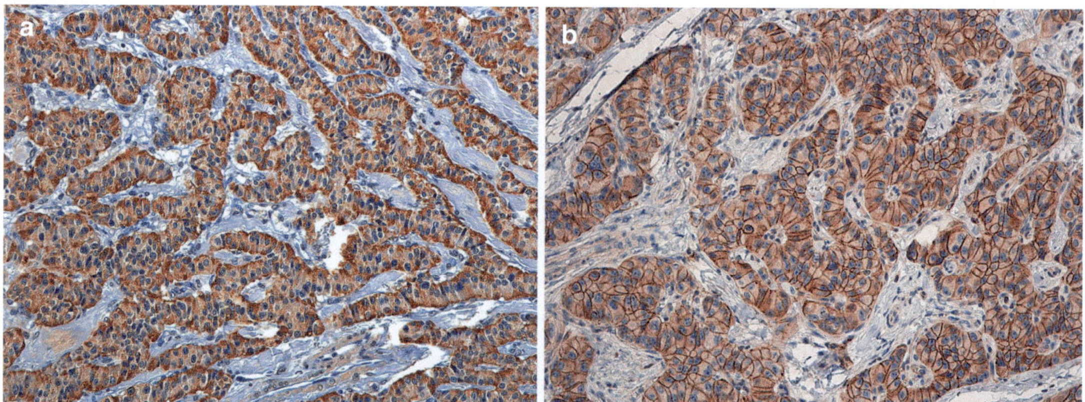

Fig. 6.6 Diffuse and intense expression of insulin (**a**) and of somatostatin receptor subtype 2A (SSTR2A) (**b**) in a functioning, insulin-producing PanNET G1 (insulinoma, same case of Figs. 6.2 and 6.5). A and B immunoperoxidase

decreases for synaptophysin, NSE, PGP 9.5, and CD56 N-CAM, all of which may stain non-neuroendocrine neoplasms. By converse, the search for cell-type-specific markers, namely, the peptide hormones like insulin, glucagon, pancreatic polypeptide, somatostatin, and ghrelin, is not required. When performed, usually it may show only a variable fraction of positive NET cells or, more rarely, a diffuse pattern of expression (Fig. 6.6a) [6]. The search for specific hormones is not mandatory for the diagnosis of NET but may be required for confirmation of a clinically functional condition. Other immunohistochemical stains may be required to answer specific clinical query or in the metastatic setting. In particular, the assessment of the somatostatin receptor subtype 2A (SSTR2A) may be requested on tissue when the in vivo assessment of lesions expressing the somatostatin receptors by nuclear medicine methods (e.g., Octreoscan® or Ga68-DOTA-NOC/TOC) is not available (Fig. 6.6b). Other markers including the nuclear transcription factors like the insulin gene enhancer protein islet-1 (ISL-1), the homeobox CDX2, and the NK2 homeobox 1 (NKX2-1), also known as thyroid transcription factor 1 (TTF-1), may be useful to determine the origin of a neuroendocrine cancer metastasis of potential pancreatic origin.

Their use and significance need to be carefully weighed according to their known tissue-specificity limits and to the clinical evidence of the specific case under study.

NECs by definition display a high proliferative fraction, though histology may reveal different features. A solid structure with some trabecular packed areas – a structure generally defined as "organoid" – is often observed, together with moderate to severe cytological atypia, sometimes with relatively abundant eosinophilic cytoplasm, polymorphic large nuclei, increased nuclear/cytoplasmic ratio, evident nucleoli, and multiple mitoses often atypical (Fig. 6.4). Such aspects may well refer to the "structures of lower or atypical differentiations" defined as Type D by Soga and Tazawa [43]. Necrosis in such cases is usually scant and spotty; however, it becomes more evident with increased large solid sheet structure and increased cell atypia with large nuclei and reduced cytoplasm, high-grade features more classically associated with large cell NECs. Not infrequently, cases showing areas with different histology of low and high grade may be observed [45]. In such cases, the highest-grade areas drive the diagnosis, according to the WHO 2010 grading rules. At immunohistochemistry, both chromogranin A and synaptophysin are widely expressed, though, while synaptophysin is usually intense, chromogranin A may be only scant and presenting as a thin rim of positive stain at cell periphery or as dots at Golgi cell site. Such features reflect the relative absence of large dense-core vesicles (LDCV) containing chromogranin A as observed at ultrastructure in NECs. Hormones in general are only rarely observed similar to SSTR2A, which however may be present in about 25–30 % of NECs [46]. Other neuroendocrine markers like NSE and CD56 N-CAM may be useful since they do not associate with neuroendocrine granules [13].

6.6 Pathological Classification: Staging

Staging is the second tool introduced by WHO 2010, following the indication by the International Union for Cancer Control (*Union Internationale*

Contre le Cancer, UICC) and aligning with the American Joint Committee on Cancer (AJCC) of the American College of Surgeons (Table 6.2) [47, 48]. In the absence of any official staging for neuroendocrine neoplasms at any anatomical side, the staging schemes for the exocrine cancer counterparts were commonly utilized in clinical practice for neuroendocrine cancer patients. However, the biological difference between the two cancer types made such practice of limited clinical value. On such bases, ENETS proposed a neuroendocrine cancer-specific staging system for any gastroenteropancreatic anatomical site [27]. The ENETS scheme for pancreas neuroendocrine neoplasm proved effective in several studies [25, 41, 49–51]. The WHO/UICC/AJCC staging system adopted for the neuroendocrine neoplasms of the pancreas is however by definition the very same as for the adenocarcinoma. This generated some concern for its clinical application [52]. Both systems are indeed effective [17, 53, 54]; however, in a head to head comparison on a large cohort of about 1,000 patients, the ENETS system described more accurately the neuroendocrine cancer disease [15].

6.7 Pathology Report

In view of their prognostic significance, the pathology report must contain all the information useful for grading and staging definitions. This may be provided in the Macroscopic and Microscopic sections of the pathology report. The amount of information that can be given varies depending on the type of examined sample, either a cytological or a small biopsy versus a major surgery histological sample. For cytological or small histological biopsy samples, the minimum information that must be given is the neuroendocrine neoplasm definition (whether NET or NEC), thus implying a rough grading category (whether G1, G2, or G3). Indeed, cytology samples usually allow the neuroendocrine family definition (NET or NEC) only, being impossible a precise grading by mitotic or Ki67 index definition (see Chap. 5 for details). In small biopsy, histological sample grading can be assessed and proved effectively informative for clinical use [32].

Table 6.2 Staging of pancreatic neuroendocrine neoplasms according to ENETS and UICC/AJCC/WHO 2010

	ENETS			UICC/AJCC/WHO 2010			
T definitions							
TX	Primary tumor cannot be assessed			Primary tumor cannot be assessed			
T0	No evidence of primary tumor			No evidence of primary tumor			
Tis	na			Carcinoma in situ			
T1	Tumor limited to the pancreas and size <2 cm			Tumor limited to the pancreas, 2 cm or less in greatest dimension			
T2	Tumor limited to the pancreas and size 2–4 cm			Tumor limited to the pancreas, more than 2 cm in greatest dimension			
T3	Tumor limited to the pancreas and size >4 cm or invading duodenum or bile duct			Tumor extends beyond the pancreas but without involvement of the celiac axis or the superior mesenteric artery			
T4	Tumor invading adjacent organs (stomach, spleen, colon, adrenal gland) or the wall of large vessels (celiac axis or the superior mesenteric artery)			Tumor involves the celiac axis or the superior mesenteric artery (unresectable primary tumor)			
N definitions							
NX	Not known			Not known			
N0	No regional lymph node metastasis			No regional lymph node metastasis			
N1	Regional lymph node metastasis			Regional lymph node metastasis			
M definitions							
MX	Not known			Not known			
M0	No distant metastasis			No distant metastasis			
M1	Distant metastasis			Distant metastasis			
Stage definitions							
Stage 0	na			Stage 0	Tis	N0	M0
Stage I	T1	N0	M0	Stage IA	T1	N0	M0
Stage IIa	T2	N0	M0	Stage IB	T2	N0	M0
Stage IIb	T3	N0	M0	Stage IIA	T3	N0	M0
Stage IIIa	T4	N0	M0	Stage IIB	T1–T3	N1	M0
Stage IIIb	Any T	N1	M0	Stage III	T4	Any N	M0
Stage IV	Any T	Any N	M1	Stage IV	Any T	Any N	M1

Modified from Rindi et al. [27], Sobin et al. [47], Edge et al. [48], Bosman and Carneiro [10]
ENETS European Neuroendocrine Tumor Society, *WHO* World Health Organization, *UICC* International Union for Cancer Control, *AJCC* American Joint Cancer Committee, *T* tumor, *N* node, *M* metastasis, *na* not available

For surgical samples, the Macroscopic section must provide the most relevant information regarding T according to common good pathology practice. The Microscopic section must provide all relevant morphological features including the invasion of nearby tissue if present, the margins status (R), and the number of lymph nodes and their status. Other features can also be reported as, for instance, angio- and neural invasion and the presence of necrosis, in light of their potential utility, though not in the current grading scheme. Other features including the pattern of tumor growth, extension of the fibrosis, angiogenesis, and apopto-sis may be reported, though it is understood that they do not have prognostic significance [55]. It is good practice to provide also the immunohisto-chemistry data on which the diagnosis is based. The mitotic and the Ki67 indexes must be reported in full to allow clinicians to tailor a patient-specific management/therapeutic strategy. Finally, the WHO stage must be provided within the pathology report, adding the ENETS stage in case of discrepancy. No matter what type of sample is analyzed, the minimum synthetic diagnosis must contain the neuroendocrine cancer definition (NET or NEC) and, when possible, the grade (G1–G3).

Acknowledgments This work was in part supported by internal university grants (line D1/2012–2014, Università Cattolica) and by the Associazione Italiana Ricerca sul Cancro – AIRC IG 2013 14696 to GR.

References

1. Oberndorfer S (1907) Karzinoide Tumoren des Dünndarms. Frankf Z Pathol Int 1:425–432
2. Williams R (1960) A metastasizing carcinoid tumour with unusual features. Br Med J 1:28–30
3. Pearse AG (1974) The APUD cell concept and its implications in pathology. Pathol Annu 9:27–41
4. Pearse AG, Polak JM (1974) Endocrine tumours of neural crest origin: neurolophomas, apudomas and the APUD concept. Med Biol 52:3–18
5. Williams ED, Siebenmann RE, Sobin LH (eds) (1980) Types hystologiques des tumeurs endocriniennes. Organisation mondiale de la Santé, Geneve
6. Solcia E, Capella C, Kloppel G (1997) Tumors of the pancreas. Armed Forces Institute of Pathology, Washington, DC
7. Solcia E, Klöppel G, Sobin LH (2000) Histological typing of endocrine tumours. Springer, New York
8. DeLellis RA, Lloyd RV, Heitz PU, Eng C (2004) World Health Organization classification of tumours, pathology and genetics of tumours of endocrine organs. IARC Press, Lyon
9. Hruban RH, Pitman MB, Klimstra DS (2007) Tumors of the pancreas. The American Registry of Pathology and the Armed Force Institute of Pathology, Washington, DC
10. Bosman F, Carneiro F (2010) World Health Organization classification of tumours, pathology and genetics of tumours of the digestive system. IARC Press, Lyon
11. Rindi G, Arnold R, Capella C, Klimstra DS, Klöppel G, Komminoth P, Solcia E (2010) Nomenclature and classification of digestive neuroendocrine tumours. In: Bosman F, Carneiro F (eds) World Health Organization classification of tumours, pathology and genetics of tumours of the digestive system. IARC Press, Lyon, pp 10–12
12. Klimstra DS, Arnold R, Capella C, Klöppel G, Komminoth P, Solcia E, Rindi G (2010) Neuroendocrine neoplasms of the pancreas. In: Bosman F, Carneiro F (eds) World Health Organization Classification of tumours, pathology and genetics of tumours of the digestive system. IARC Press, Lyon, pp 322–330
13. Rindi G, Leiter AB, Kopin AS, Bordi C, Solcia E (2004) The "normal" endocrine cell of the gut: changing concepts and new evidences. Ann N Y Acad Sci 1014:1–12
14. Mansour JC, Chen H (2004) Pancreatic endocrine tumors. J Surg Res 120:139–161
15. Rindi G, Falconi M, Klersy C, Albarello L, Boninsegna L, Buchler MW, Capella C, Caplin M, Couvelard A, Doglioni C, Delle Fave G, Fischer L, Fusai G, de Herder WW, Jann H, Komminoth P, de Krijger RR, La Rosa S, Luong TV, Pape U, Perren A, Ruszniewski P, Scarpa A, Schmitt A, Solcia E, Wiedenmann B (2012) TNM staging of neoplasms of the endocrine pancreas: results from a large international cohort study. J Natl Cancer Inst 104:764–777
16. Falconi M, Bartsch DK, Eriksson B, Kloppel G, Lopes JM, O'Connor JM, Salazar R, Taal BG, Vullierme MP, O'Toole D (2012) ENETS consensus guidelines for the management of patients with digestive neuroendocrine neoplasms of the digestive system: well-differentiated pancreatic non-functioning tumors. Neuroendocrinology 95:120–134
17. Ellison TA, Wolfgang CL, Shi C, Cameron JL, Murakami P, Mun LJ, Singhi AD, Cornish TC, Olino K, Meriden Z, Choti M, Diaz LA, Pawlik TM, Schulick RD, Hruban RH, Edil BH (2014) A single institution's 26-year experience with nonfunctional pancreatic neuroendocrine tumors: a validation of current staging systems and a new prognostic nomogram. Ann Surg 259:204–212
18. Yao JC, Hassan M, Phan A, Dagohoy C, Leary C, Mares JE, Abdalla EK, Fleming JB, Vauthey JN, Rashid A, Evans DB (2008) One hundred years after "carcinoid": epidemiology of and prognostic factors for neuroendocrine tumors in 35,825 cases in the United States. J Clin Oncol 26:3063–3072
19. Garcia-Carbonero R, Capdevila J, Crespo-Herrero G, Diaz-Perez JA, Martinez Del Prado MP, Alonso Orduna V, Sevilla-Garcia I, Villabona-Artero C, Beguiristain-Gomez A, Llanos-Munoz M, Marazuela M, Alvarez-Escola C, Castellano D, Vilar E, Jimenez-Fonseca P, Teule A, Sastre-Valera J, Benavent-Vinuelas M, Monleon A, Salazar R (2010) Incidence, patterns of care and prognostic factors for outcome of gastroenteropancreatic neuroendocrine tumors (GEP-NETs): results from the National Cancer Registry of Spain (RGETNE). Ann Oncol 21:1794–1803
20. Scherubl H, Streller B, Stabenow R, Herbst H, Hopfner M, Schwertner C, Steinberg J, Eick J, Ring W, Tiwari K, Zappe SM (2013) Clinically detected gastroenteropancreatic neuroendocrine tumors are on the rise: epidemiological changes in Germany. World J Gastroenterol 19:9012–9019
21. Ito T, Igarashi H, Nakamura K, Sasano H, Okusaka T, Takano K, Komoto I, Tanaka M, Imamura M, Jensen RT, Takayanagi R, Shimatsu A (2014) Epidemiological trends of pancreatic and gastrointestinal neuroendocrine tumors in Japan: a nationwide survey analysis. J Gastroenterol 50:58–64
22. Larghi A, Capurso G, Carnuccio A, Ricci R, Alfieri S, Galasso D, Lugli F, Bianchi A, Panzuto F, De Marinis L, Falconi M, Delle Fave G, Doglietto GB, Costamagna G, Rindi G (2012) Ki-67 grading of nonfunctioning pancreatic neuroendocrine tumors on histologic samples obtained by EUS-guided fine-needle tissue acquisition: a prospective study. Gastrointest Endosc 76:570–577

23. EUCERD recommendations on quality criteria for centres of expertise for rare diseases in member states. http://www.EUCERD.eu/upload/file/EUCERDRecommendationCE.pdf. Accessed 24 Oct 2011

24. EURORDIS Policy fact sheet – European references networks. http://www.eurordis.org

25. Scarpa A, Mantovani W, Capelli P, Beghelli S, Boninsegna L, Bettini R, Panzuto F, Pederzoli P, delle Fave G, Falconi M (2010) Pancreatic endocrine tumors: improved TNM staging and histopathological grading permit a clinically efficient prognostic stratification of patients. Mod Pathol 23:824–833

26. Allegranza A, Girlando S, Arrigoni GL, Veronese S, Mauri FA, Gambacorta M, Pollo B, Dalla Palma P, Barbareschi M (1991) Proliferating cell nuclear antigen expression in central nervous system neoplasms. Virchows Arch A Pathol Anat Histopathol 419:417–423

27. Rindi G, Kloppel G, Alhman H, Caplin M, Couvelard A, de Herder WW, Erikssson B, Falchetti A, Falconi M, Komminoth P, Korner M, Lopes JM, McNicol AM, Nilsson O, Perren A, Scarpa A, Scoazec JY, Wiedenmann B (2006) TNM staging of foregut (neuro)endocrine tumors: a consensus proposal including a grading system. Virchows Arch 449:395–401

28. Rindi G, Kloppel G, Couvelard A, Komminoth P, Korner M, Lopes JM, McNicol AM, Nilsson O, Perren A, Scarpa A, Scoazec JY, Wiedenmann B (2007) TNM staging of midgut and hindgut (neuro) endocrine tumors: a consensus proposal including a grading system. Virchows Arch 451:757–762

29. Joensuu H, Eriksson M, Hall KS, Hartmann JT, Pink D, Schutte J, Ramadori G, Hohenberger P, Duyster J, Al-Batran SE, Schlemmer M, Bauer S, Wardelmann E, Sarlomo-Rikala M, Nilsson B, Sihto H, Ballman KV, Leinonen M, DeMatteo RP, Reichardt P (2014) Risk factors for gastrointestinal stromal tumor recurrence in patients treated with adjuvant imatinib. Cancer 120:2325–2333

30. Pelosi G, Zamboni G, Doglioni C, Rodella S, Bresaola E, Iacono C, Serio G, Iannucci A, Scarpa A (1992) Immunodetection of proliferating cell nuclear antigen assesses the growth fraction and predicts malignancy in endocrine tumors of the pancreas. Am J Surg Pathol 16:1215–1225

31. Couvelard A, Deschamps L, Ravaud P, Baron G, Sauvanet A, Hentic O, Colnot N, Paradis V, Belghiti J, Bedossa P, Ruszniewski P (2009) Heterogeneity of tumor prognostic markers: a reproducibility study applied to liver metastases of pancreatic endocrine tumors. Mod Pathol 22:273–281

32. Yang Z, Tang LH, Klimstra DS (2011) Effect of tumor heterogeneity on the assessment of Ki67 labeling index in well-differentiated neuroendocrine tumors metastatic to the liver: implications for prognostic stratification. Am J Surg Pathol 35:853–860

33. Tang LH, Gonen M, Hedvat C, Modlin IM, Klimstra DS (2012) Objective quantification of the Ki67 proliferative index in neuroendocrine tumors of the gastro-enteropancreatic system: a comparison of digital image analysis with manual methods. Am J Surg Pathol 36:1761–1770

34. Goodell PP, Krasinskas AM, Davison JM, Hartman DJ (2012) Comparison of methods for proliferative index analysis for grading pancreatic well-differentiated neuroendocrine tumors. Am J Clin Pathol 137:576–582

35. McCall CM, Shi C, Cornish TC, Klimstra DS, Tang LH, Basturk O, Mun LJ, Ellison TA, Wolfgang CL, Choti MA, Schulick RD, Edil BH, Hruban RH (2013) Grading of well-differentiated pancreatic neuroendocrine tumors is improved by the inclusion of both Ki67 proliferative index and mitotic rate. Am J Surg Pathol 37:1671–1677

36. Reid MD, Bagci P, Ohike N, Saka B, Erbarut Seven I, Dursun N, Balci S, Gucer H, Jang KT, Tajiri T, Basturk O, Kong SY, Goodman M, Akkas G, Adsay V (2014) Calculation of the Ki67 index in pancreatic neuroendocrine tumors: a comparative analysis of four counting methodologies. Mod Pathol, in press, available on-line

37. Scoazec JY, Couvelard A, Monges G, Leteurtre E, Belleanee G, Guyetant S, Duvillard P, Danjoux M, Parot X, Lepage C (2012) Well-differentiated grade 3 digestive neuroendocrine tumors: myth or reality? The PRONET study group. J Clin Oncol 30:(15S). Abstract 4129 pp

38. Sorbye H, Welin S, Langer SW, Vestermark LW, Holt N, Osterlund P, Dueland S, Hofsli E, Guren MG, Ohrling K, Birkemeyer E, Thiis-Evensen E, Biagini M, Gronbaek H, Soveri LM, Olsen IH, Federspiel B, Assmus J, Janson ET, Knigge U (2012) Predictive and prognostic factors for treatment and survival in 305 patients with advanced gastrointestinal neuroendocrine carcinoma (WHO G3): the NORDIC NEC study. Ann Oncol 24:152–160

39. Velayoudom-Cephise FL, Duvillard P, Foucan L, Hadoux J, Chougnet CN, Leboulleux S, Malka D, Guigay J, Goere D, Debaere T, Caramella C, Schlumberger M, Planchard D, Elias D, Ducreux M, Scoazec JY, Baudin E (2013) Are G3 ENETS neuroendocrine neoplasms heterogeneous? Endocr Relat Cancer 20:649–657

40. Basturk O, Yang Z, Tang LH, Hruban RH, Adsay V, McCall CM, Krasinskas AM, Jang KT, Frankel WL, Balci S, Sigel C, Klimstra DS (2015) The high-grade (WHO G3) pancreatic neuroendocrine tumor category is morphologically and biologically heterogenous and includes both well differentiated and poorly differentiated neoplasms. Am J Surg Pathol, in press, available on-line

41. La Rosa S, Klersy C, Uccella S, Dainese L, Albarello L, Sonzogni A, Doglioni C, Capella C, Solcia E (2009) Improved histologic and clinicopathologic criteria for prognostic evaluation of pancreatic endocrine tumors. Hum Pathol 40:30–40

42. Jann H, Roll S, Couvelard A, Hentic O, Pavel M, Muller-Nordhorn J, Koch M, Rocken C, Rindi G, Ruszniewski P, Wiedenmann B, Pape UF (2011)

Neuroendocrine tumors of midgut and hindgut origin: tumor-node-metastasis classification determines clinical outcome. Cancer 117:3332–3341

43. Soga J, Tazawa K (1971) Pathologic analysis of carcinoids; histologic reevaluation of 62 cases. Cancer 28:990–998

44. Rindi G, Terenghi G, Westermark G, Westermark P, Moscoso G, Polak JM (1991) Islet amyloid polypeptide in proliferating pancreatic B cells during development, hyperplasia, and neoplasia in humans and mice. Am J Pathol 138:1321–1334

45. Rindi G, Petrone G, Inzani F (2014) The 2010 WHO classification of digestive neuroendocrine neoplasms: a critical appraisal four years after its introduction. Endocr Pathol 25:186–192

46. Volante M, Brizzi MP, Faggiano A, La Rosa S, Rapa I, Ferrero A, Mansueto G, Righi L, Garancini S, Capella C, De Rosa G, Dogliotti L, Colao A, Papotti M (2007) Somatostatin receptor type 2A immunohistochemistry in neuroendocrine tumors: a proposal of scoring system correlated with somatostatin receptor scintigraphy. Mod Pathol Off J U S Can Acad Pathol Inc 20:1172–1182

47. Sobin L, Gospodarowicz M, Wittekind C (2009) TNM classification of malignant tumours. Wiley Blackwell, Bognor Regis

48. Edge SB, Byrd DR, Compton CC, Fritz AG, Greene FL, Trotti A (2010) AJCC cancer staging manual. Springer, New York

49. Fischer L, Kleeff J, Esposito I, Hinz U, Zimmermann A, Friess H, Buchler MW (2008) Clinical outcome and long-term survival in 118 consecutive patients with neuroendocrine tumours of the pancreas. Br J Surg 95:627–635

50. Pape UF, Jann H, Muller-Nordhorn J, Bockelbrink A, Berndt U, Willich SN, Koch M, Rocken C, Rindi G, Wiedenmann B (2008) Prognostic relevance of a novel TNM classification system for upper gastroenteropancreatic neuroendocrine tumors. Cancer 113:256–265

51. Ekeblad S, Skogseid B, Dunder K, Oberg K, Eriksson B (2008) Prognostic factors and survival in 324 patients with pancreatic endocrine tumor treated at a single institution. Clin Cancer Res 14:7798–7803

52. Kloppel G, Rindi G, Perren A, Komminoth P, Klimstra DS (2010) The ENETS and AJCC/UICC TNM classifications of the neuroendocrine tumors of the gastrointestinal tract and the pancreas: a statement. Virchows Arch 456:595–597

53. Strosberg JR, Cheema A, Weber J, Han G, Coppola D, Kvols LK (2011) Prognostic validity of a novel American joint committee on cancer staging classification for pancreatic neuroendocrine tumors. J Clin Oncol 29:3044–3049

54. Strosberg JR, Cheema A, Weber JM, Ghayouri M, Han G, Hodul PJ, Kvols LK (2012) Relapse-free survival in patients with nonmetastatic, surgically resected pancreatic neuroendocrine tumors: an analysis of the AJCC and ENETS staging classifications. Ann Surg 256:321–325

55. Klimstra DS (2013) Pathology reporting of neuroendocrine tumors: essential elements for accurate diagnosis, classification, and staging. Semin Oncol 40:23–36

Immunohistochemical Approach to the Diagnosis and Prognostic Evaluation of Pancreatic Neuroendocrine Neoplasms

Ricardo V. Lloyd, Jason N. Rosenbaum, and Lori A. Erickson

7.1 Normal Adult Pancreas

The normal adult pancreatic islets are mostly round to ovoid structures distributed in the head, body, and tail of the pancreas [1–5]. The principal hormones in the human pancreas (Fig. 7.1a–d) include insulin-producing beta cells which make up between 60 and 70 % of the endocrine mass (Fig. 7.1a), glucagon-producing alpha cells (Fig. 7.1b) which make up about 15–20 % of the endocrine mass, somatostatin-producing delta cells which make up around 5–10 % of the endocrine mass (Fig. 7.1c), and pancreatic polypeptide (PP)-producing cells which constitute about 2–5 % of the endocrine mass (Fig. 7.1d). The islets in the posterior portion of the head of the pancreas are more irregular in shape and are composed mainly of PP-producing cells (about 70 % of the endocrine mass in the posterior portion of the head of the pancreas) [2]. In addition to the classical hormones, recent studies have found ghrelin in a small percentage of islet cells [6]. Ghrelin-producing cells are present in the

mantle of the islets in the adult human pancreas. Although some hormones such as gastrin and vasoactive intestinal polypeptide (VIP) are present in pancreatic neuroendocrine tumors (PanNETs), they are not found in the normal adult islets. These hormones have been reported in fetal islet tissues [1, 2]. Islet cell hormones are present in pancreatic duct cells close to islets, and during the pathological process of nesidioblastosis, these cells may give rise to hormone-producing cells such as insulin. These cells or other precursor cells may be the precursors for pancreatic endocrine neoplasms (PanNETs) in the adult pancreas.

7.1.1 Transcription Factors in Pancreatic Neuroendocrine Tissues

A large number of transcription factors (TFs) that are critical for development of the normal pancreas have been identified in PanNETs. The four principal TFs include islet 1 gene product (ISL1) (Fig. 7.2), pancreatico-duodenal homeobox 1 gene product (PDX1), neurogenin 3 gene product (NGN3), and CDX2 homeobox gene product (CDX2) [7–14]. Studies have been done to correlate the PanNET hormonal profile with specific TFs. Insulin-positive tumors usually express ISL1. In a recent study, 90 % of primary PanNETs were positive for ISL1, while only 76 % of

R.V. Lloyd, MD, PhD (✉) • J.N. Rosenbaum, MD
Department of Pathology, University of Wisconsin
School of Medicine and Public Health,
600 Highland Ave, Madison, WI 53792, USA
e-mail: rvlloyd@wisc.edu

L.A. Erickson, MD
Department of Laboratory Medicine and Pathology,
Mayo Clinic College of Medicine, 200 First St SW,
Rochester, MN 55905, USA

S. La Rosa, F. Sessa (eds.), *Pancreatic Neuroendocrine Neoplasms: Practical Approach to Diagnosis, Classification, and Therapy*, DOI 10.1007/978-3-319-17235-4_7,
© Springer International Publishing Switzerland 2015

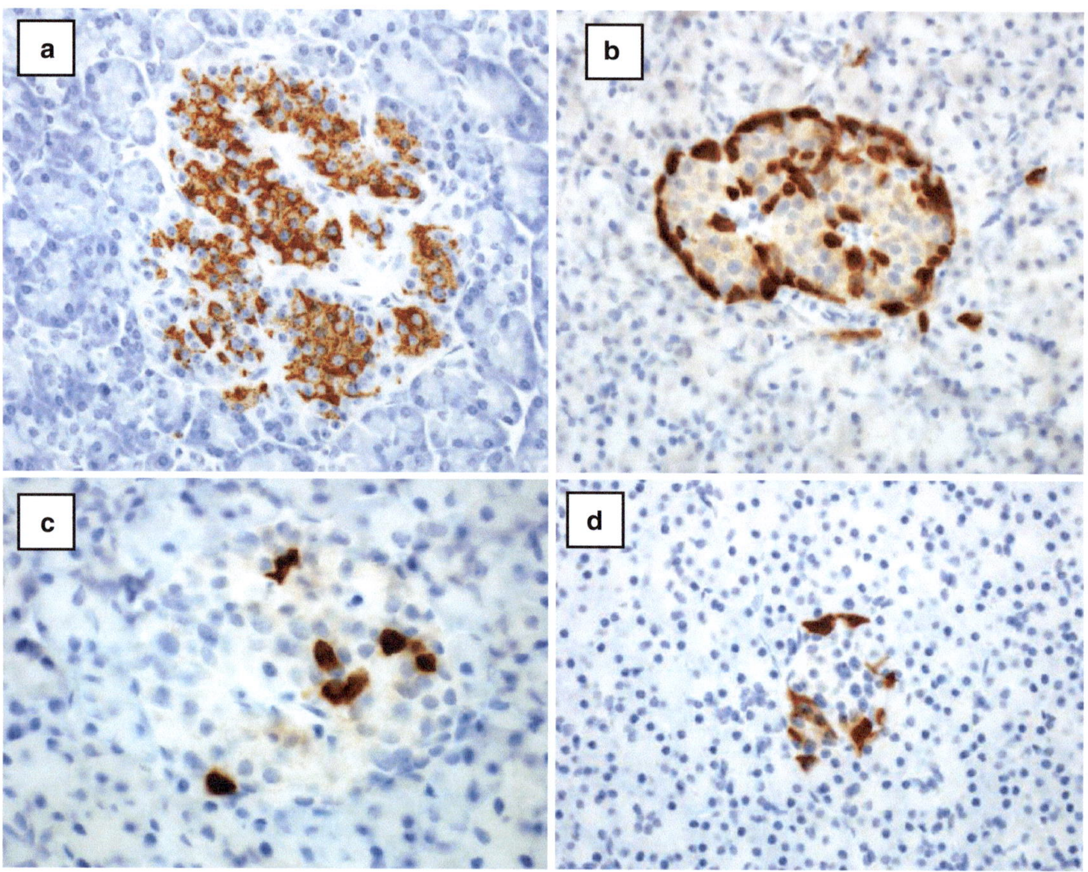

Fig. 7.1 Immunohistochemical localization of islet cell hormones in normal islets. (**a**) Insulin localization in approximately 60–70 % of islet cells. (**b**) Glucagon localization in the periphery of the islets in approximately 15–20 % of islet cells. (**c**) Somatostatin localization in approximately 5–10 % of islet cells. (**d**) Human pancreatic polypeptide is present in 2–5 % of islet cells in the body of the pancreas

metastatic PanNETs were positive indicating loss of expression in the malignant tumors [12]. Glucagon-positive tumors express ISL1 and are usually negative for most of the other principal TFs. Gastrin-producing tumors express PDX1, ISL1, and NGN3. CDX2 is often found in gastrin-producing cells. Somatostatin-producing cells often express ISL1, PDX1, and NGN3. There is usually not an association between TF patterns of expression and PanNET features such as grade, size, location, presence of metastases, and functional activity. Studies in experimental animals, especially knockout mice, have shown the functional role of many TFs in pancreatic development [2]. For example, animals lacking NGN3 fail to develop endocrine cells. Other TFs like

PAX4 are involved in the early phases of development of endocrine lineages, while others like PAX6 are involved in the maturation of committed endocrine cells [2].

INSM1 is a zinc-finger TF expressed transiently in developing embryonic and regenerating adult neuroepithelial tissue. INSM1 was originally isolated from human insulinoma and glucagonoma tissues, from which it took its name (*insulinoma*-associated protein 1). INSM1 coordinates differentiation of neuroendocrine and neuroepithelial cells with termination of cell division and is thought to have critical regulatory roles during neuroendocrine differentiation. It has been detected in many neuroendocrine tissues in rodents and other animals. In human adult

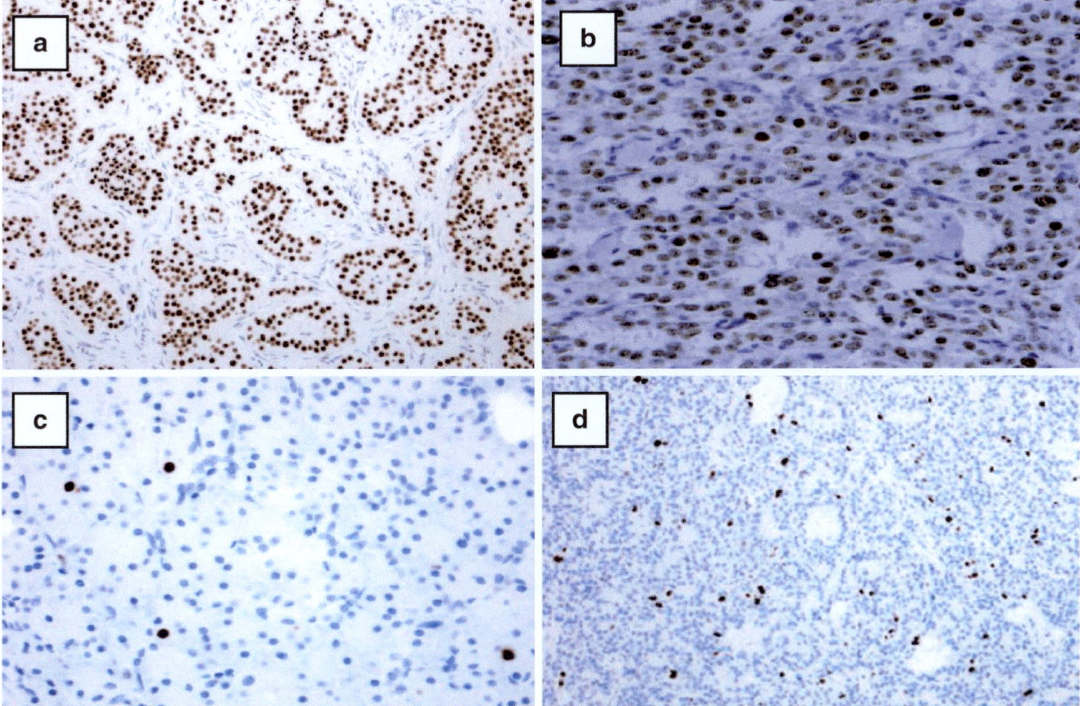

Fig. 7.2 (**a**) Localization of ISL1 in an insulin-producing pancreatic neuroendocrine tumor. (**b**) Localization of INSM1 in an insulin-producing pancreatic neuroendocrine tumor. (**c**) Immunostaining for Ki-67 in a grade 1 pancreatic neuroendocrine tumor with a labeling index of 2 %. (**d**) Immunostaining for Ki-67 in a grade 2 pancreatic neuroendocrine tumor with a labeling index of 10 %

tissues, INSM1 has been identified in multiple tumors of NE or of neuroepithelial origin. Recent studies have shown that INSM1 is widely distributed in normal islet cells, and it has been detected in many different types of islet cell tumors (Fig. 7.2b) [15, 16].

7.1.2 Ki-67 in Pancreatic Neuroendocrine Neoplasms

Immunohistochemical staining for Ki-67 (Figs. 7.1c and 7.2d) along with mitotic counts is critical for the grading of PanNETs [17–19]. Grade I (G1) tumors usually have a Ki-67 index of less than 3 % and less than two mitoses per ten high power fields (HPF). G2 tumors have a Ki-67 index of 3–20 % or 2–20 mitoses per 10 HPF. G3 or poorly differentiated pancreatic endocrine carcinomas have a Ki-67 index greater than 20 % and >20 mitoses per 10 HPF [19]. It

is recommended that at least 500 tumor cells be counted in tumor hot spots for calculation of the Ki-67 index. If there is discordance between the Ki-67 index and mitotic count, the higher grade should be used (Table 7.1).

One potential source of variation between laboratories with the Ki-67 index is the method used to obtain and to analyze the data. There are a limited number of monoclonal antibodies (MIB1) used for immunostaining. Most of these produce highly reproducible results—especially with automated staining—so the method of immunostaining is usually not a significant problem. Visually estimating the percentage of positive cells with the "eyeballing" method is usually not reproducible [17]; in contrast, automated counting is more reliable, but may show some operator variability depending on the experience of the operator and the quality of the software used in the analysis. Tumor heterogeneity and subjectivity in determining the hot

Table 7.1 Immunohistochemical markers for islet cells and pancreatic neuroendocrine tumors

Secretory granule-associated proteins
Chromogranins A and B, secretogranins I and II and 7B2
Prohormone convertases PC1/3 and PC2
Membrane-related proteins
Synaptophysin
Synaptic vesicle proteins 2
Synaptotagmins
Vesicular monoamine transporters
Vesicle-associated membrane protein
Cytoplasmic proteins
CD56
Neuron-specific enolase
PGP 9.5
Proliferation markers
Ki-67
Cell membrane -associated protein
Somatostatin receptors

spots for analyses probably contribute to variation in proliferation indices between different laboratories.

7.1.3 Broad-Spectrum Immunohistochemical Staining of PanNETs

PanNETs are characterized by the presence of secretory granules and membrane-bound vesicles. The chromogranins, including chromogranin A and chromogranin B, and secretogranins are present in secretory granules. Chromogranin A is widely used to characterize PanNETs (Fig. 7.3a) [20–23]. It is a very specific neuroendocrine marker, but is not as sensitive as some other markers. The sensitivity is most likely

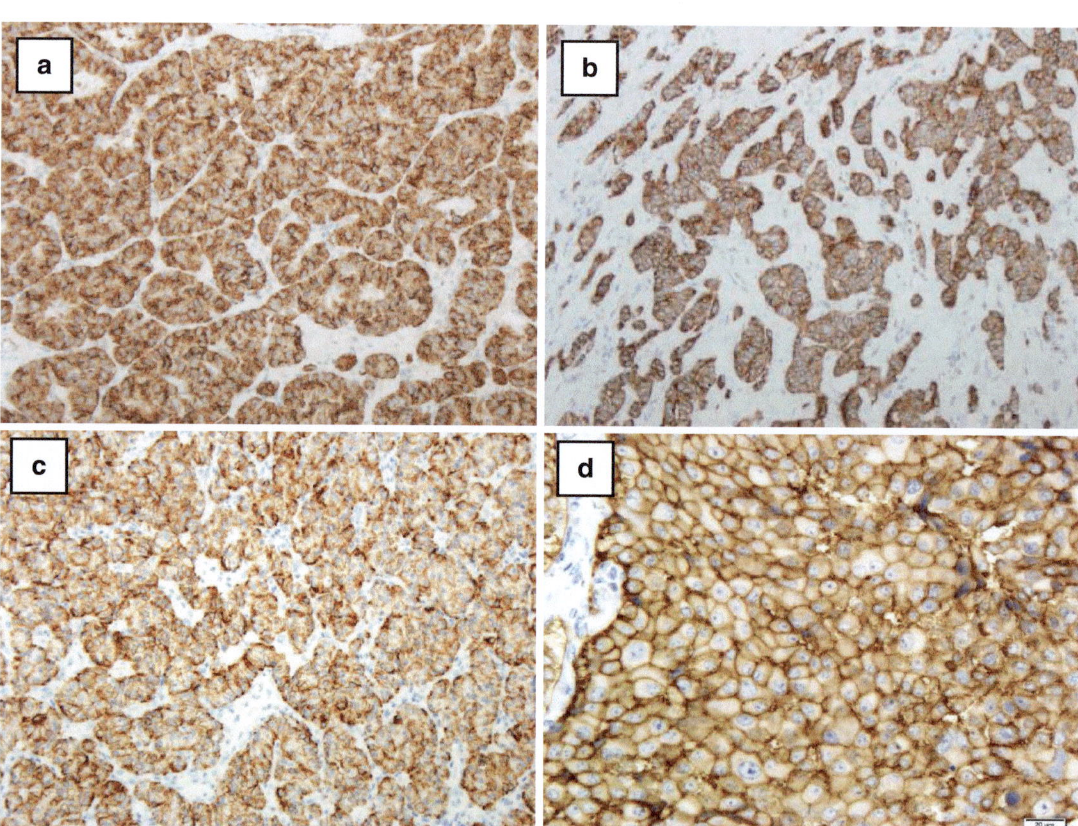

Fig. 7.3 (**a**) Chromogranin A expression in a pancreatic neuroendocrine tumor. There is diffuse staining for chromogranin A which labels the protein in the dense core secretory granules. (**b**) Localization of synaptophysin in membrane-related vesicles in a pancreatic endocrine tumor showing diffuse cytoplasmic staining. (**c**) Localization of cytokeratin 19 in an insulin-producing pancreatic endocrine tumor. (**d**) Localization of somatostatin receptor protein type 2 in a pancreatic endocrine carcinoma with a Ki-67 labeling index of 2 1% showing distinct cytoplasmic membrane staining (Courtesy of Dr RY Osamura)

related to the number of secretory granules in the neoplasm. Synaptophysin (Fig. 7.3b) which is associated with cytoplasmic membrane vesicles is highly sensitive [24], but not as specific as chromogranin A, since some non-neuroendocrine tumors, such as the adrenal cortex, also express synaptophysin.

CD56, a broad-spectrum neuroendocrine marker, directed against cell adhesion molecules, is the least specific of these three principal neuroendocrine markers, but is used in practice when the differential diagnosis includes a neuroendocrine tumor and chromogranin A and synaptophysin are negative [22]. Protein Gene Product 9.5 (PGP 9.5) belongs to the carboxy-terminal hydrolase family and is involved in the degradation of cytosolic and nuclear proteins through an ATP- and ubiquitin-dependent mechanism. It has a role in the regulation of the cell cycle. Although it is expressed in the normal pancreatic islets and in PanNETs, PGP9.5 is also expressed by the exocrine pancreas, so it is not a specific marker for PanNETs [22]. Neuron-specific enolase (NSE) was historically the first broad-spectrum neuroendocrine marker, but because of the relative lack of specificity is not used frequently in many diagnostic pathology laboratories [25]. Other broad-spectrum markers that may also be positive in PanNETs include prohormone convertases (PCs), PC2 and PC1/PC3 [22]. Additional membrane-related proteins in addition to synaptophysin such as synaptic vesicle protein, synaptotagmins, vesicular monoamine transporters, and vesicle-associated membrane proteins are also potentially useful broad-spectrum neuroendocrine markers, but they are not widely used [22].

7.1.4 Miscellaneous Broad-Spectrum Markers

Cytokeratin 19 (CK19) may be expressed by some PanNETs (Fig. 7.3c). Some reports indicated that CK 19 was a marker for some aggressive PanNETs [26, 27]. CD117 (C-Kit) has been reported to be a marker with prognostic significance in PanNETs. It was found to be an independent prognostic marker in more aggressive PanNETs [28].

The gene products of the death domain-associated proteins DAXX and ATR-X which encode proteins involved in chromatin remodeling have been detected in 40 % of PanNETs. The expression of these markers has been associated with activation of alternative lengthening of telomeres [29]. DAXX and ATR-X protein loss have been associated with tumor stage and metastasis, reduced time of relapse-free survival, and decreased time of tumor-associated survival. Marinoni et al. have suggested that mutations of DAXX and ATRX along with chromosome instability have been associated with PanNET progression [29].

7.2 Somatostatin Receptors

Somatostatin receptors are members of the seven-transmembrane G-protein coupled receptor superfamily which are widely distributed throughout the body. There are five subtypes of somatostatin receptors (SSTs) [30, 31]. The main function of somatostatin is the inhibition of secretion of various hormones. This function is mediated through SSTs 2. Suppression of cell growth is carried out by SSTS 1, 2, and 5. The presence of SSTs indicates whether tumors will respond to somatostatin analog therapy, which usually acts on SST subtypes 2, 3, and 5. The presence of the SST subtypes has been studied by receptor autoradiography, in situ hybridization, polymerase chain reactions, and immunohistochemistry (Fig. 7.3d) with subtype-specific antibodies [30, 31]. All five SSTs have been identified in the normal islets. SST 5 was not present in normal PP cells. The expression may vary with different types of PanNETs. For example, insulinomas may not express some SST subtypes. This correlates with the observation that around 20–50 % of insulinomas are unresponsive to somatostatin analog treatment [2]. This emphasizes the importance of determining the presence of and specific subtypes of SSTs before treatment of pancreatic PanNETs with somatostatin analog therapy (Table 7.2).

Table 7.2 Hormones produced by pancreatic neuroendocrine tumors

Functioning tumors
Insulinoma
Glucagonoma
Somatostatinoma
Vasoactive intestinal polypeptide (VIPoma)
Gastrinoma
Enterochromaffin-cell tumors (serotonin)
Nonfunctioning tumors
Pancreatic polypeptide
Ectopic hormone production-functioning tumors
Growth hormone releasing hormone (GHRH)
Growth hormone (GH)
Ghrelin
Corticotropin-releasing hormone (CRH)
Adrenocorticotropin hormone (ACTH)
Parathyroid hormone (PTH)
Parathyroid hormone-related peptide (PTHrp)
Ectopic hormone-nonfunctioning tumors
Calcitonin

7.2.1 Hormone Producing Functioning PanNETs

7.2.1.1 Insulinomas

Insulinomas are the most common functioning PanNETs. They occur most frequently between 30 and 60 years of age [32–34]. Insulinomas are generally small with an average diameter of 1.5 cm. Patients with insulinomas usually present with symptoms including hypoglycemia, headaches, weakness, dizziness incoherence, convulsions, or coma. Insulinomas occur most frequently in the body and tail of the pancreas as solitary benign tumors which are usually treated by surgical resection or enucleation. They may show different patterns of growth including trabecular-gyriform, lobular, and solid patterns. Amyloid (composed of amylin protein) may be present in insulin-producing islet cells and in insulinomas (Fig. 7.4a). After Congo Red staining and examination with polarized light, amyloid in insulinoma shows the characteristic green birefringence. Insulin immunostaining is present in almost all insulinomas (Fig. 7.4b). Many tumors are also positive for proinsulin and for amylin. About half of insulinomas are multihormonal with cells also positive for glucagon, somatostatin, gastrin, and PP. Most insulinomas are benign (90–95 %). Malignant insulinomas are diagnosed by metastatic or locally invasive disease. Patients with malignant insulinomas have a median survival of only 4 years [2, 33].

7.2.1.2 Glucagonomas

Glucagonomas are usually well-differentiated PanNETs derived from the alpha cells. Patients may present with dermatitis (also known as necrolytic migratory erythema), stomatitis, diabetes, weight loss, and anemia [34–38]. They are uncommon even for pancreatic endocrine tumors and represent about 8 % of functioning PanNETs. Most tumors are solitary and are localized in the body and tail region with a mean diameter of around 7.6 cm. Most glucagonomas are malignant and patients may have local invasion or metastases to the liver, regional lymph nodes, bone, lungs, and adrenals. Glucagonomas are characterized by a trabecular and diffuse pattern of growth. Vascular and perineural invasion are common. Immunohistochemical stains are positive for glucagon (Fig. 7.4c) and for peptides derived from proglucagon, such as glicentin, and glucagon-like peptides. Glucagonomas may also express other pancreatic islet cell hormones. About 80 % of glucagonomas are malignant and approximately 70 % of patients have metastases at the time of diagnosis. Like many PanNETs, glucagonomas grow slowly and patients may survive for many years after surgical resection [2, 33].

7.2.1.3 Somatostatinomas

Somatostatinomas are PanNETs associated with the somatostatinoma syndrome which includes diabetes mellitus, cholelithiasis, diarrhea with or without steatorrhea, weight loss, hypochlorhydria, and anemia [2, 33]. The tumors are commonly located in the head of the pancreas, but may arise anywhere in the pancreas. Somatostatinomas are more common in the duodenum than in the pancreas. They are generally large tumors ranging in average diameter from 5 to 6 cm. The histological spectrum of somatostatinomas may range from trabecular and acinar

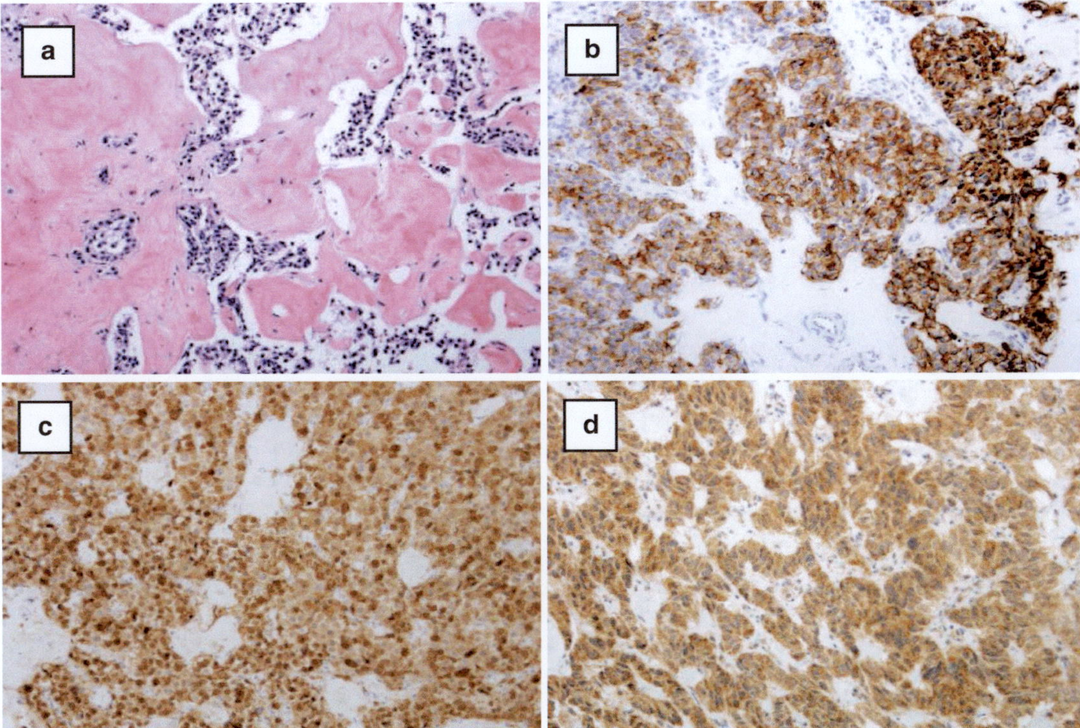

Fig. 7.4 (**a**) Congo red staining showing staining positive reaction for amyloid in an insulinoma. (**b**) Immunohistochemical staining for insulin showing diffuse positive staining in the tumor. (**c**) Pancreatic glucagonoma showing strong positive staining for glucagon in the tumor cells. (**d**) Pancreatic VIPoma showing strong positive staining in the tumor cells

patterns to solid sheets of tumor cells growing in a diffuse manner. Tumors frequently show angioinvasion and perineural invasion. Psammoma bodies, which are frequently found in duodenal tumors, are rare in pancreatic tumors. Immunohistochemical staining for somatostatin can be quite variable. Immunoreactivity for other hormones including gastrin and calcitonin may be present [2].

7.2.1.4 Vasoactive Intestinal Polypeptide-Producing Tumors (VIPomas)

VIPomas occur mainly in the pancreas and are associated with the Verner-Morrison syndrome which includes watery diarrhea, hypokalemia, and achlorhydria (WHDA) due to the secretion of vasoactive intestinal polypeptide (VIP), peptide histidine methionine (PHM), and related hormone-like substances [39]. VIPomas are rare

pancreatic endocrine tumors. Most VIPomas are solitary tumors, and they are most frequent in the tail of the pancreas. Tumors have an average size of 5 cm. The metastatic rate ranges from 40 to 70 % [2]. The tumors may grow as solid, trabecular, or tubulo-acinar patterns and microcysts may be present. Vascular and perineural invasion is a common finding. Immunoreactivity for VIP is usually detected (Fig. 7.4d), and the tumors may also be positive for PHM, PP, or somatostatin. Around 80 % of VIPomas may be metastatic at the time of diagnosis. If surgery is not effective, treatment with long-acting somatostatin analogs may help to control WHDA symptoms in some patients [2, 33].

7.2.1.5 Gastrinomas

Gastrinomas occur in the pancreas as well as several other locations including the duodenum, upper jejunum, and stomach. The tumors are frequently associated with the Zollinger-Ellison syndrome (ZES) which includes peptic ulcers, due to excessive gastrin production [2, 33]. Gastrinomas are the second most common functioning PanNETs after insulinomas. Approximately 20 % of patients with pancreatic gastrinomas have MEN1. Gastrinomas are most frequently found in the head of the pancreas. A trabecular pattern of growth is most common, but tumors may also show a solid or pseudo acinar pattern. Most gastrinomas are positive for gastrin. Antibodies against the C-terminus or N-terminus of gastrin-34 as well as against gastrin 17 are used in establishing the diagnosis. Gastrinomas may also be positive for glucagon, insulin somatostatin, or PP. Most pancreatic gastrinomas are malignant, and the tumors metastasize to the liver and lymph nodes. Liver metastasis, but not lymph node metastases, is associated with patient survival [2].

7.2.1.6 Enterochromaffin-Cell (Serotonin-Producing) Tumors

Enterochromaffin (EC) cell- or serotonin-producing tumors are extremely uncommon [2, 40]. They are usually well-differentiated carcinomas, although small tumors causing carcinoid syndrome without metastases have been reported. The tumors are usually composed of solid nests or trabecular patterns of growth.

7.2.2 Ectopic Hormone-Producing Functioning PanNETs

Ectopic hormone-producing functioning PanNETs include tumors producing growth hormone (GH) and growth-hormone-releasing hormone (GHRH), and Ghrelin-producing, adrenocorticotropin-producing hormone (ACTH), and parathyroid hormone-secreting tumors (PTH).

7.2.2.1 GHRH, GH, and Ghrelin-Producing Tumors

The GHRH and GH-producing tumors are extremely rare tumors that usually occur in younger patients are associated with acromegaly and are almost always malignant [41–44]. When the tumors produce GHRH, this stimulates the pituitary gland leading to pituitary GH cell hyperplasia and excessive GH secretion. The tumors are usually large and metastases to the liver and lymph nodes may be seen. Some patients may have MEN1 or ZES. A rare case of a malignant ghrelin-producing PanNETs has been reported, but the patient did not have acromegaly [45].

7.2.2.2 Adrenocorticotropic Hormone (ACTH)-Producing PanNETs

These tumors cause around 10 % of ectopic Cushing's syndrome. They are more common in young women, but may have also been reported in a few children [2, 46, 47]. The tumors are almost always malignant with metastases to liver, lymph nodes, kidney, thyroid, and bone. Rare cases of small-cell neuroendocrine carcinomas producing ACTH and causing Cushing's syndrome in the pancreas have also been reported [47].

7.2.2.3 Parathyroid Hormone-Secreting Tumors

Parathyroid hormone (PTH)- or parathyroid hormone-related peptide (PTHrp)-producing tumors associated with hypercalcemia and hyperparathyroidism are very uncommon. PTHrp has been detected in normal islets and is commonly detected in other PanNETs [48–51]. The presence of scattered immunoreactive cells is not associated with hypercalcemia.

7.2.3 Nonfunctioning Well-Differentiated PanNETs

These are tumors showing endocrine differentiation without evidence of clinical endocrine syndrome [2, 33, 52, 53]. Immunohistochemical studies are usually positive for broad-spectrum endocrine markers such as chromogranin A and synaptophysin. They may also express other hormones focally by immunohistochemical staining. These nonfunctioning tumors have been detected in 0.3–1.6 % of unselected autopsy cases and in up to 10 % of cases in which the pancreas was carefully examined grossly and microscopically [2]. Nonfunctioning PanNETs represent 30–40 % of resected pancreatic neuroendocrine tumors. The majority of cases from surgical resection are malignant tumors with metastatic disease, and patients usually present with an expanding pancreatic mass or with mass occupying lesion from metastatic disease. The tumors are more common in the head of the pancreas and average about 5 cm in diameter. The histological appearance is similar to functioning tumors with a trabecular or solid pattern of growth. Malignant tumors usually have increased mitotic activity with vascular and/or perineural invasion [2, 52, 53].

Hormones such as PP, glucagon, somatostatin, and insulin are frequently detected in a variable number of cells in the tumors. Insulin-producing cells are quite rare. Gastrin and VIP have not been reported in these tumors [2]. Small incidental nonfunctioning well-differentiated tumors usually have an excellent prognosis, while the large symptomatic nonfunctioning well-differentiated tumors have a poor prognosis with a mean survival between 23 months and 4.3 years [2, 33].

7.2.3.1 Pancreatic Polypeptide-Producing Tumors

Endocrine tumors composed predominantly of PP-immunoreactive cells are very uncommon. About 50 % of patients with PanNETs have elevated serum levels of PP. No defined endocrine function associated with PP hypersecretion has been reported to date, so PanNETs with elevated serum levels of PP are usually considered as nonfunctioning tumors. Malignant PP-producing tumors are usually large with a mean diameter of 8 cm, and they usually show a solid growth pattern. Most tumors are present in the head of the pancreas. The diagnosis of a PP-producing tumor usually requires that PP is present in at least 50 % of the tumor cells [2].

7.2.4 Ectopic Hormone-Producing Nonfunctioning PanNETs

7.2.4.1 Calcitonin-Producing Tumors

Calcitonin immunoreactivity may be detected in a variety of PanNETs such as VIP- and somatostatin-producing tumors. However, pure calcitonin-producing tumors are rare in the pancreas. Because the physiological function of calcitonin in the human body has not been clearly elucidated and excessive production of calcitonin as in medullary thyroid carcinomas is not associated with any specific syndromes, these tumors are considered nonfunctioning. Despite this, some patients may have diarrhea and abdominal pain which disappear after surgical excision of the tumor [2, 33, 54]. Calcitonin-producing tumors are generally large with a mean diameter of 6.3 cm, but may be to 20 cm in diameter. The tumors are usually solitary and may be present in the head, body, or tail of the pancreas. Most of the tumors are malignant with metastatic disease to the liver or lymph nodes at the time of diagnosis. The tumors may also metastasize to the brain and bone. In contrast with medullary thyroid carcinomas, amyloid deposits have not been reported in calcitonin-producing PanNETs. In addition to calcitonin immunoreactivity, the tumors may also be positive for somatostatin and PP [2].

7.2.5 Poorly Differentiated Endocrine Carcinomas (PDECs)

PDECs are highly malignant neoplasms composed of small to large cells with endocrine features [2, 33, 55]. They are more common in men and most of the carcinomas are nonfunctioning. Paraneoplastic syndrome is uncommon in pancreatic PDECs. They are usually large tumors with a mean diameter of 4.2 cm and may show areas of hemorrhage and necrosis. The cells range from small to intermediate size with occasional large-cell tumors.

The mitotic index is greater than 20 per 10 HPF and the Ki-67 index is greater than 20 %. The tumors are positive for chromogranin, NSE, and synaptophysin. Immunohistochemical detection of hormones is usually negative, but a few tumors may be positive for calcitonin, somatostatin, or ACTH. Immunoreactivity for p53 is usually positive. These tumors metastasize to liver, regional lymph nodes, and to extra-abdominal sites including lung and bone [2, 33].

7.3 Mixed Adenoneuroendocrine Carcinoma (MANEC)

These tumors (previously designated as mixed exocrine-endocrine tumors) are epithelial neoplasms with a predominant exocrine growth pattern and an endocrine component. The endocrine component should represent at least a third of the tumor cell population [56–59]. The exocrine component is usually malignant such as ductal adenocarcinoma or acinar cell carcinoma, but it can also be benign [57]. Immunohistochemical staining for keratins, epithelial membrane antigen, CEA, CA19.9, trypsin, amylase, lipase, and other markers of specific exocrine differentiation as well as for markers of endocrine differentiation such as chromogranin A, synaptophysin, and NSE is useful in establishing the diagnosis. The biological behavior of the malignant tumors is determined by the exocrine component [2].

References

1. Jürgensen A, Klöppel G (2000) Ontogeny, differentiation and growth of the endocrine pancreas. Virchows Arch 436:527–538
2. LaRosa S, Furlan D, Sessa F, Capella C (2010) The endocrine pancreas. In: Lloyd RV (ed) Endocrine pathology, differential diagnosis and molecular advances. Springer, New York, pp 367–418
3. Okada N, Takaki R, Kitagawa M (1967) Histological and immunofluorescence studies on the site of origin of glucagon in mammalian pancreas. J Histochem Cytochem 16:405–409
4. Orci L, Baetens D, Dubois MP et al (1975) Evidence for D-cell of the pancreas secreting somatostatin. Horm Metab Res 7:400–402
5. Fiocca R, Sessa F, Tenti P et al (1983) Pancreatic polypeptide (PP) cells in the PP-rich lobe of the human pancreas are identified ultrastructurally and immunocytochemically as F cells. Histochemistry 77:511–523
6. Andralojc KM, Mercalli A, Nowak KW et al (2009) Ghrelin-producing epsilon cells in the developing and adult human pancreas. Diabetologia 52:486–493
7. Gu G, Dubauskaite J, Melton DA (2002) Direct evidence for the pancreatic lineage: NGN3+ cells are islet progenitors and are distinct from duct progenitors. Development 129:2447–2457
8. Ashizawa S, Brunicardi FC, Wang XP (2004) PDX-1 and the pancreas. Pancreas 28:109–120
9. Ahlgren U, Pfaff SL, Jessel TM et al (1997) Independent requirement for ISL1 in formation of pancreatic mesenchyme and islet cells. Nature 385:257–260
10. Gradwohl G, Dierich A, LeMeur M et al (2000) Neurogenin3 is required for the development of the four endocrine cell lineages of the pancreas. Proc Natl Acad Sci U S A 97:1607–1611
11. Graham RP, Shrestha B, Caron BL et al (2013) Islet-1 is a sensitive but not entirely specific marker for pancreatic neuroendocrine neoplasms and their metastases. Am J Surg Pathol 37:399–405
12. Hermann G, Konukiewitz B, Schmitt A et al (2011) Hormonally defined pancreatic and duodenal neuroendocrine tumors differ in their transcription factor signatures: expression of ISL1, PDX1, NGN3, and CDX2. Virchows Arch 459:147–154
13. Erickson LA, Papouchado B, Dimashkieh H et al (2004) Cdx2 as a marker for neuroendocrine tumors of unknown primary sites. Endocr Pathol 15:247–252
14. Agaimy A, Erlenbach-Wünsch K, Konukiewitz B et al (2013) ISL1 expression is not restricted to pancreatic well-differentiated neuroendocrine neoplasms, but is also commonly found in well and poorly differentiated neuroendocrine neoplasms of extrapancreatic origin. Mod Pathol 26:995–1003
15. Lan MS, Breslin MB (2009) Structure, expression, and biological function of INSM1 transcription factor in neuroendocrine differentiation. FASEB J 23:2024–2033
16. Rosenbaum JN, Guo Z, Baus RM et al (2015) INSMI: a novel immunohistochemical and molecular marker for neuroendocrine and neuroepithelial neoplasms. Am J Clin Pathol (in press)
17. Tang LH, Gonen M, Hedvat C et al (2012) Objective quantification of the Ki67 proliferative index in neuroendocrine tumors of the gastroenteropancreatic system: a comparison of digital image analysis with manual methods. Am J Surg Pathol 36:1761–1767
18. McCall CM, Shi C, Cornish TC et al (2013) Grading of well-differentiated pancreatic neuroendocrine tumors is improved by the inclusion of both Ki67 proliferative index and mitotic rate. Am J Surg Pathol 37:1671–1677
19. Klöppel G, Perren A, Heitz PU (2004) The gastroenteropancreatic neuroendocrine cell system and its tumors: the WHO classification. Ann NY Acad Sci 1014:13–27
20. Lloyd RV, Wilson BS (1983) Specific endocrine tissue marker defined by a monoclonal antibody. Science 222:628–630
21. Lloyd RV, Mervak T, Schmidt K et al (1984) Immunohistochemical detection of chromogranin and neurone specific enolase in pancreatic endocrine neoplasms. Am J Surg Pathol 8:607–614
22. Portela-Gomes GM, Hacker GW, Weitgasser R (2004) Neuroendocrine cell markers for pancreatic islets and tumors. Appl Immunohistochem Morphol 12:183–192
23. Portela-Gomes GM, Stridsberg M (2001) Selective processing of chromogranin A in the different islet cells in human pancreas. J Histochem Cytochem 49:483–490

24. Wiedenmann B, Franke WW (1985) Identification and localization of synaptophysin, an integral membrane glycoprotein of MW 38,000 characteristic of presynaptic vesicles. Cell 41:1017–1028
25. Schmechel D, Marango PJ, Brightman M (1978) Neuron specific enolase is a molecular marker for peripheral and central neuroendocrine cells. Nature 276:834–836
26. Desphande V, Fernandez-del Castillo C, Muzikansky A et al (2004) Cytokeratin 19 is a powerful predictor of survival in pancreatic endocrine tumors. Am J Surg Pathol 28:1145–1153
27. La Rosa S, Rigoli E, Uccella S et al (2007) Prognostic and biological significance of cytokeratin 19 in pancreatic endocrine tumours. Histopathology 50:597–606
28. Zhang L, Smyrk TC, Oliveira AM et al (2009) KIT is an independent prognostic marker for pancreatic endocrine tumors: a finding derived from analysis of islet cell differentiation markers. Am J Surg Pathol 33:1562–1569
29. Marinoni I, Kurrer AS, Vassella E et al (2014) Loss of DAXX and ATRX are associated with chromosome instability and reduced survival of patients with pancreatic neuroendocrine tumors. Gastroenterology 146:453–460
30. Reubi JC, Kappeler A, Waser B et al (1998) Immunohistochemical localization of somatostatin receptor sst2A in human tumors. Am J Pathol 153:233–245
31. Papotti M, Bongiovanni M, Volante M et al (2002) Expression of somatostatin receptor types 1–5 in 81 cases of gastrointestinal and pancreatic endocrine tumors, A correlative immunohistochemical and reverse-transcriptase polymerase chain reaction analysis. Virchows Arch 440:461–475
32. Reid MD, Balci S, Saka B et al (2014) Neuroendocrine tumors of the pancreas: current concepts and controversies. Endocr Pathol 25:65–79
33. Oberg K (2010) Pancreatic endocrine tumors. Semin Oncol 37:594–618
34. La Rosa S, Klersy C, Uccella S et al (2009) Improved histologic and clinicopathologic criteria for prognostic evaluation of pancreatic endocrine tumors. Hum Pathol 40:30–40
35. Soga J, Yakuwa Y (1998) Glucagonoma/diabetico-dermatogenic syndrome (DDS): a statistical evaluation of 407 reported cases. J Hepatobiliary Pancreat Surg 5:312–319
36. Ruttman E, Klöppel G, Klehn M et al (1980) Pancreatic glucagonoma with and without the syndrome. Immunocytochemical study of 5 tumor cases and review of the literature. Virchows Arch A Pathol Anat Histopathol 388:51–67
37. DeLellis RA, Lloyd RV, Heitz PU et al (2004) World Health Organization classification of tumours. Pathology & genetics of tumours of endocrine organs. IARC, Lyon
38. Thompson GB, van Heerden JA, Grant CS et al (1988) Islet cell carcinomas of the pancreas: a twenty-year experience. Surgery 104:1011–1017
39. Capella C, Polak JM, Buffa et al (1983) Morphologic patterns and diagnostic criteria of VIP-producing endocrine tumors. A histologic, histochemical, ultrastructural and biochemical study of 32 cases. Cancer 52:1860–1874
40. McCall CM, Shi C, Klein AP et al (2012) Serotonin expression in pancreatic neuroendocrine tumors correlates with a trabecular histologic pattern and large duct involvement. Hum Pathol 43:1169–1176
41. Sanno N, Teramoto A, Osamura RY et al (1997) A growth hormone-releasing hormone-producing pancreatic islet cell tumor metastasized to the pituitary is associated with pituitary somatotroph hyperplasia and acromegaly. J Clin Endocrinol Metab 82:2731–2737
42. Ezzat S, Ezrin C, Yamashita S et al (1993) Recurrent acromegaly resulting from ectopic growth hormone gene expression by a metastatic pancreatic tumor. Cancer 71:66–70
43. Dayal Y, Lin HD, Tallberg K et al (1986) Immunocytochemical demonstration of growth hormone – releasing factor in gastrointestinal and pancreatic endocrine tumors. Am J Clin Pathol 85:13–20
44. Asa SL, Kovacs K, Thoner MD et al (1985) Immunohistological localization of growth-hormone-releasing hormone in human tumors. J Clin Endocrinol Metab 60:423–427
45. Volante M, Allia E, Gugliotta P (2002) Expression of ghrelin and of the GH secretagogue receptors by pancreatic islet cells and related endocrine tumors. J Clin Endocrinol Metab 87:1300–1308
46. Clark ES, Carney JA (1984) Pancreatic islet cell tumor associated with Cushing syndrome. Am J Surg Pathol 8:917–924
47. Corrin B, Gilby ED, Jones NF et al (1973) Oat cell carcinoma of the pancreas with ectopic ACTH secretion. Cancer 31:1523–1527
48. Arps H, Dietel M, Schulz A et al (1986) Pancreatic endocrine carcinoma with ectopic PTH-production and paraneoplastic hypercalcemia. Virchows Arch A Pathol Anat Histopathol 408:497–503
49. Ratcliffe WA, Bowden SJ, Dunne FP et al (1994) Expression and processing of parathyroid hormone related protein in a pancreatic endocrine cell tumour associated with hypercalcemia. Clin Endocrinol 40:679–686
50. Miraliakbari BA, Asa SL, Boudreau SF (1992) Parathyroid hormone-like peptide in pancreatic endocrine carcinoma and adenocarcinoma associated with hypercalcemia. Hum Pathol 23:884–887
51. Rizzoli R, Sappino AP, Bonjour JP (1990) Parathyroid hormone-related protein and hypercalcemia in pancreatic neuroendocrine tumors. Int J Cancer 46:394–398
52. Eckhauser FE, Cheung PS, Vinik AI et al (1986) Nonfunctioning malignant neuroendocrine tumors of the pancreas. Surgery 100:978–988
53. Evans DB, Skibber JM, Lee JE et al (1993) Nonfunctioning islet cell carcinoma of the pancreas. Surgery 114:1175–1182

54. La Rosa S, Sessa F, Uccella S et al (1997) Histological and immunohistochemical study of calcitonin-cell tumors of the pancreas. Digestion 58(Suppl 2):19

55. La Rosa S, Sessa F, Capella C et al (1996) Prognostic criteria in nonfunctioning pancreatic endocrine tumors. Virchows Arch 429:323–333

56. Klöppel G (2000) Mixed exocrine-endocrine tumors of the pancreas. Semin Diagn Pathol 17:104–108

57. Keel SB, Zukerberg L, Graeme-Cook F et al (1996) A pancreatic endocrine tumor arising within a serous cystadenoma of the pancreas. Am J Surg Pathol 20:471–475

58. Klimstra DS, Rosai J, Heffess CS (1994) Mixed acinar-endocrine carcinomas of the pancreas. Am J Surg Pathol 18:765–778

59. Klöppel G (2011) Classification and pathology of gastroenteropancreatic neuroendocrine neoplasms. Endocrinol Relat Cancer 18(Suppl 1):S1–S16

Insulinoma

8

Jean-Yves Scoazec

Insulinomas are functioning neuroendocrine tumors (NETs), associated with, and usually revealed by, clinical and biological symptoms secondary to insulin overproduction by neoplastic cells [1]. Insulinomas form a well-defined subset among neuroendocrine neoplasms because of their distinctive biology, their characteristic clinical and biological presentation, and their rather uniform morphological features. Most of them are well-differentiated, slowly evolving neoplasms, almost invariably located in the pancreas. In this chapter, we will review the historical background, epidemiology, diagnosis, morphological, immunohistochemical, and genetic features and prognosis of this clinicopathological entity. Finally, we will briefly address the role of the pathologist in the diagnosis of other etiologies of endogenous hyperinsulinism.

J.-Y. Scoazec
Services de Pathologie morphologique et moléculaire, Département de Biopathologie et Unité AMMICa INSERM US23, CNRS UMS3655, Gustave Roussy Cancer Campus, 114 rue Edouard Vaillant, 94805 Villejuif Cedex, France

Faculté de Médecine, Université Paris Sud, Le Kremlin-Bicêtre, Paris 94276, France
e-mail: jean-yves.scoazec@gustaveroussy.fr

8.1 Historical Background

The endocrine islets located in the pancreas were first described in detail by Virchow's student Paul Langerhans in his thesis in 1869, but the term "Langerhans islet" was coined only in 1893 [2]. The first case of "islet cell adenoma" was reported in 1902 by AG Nicholls. The first recognition of a pancreatic tumor as a source of uncontrolled insulin production and the first attempt to operate a case of malignant insulinoma (which unfortunately proved to be unresectable), were made in 1927 by WJ Mayo and his group in Rochester [2]. The first successful resection of a benign insulinoma was performed in 1929 in Toronto by R Graham [2]. The so-called Whipple triad, essential for the clinical diagnosis of insulinoma, was described by Whipple and Frantz in 1938. The first ultrastructural description of normal and neoplastic beta cells and the description of the typical appearance of insulin-loaded secretory granules, which have remained for a long time the unique method available for the definitive identification of normal and neoplastic beta cells, were provided by Lacy in 1957 [3]; the same author reported the first localization of insulin by immunofluorescence in pancreatic tissues as soon as 1957, much before the large diffusion of immunohistochemistry in research and diagnostic laboratories [4].

S. La Rosa, F. Sessa (eds.), *Pancreatic Neuroendocrine Neoplasms: Practical Approach to Diagnosis, Classification, and Therapy*, DOI 10.1007/978-3-319-17235-4_8,
© Springer International Publishing Switzerland 2015

8.2 Epidemiology

Like other NET subsets, insulinomas are rare tumors with a low incidence but a comparatively high prevalence, because of the long survival of most patients [1]. The annual incidence of insulinoma in a well-defined population (Olmsted County, Southeastern Minnesota) was shown to be 0.4 per 100,000 persons; other reports have found annual incidence rates ranging from 0.07 to 0.12/100,000 in less well-defined populations [5]. The incidence in European countries is usually assumed to be between one and three per million per year [1].

Insulinomas can be diagnosed over a large age range, but there is an age-specific incidence peak in the fifth decade of life; a slight female predominance (60:40) is usually observed. Despite their rarity, insulinomas are the most frequent type of functioning neuroendocrine neoplasms of the pancreas: they account up to 50–70 % of cases according to the series, followed by gastrinomas [1]. Malignant insulinomas are exceedingly rare: less than 10 % of cases show objective features of malignancy; they occur later than benign insulinomas and are associated with a male predominance. Five to 10 % of insulinomas are associated with the MEN-1 syndrome; such tumors are usually multiple and may be malignant in up to 25 % of cases [1, 5].

It must be underlined that available epidemiological data are in need of reevaluation. On one hand, many recent studies, coming from different countries, have shown that the apparent incidence of neuroendocrine neoplasms is rapidly increasing. On the other hand, the proportion of functioning neuroendocrine tumors now observed in clinical practice is much lower than in the past, likely as a result of the progress made in diagnostic and functional imaging procedures. Finally, some data suggest that the geographical distribution of insulinoma may be uneven and that this tumor subset may be more frequent in some areas, such as China, than in Western countries.

8.3 Diagnosis

By definition, insulinoma is associated with clinical symptoms and biological abnormalities due to endogenous hyperinsulinism. The key diagnostic feature is the Whipple triad, which associates symptoms of hypoglycemia, concomitant of plasma glucose levels ≤ 2.2 mmol/l, resolving after glucose intake [1]. Once Whipple triad is firmly established, the following tight biological criteria are required for a diagnosis of insulinoma: low blood glucose levels (≤ 2.2 mmol/l), with concomitant high insulin levels ≥ 6 µU/l, C-peptide levels $\geq 6,200$ pmol/l, and proinsulin levels ≥ 5 pmol/l, along with beta-hydroxybutyrate levels ≤ 2.7 mmol/l and absence of sulfonylurea (metabolites) in the plasma and/or urine. Controlled testing during a 72-h fast remains the gold standard and might be required in some cases to achieve a definitive diagnosis [1].

The next diagnostic step is the localization of the tumor. Insulinomas are evenly distributed within the three main parts of the pancreas, head, body, and tail. Macroscopically, they are usually solitary, well circumscribed, and small tumors: about 90 % (85–99 % according to the series) are less than 2.5 cm in diameter when detected. These characteristics explain why it is sometimes difficult to achieve a precise preoperative localization of the lesion. CT and MRI are limited in their capacity to identify small tumors. The same is true for functional imaging, and especially for octreotide scintigraphy, which detects only 20–50 % of tumors. Endoscopic ultrasound, in experienced hands, is currently one of the most specific and sensitive examination to detect small tumors [1]. It must be noted that exceptional cases of insulinomas have been described in ectopic pancreata [6] or even in extrapancreatic locations, including the small intestine, lung, cervix, and ovary [7].

The definitive preoperative pathological diagnosis is rarely achieved for primary tumors, since guided biopsy or fine-needle aspirates are difficult to obtain from most lesions, especially when they are small and difficult to localize. Cytology is not recommended as a standard procedure [1]. The main interest of cytology or biopsy is to confirm the nature of a suspected metastasis in the context of a possible or definite malignant insulinoma.

The pathological diagnosis will therefore be usually achieved through the examination of a surgical specimen. Different surgical strategies can be considered. For localized insulinomas of the head or for multiple tumors, surgical enucleation remains recommended [1]. When the tumor is located in the neck, body, or tail of the pancreas and is anatomically unsuitable for enucleation, central or distal pancreatectomy must be performed. The pathological examination of the lesion must be done according to the general recommendations available for all neuroendocrine tumors [8]. The pathological diagnosis must rely on both morphological and immunohistochemical arguments; the neuroendocrine nature of the tumor must be confirmed by the use of general neuroendocrine markers, such as chromogranin A and synaptophysin. The morphological differentiation must be evaluated. Histological grading (G1/G2/G3) must be performed according to ENETS and WHO recommendations, on the basis of both mitotic count and Ki67 index. The lesion must then be classified according to the 2010 WHO classification [9]. When possible, the pTNM stage must be provided. Two main staging systems exist for neuroendocrine tumors, including insulinomas: ENETS proposals [10] and UICC staging system [11]. These two systems are similar for many NET subsets but significantly different for pancreatic NETs; however, both have been shown to be of prognostic relevance. Whereas no specific comparison has been performed for insulinomas, it can therefore be assumed that the two systems can therefore be used for this NET subset, providing the pathologist clearly indicates which system has been used.

8.4 Morphology, Immunohistochemistry, and Genetics

The great majority of pancreatic insulinomas are well-differentiated neuroendocrine neoplasms, with low proliferative capacities: they can be therefore classified as NET/NEN G1 in the 2010 WHO classification. Rare cases are G2 or even G3 tumors [1].

8.4.1 Morphology

The microscopic appearance of most insulinomas is therefore that of most well-differentiated neuroendocrine tumors. The growth pattern is mostly trabecular or solid. Neoplastic cells are monomorphic, with low nucleocytoplasmic ratio, a large eosinophilic cytoplasm, and an ovoid, regular nucleus-containing salt-and-pepper chromatin with well visible nucleoli. There are no or little atypia. Mitotic figures are rare. Necrosis is absent. In most cases, the stroma is poorly developed but contains numerous capillary vessels. Much more rarely, atypia is prominent and mitoses are frequent.

In a proportion of cases, the microscopic appearance is more suggestive, because of the presence of amyloid deposits in the stroma (Figs. 8.1 and 8.2). Amyloid fibrils are present in large amounts in about 5 % of cases, but focal deposits can be detected by Congo red staining in up to 65 % of cases. Insulinoma-associated amyloid fibrils are made of deposits of islet amyloid polypeptide (IAPP), also called amylin [12]. IAPP is produced by beta cells; its precursor, proIAPP, is stored in the same secretory granules than insulin; the mature form is co-secreted with insulin and behaves as a hormone involved in glycemic control. Amyloid formation initiates within beta cells, through the aggregation of proIAPP within the secretory granules themselves; these aggregates are able to collect mature IAPP molecules; the same process continues after the aggregates are released outside the cell into the extracellular matrix, promoting the progressive growth of amyloid

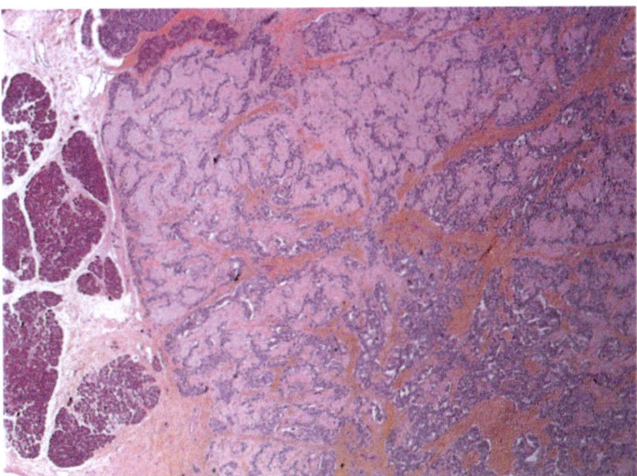

Fig. 8.1 Large pancreatic insulinoma with amyloid stroma (hematoxylin eosin saffron, original magnification ×120)

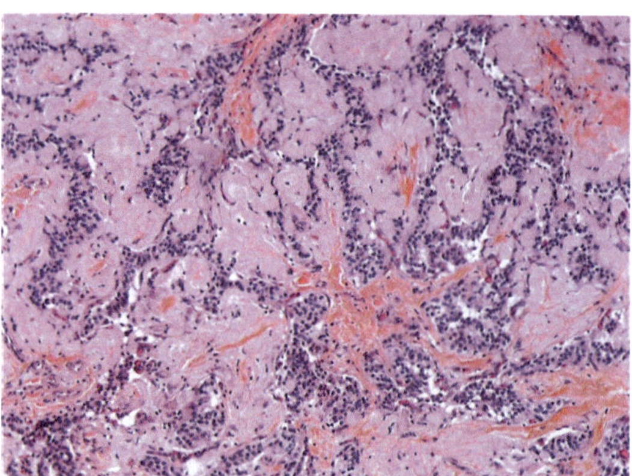

Fig. 8.2 Higher magnification showing well-differentiated neuroendocrine cells, without mitotic figures (hematoxylin eosin saffron, original magnification ×260)

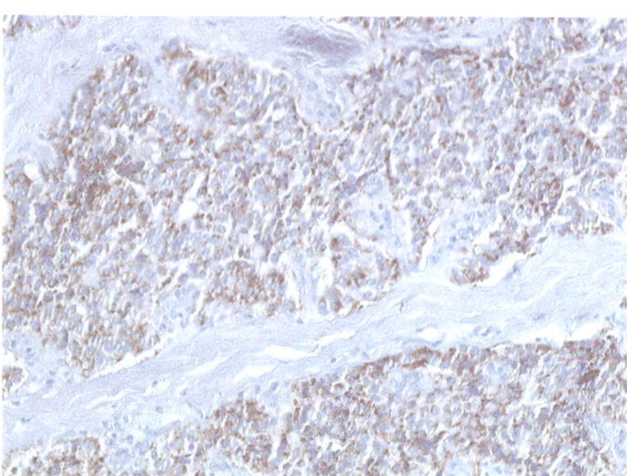

Fig. 8.3 Insulin expression with pericellular cytoplasmic distribution (indirect immunoperoxidase, original magnification ×260)

masses which eventually become detectable by light microscopy.

Associated lesions should be looked for in surrounding tissue if the type of resection allows (a) other endocrine or non-endocrine tumors or (b) endocrine microadenomatosis, defined by an increase in the number and size of pancreatic insular structures, which retain diameters less than 5 mm. Such lesions might suggest a syndrome of familial predisposition to pancreatic endocrine tumor, especially the MEN-1 syndrome, but are not specific. In many cases, islet cell enlargement is only adaptive to repeated and/or prolonged insulin-induced hypoglycemias.

8.4.2 Immunohistochemistry

In almost all cases of insulinomas, it is possible to demonstrate the presence of insulin- and proinsulin-producing cells, but with a variable intensity of staining, from weak to strong. Some insulinomas do not react positively despite a correct diagnosis, likely as a result of a rapid release of the hormone from insulin-producing cells [1]. The subcellular distribution of hormonal products is variable [13]. In many cases, a normal pattern of intracellular distribution is retained: insulin is predominantly detected as granular deposits along the basal (secretory) pole of neoplastic cells, whereas proinsulin is predominantly

detected in their perinuclear area. In other cases, insulin and proinsulin are diffusely detected all over the cytoplasm of neoplastic cells; this abnormal distribution pattern is associated with abnormalities in the proinsulin to insulin conversion. IAPP is also commonly detected in most insulinomas. It must be underlined that, in addition to insulin and proinsulin, it is not exceptional to detect other hormones in minor populations of neoplastic cells (Fig. 8.3).

The demonstration of insulin or proinsulin in neoplastic cells is not absolutely required for a definitive diagnosis of insulinoma [1]. The main interest of insulin or proinsulin staining is to confirm the nature of a resected tumor, when multiple tumors are present in the same patient, or to confirm the nature of a possible metastatic deposit from a potentially malignant insulinoma.

The expression of several transcription factors associated with beta-cell lineage development, such as PDX1 and Islet-1, also termed ISL1, has been recently studied [14]. PDX1 is required for pancreatic development and beta-cell maturation; ISL1 is involved in endocrine islet embryogenesis and in beta-cell maturation. Insulinomas express only PDX1 and ISL1, but these two transcription factors can be expressed in all other pancreatic NET subsets, including gastrin-, glucagon-, and somatostatin-producing tumors. These markers are therefore a clue to the pancreatic origin of a neuroendocrine tumor, but their specificity is much lower than that of hormonal products for the identification of insulinomas in tissue sections.

It has been verified that insulinomas usually express, like other pancreatic NETs, several somatostatin receptors, including sst-2 and sst-5. However, somatostatin receptors are not detectable in no less than 30 % of insulinomas [15]: this proportion is high as compared to most other well- or very well-differentiated NETs. This is one of the reasons explaining the poor sensitivity of octreotide scintigraphy in this indication.

8.4.3 Genetics

Insulinomas are one of the most frequent tumor subset observed in the MEN-1 syndrome (Fig. 8.4). Rare cases of insulinomas have been also described in two other genetic predisposition syndromes, neurofibromatosis type 1 and tuberous sclerosis [1]. Von Hippel-Lindau (VHL) syndrome has not been described as being associated with insulinoma or with other forms of secreting NET.

Despite the strong association between insulinomas and genetic predisposition syndromes, alterations in the corresponding genes are extremely rare in sporadic insulinomas: only a few cases have been reported in the literature. In the same way, genes frequently altered in sporadic nonfunctioning pancreatic NETs, such as *MEN-1*, *DAXX*, and *ATRX*, are only very rarely mutated in sporadic

insulinomas. A recent study, using whole-exome sequencing, has pointed out to the possible involvement of *YY1* gene in the pathogenesis of sporadic insulinomas [16]: T372R mutation of *YY1* gene has been detected in 30 % of cases tested. *YY1* encodes the Ying yang 1 protein involved in the regulation of mitochondrial function and insulin/IGF signaling within the pancreatic beta cell, in close interaction with the mTOR pathway. Further studies are required to confirm the degree of involvement of this gene and to identify other possible driver genes in sporadic insulinomas.

8.5 Prognosis

The vast majority of insulinomas are benign lesions. Less than 10 % in Western series behave as malignant tumors [1]. Criteria of malignancy are the same as for other NETs: they include signs of local, extrapancreatic, invasion, and/or evidence of metastatic dissemination. Angioinvasion and perineural invasion are not sufficient to establish malignancy but are alarm signals calling for particular surveillance. In the same way, the rare cases of insulinomas without objective signs of malignancy but of histological grades other than G1 must be closely followed up [1].

8.6 Other Pathological Entities Associated with Endogenous Hyperinsulinism

Insulinoma is, by far, the most frequent cause of endogenous hyperinsulinism. Other diagnoses had to be considered, especially if no tumor mass can be detected at macroscopical examination of a surgical specimen. In this situation, the entire specimen should be included, in thin sagittal cross-sections. However, a very small tumor is unlikely to underlie the clinical symptoms associated with hormonal hypersecretion: it is more likely that another etiology of beta-cell hyperplasia is involved. Two main syndromes may be encountered: (a) adult nesidioblastosis, found in 3–5 % of adults with hyperinsulinism,

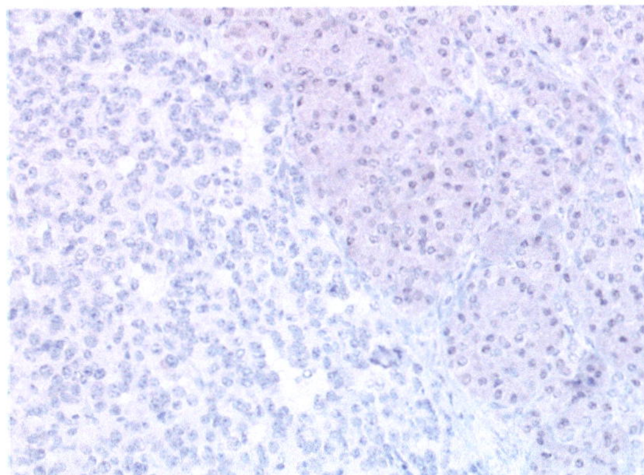

Fig. 8.4 Lack of detectable menin expression in insulinoma cells from a MEN-1 patient (indirect immunoperoxidase, original magnification ×350)

defined by the presence of abnormal Langerhans islets with hypertrophic beta cells [17]; (b) insulinomatosis, a rare and recently described condition, characterized by the presence of multiple microadenomas (size by definition <5 mm) expressing only insulin, sometimes associated with a few numbers of adenomas larger than 5 mm [18].

References

1. De Herder WW, Niederle B, Scoazec JY et al (2006) Well-differentiated pancreatic tumor/carcinoma: insulinoma. Neuroendocrinology 84:183–188
2. Shin JJ, Gorden P, Libutti SK (2010) Insulinoma: pathophysiology, localization and management. Future Oncol 6:229–237
3. Lacy PE (1957) Electron microscopic identification of different cell types in the islets of Langerhans of the guinea pig, rat, rabbit and dog. Anat Rec 128: 255–267
4. Lacy PE, Davies J (1957) Preliminary studies on the demonstration of insulin in the islets by the fluorescent antibody technic. Diabetes 6:354–357
5. Halfdanarson TR, Rubin J, Farnell MB et al (2008) Pancreatic endocrine neoplasms: epidemiology and prognosis of pancreatic endocrine tumors. Endocr Relat Cancer 15:409–427
6. Cárdenas CM, Domínguez I, Campuzano M et al (2009) Malignant insulinoma arising from intrasplenic heterotopic pancreas. JOP 10:321–323
7. La Rosa S, Pariani D, Calandra C et al (2013) Ectopic duodenal insulinoma: a very rare and challenging tumor type. Description of a case and review of the literature. Endocr Pathol 24:213–219
8. Klöppel G, Couvelard A, Perren A et al (2009) ENETS consensus guidelines for the standards of care in neuroendocrine tumors: towards a standardized approach to the diagnosis of gastroenteropancreatic neuroendocrine tumors and their prognostic stratification. Neuroendocrinology 90:162–166
9. Rindi G, Klimstra DS, Arnold R et al (2010) Nomenclature and classification of neuroendocrine neoplasms of the digestive system. In: Bosman FT, Carneiro F, Hruban RH, Theise ND (eds) WHO classification of tumours of the digestive system. IARC Press, Lyon, pp 13–14
10. Rindi G, Kloppel G, Alhman H et al (2006) TNM staging of foregut (neuro)endocrine tumors: a consensus proposal including a grading system. Virchows Arch 449:395–401
11. Sobin LH, Gospodarowicz MK, Wittekind C (2009) TNM classification of malignant tumours, 7th edn. Wiley, New York
12. Westermark P, Engström U, Johnson KH et al (1990) Islet amyloid polypeptide: pinpointing amino acid residues linked to amyloid fibril formation. Proc Natl Acad Sci U S A 87:5036–5040
13. Roth J, Klöppel G, Madsen OD et al (1992) Distribution patterns of proinsulin and insulin in human insulinomas: an immunohistochemical analysis in 76 tumors. Virchows Arch [B] Cell Pathol 63:51–61
14. Hermann G, Konukiewitz B, Schmitt A et al (2011) Hormonally defined pancreatic and duodenal neuroendocrine tumors differ in their transcription factor signatures: expression of ISL1, PDX1, NGN3, and CDX2. Virchows Arch 459:147–154
15. Bertherat J, Tenenbaum F, Perlemoine K et al (2003) Somatostatin receptors 2 and 5 are the major somatostatin receptors in insulinomas: an in vivo and in vitro study. J Clin Endocrinol Metab 88: 5353–5360
16. Cao Y, Gao Z, Li L et al (2013) Whole exome sequencing of insulinoma reveals recurrent T372R mutations in YY1. Nat Commun 4:2810
17. Anlauf M, Wieben D, Perren A et al (2005) Persistent hyperinsulinemic hypoglycemia in 15 adults with diffuse nesidioblastosis: diagnostic criteria, incidence, and characterization of beta-cell changes. Am J Surg Pathol 29:524–533
18. Anlauf M, Bauersfeld J, Raffel A et al (2009) Insulinomatosis: a multicentric insulinoma disease that frequently causes early recurrent hyperinsulinemic hypoglycemia. Am J Surg Pathol 33:339–346

Glucagonoma

Anne Couvelard and Olivia Hentic

9.1 Historical Background

Since the description in 1942 by Becker et al. of cutaneous manifestations due to a pancreatic neoplasm, McGavran et al. described in 1966 the first case of glucagon secretion by an alpha-cell carcinoma of the pancreas in a 42-year-old woman [1, 2]. The typical skin lesions called necrolytic migratory erythema were described by Wilkinson et al. in 1971 [3]. Mallinson et al. published in 1974 the first series of nine patients with a glucagonoma syndrome and a pancreatic tumor with characters of well-differentiated islet-cell tumors for eight of them [4]. It's only in 1982 that Guillausseau et al. presented a general review of 130 glucagonomas [5].

9.2 Epidemiology

The glucagonoma functional syndrome is due to a very rare pancreatic neuroendocrine tumor (PanNET) which secretes glucagon. Indeed, most (70–85 %) glucagon-secreting PanNETs are nonfunctioning [6, 7]. Glucagonoma represents 2 % of PanNETs and is the fourth functioning PanNET type after insulinoma, gastrinoma, and VIPoma [7, 8]. Their precise number is difficult to know, but the annual incidence is approximately 1 per 20 million population. The average age at diagnosis is 52.5 years and sex ratio is 0.8 [9]. Association with a multiple endocrine neoplasia type 1 occurs in 1–20 % of the glucagonoma syndrome [8, 9].

9.3 Diagnosis

In old series, the definition of glucagonoma included patients with PanNET positive for glucagon immunohistochemistry on pathologic specimen, without specific symptoms. Among the 407 cases reported by Soga et al., only 233 (57.2 %) had the typical glucagonoma diabetico-dermatogenic syndrome with a PanNET, but 284/300 (94.7 %) had glucagonemia, and 227/236 (96.2 %) had a positive immunohistochemistry for glucagon [9]. Currently, functioning NETs are tumors with specific clinical symptoms due to the raised hormone; in case of plasmatic secretion and/or positive immunohistochemistry without specific symptoms, they are not defined as functioning. According to the WHO classification of digestive NET, glucagonomas should be differentiated from nonfunctioning pancreatic alpha-cell

A. Couvelard (✉)
Pathology Department, Bichat Hospital, University Paris Diderot, 46 rue Henri Huchard,
Paris 75018, France
e-mail: anne.couvelard@bch.aphp.fr

O. Hentic
Gastroenterology and Pancreatology Department, Beaujon Hospital, University Paris Diderot,
100 Boulevard Leclerc, Clichy 92110, France
e-mail: olivia.hentic@bjn.aphp.fr

S. La Rosa, F. Sessa (eds.), *Pancreatic Neuroendocrine Neoplasms: Practical Approach to Diagnosis,
Classification, and Therapy*, DOI 10.1007/978-3-319-17235-4_9,
© Springer International Publishing Switzerland 2015

glucagon-positive tumors; indeed, part of the patients with nonfunctioning NET can present glucagon-secreting tumors without symptoms [10]. The discrepancies between glucagon secretion and the glucagon clinical syndrome probably resulted in overdiagnosis of glucagonomas in retrospective studies.

The diagnosis of glucagonoma is clinical with a typical triad: necrolytic migratory erythema, worsening or onset of diabetes mellitus, and weight loss. It should be confirmed biologically with plasmatic dosage of glucagon.

Cutaneous manifestations represent a substantial portion of diseases. Necrolytic migratory erythema is an initial feature in approximately 70 % of the patients [9, 11–13]. This is a superficial epidermal necrosis mainly located at interdigital areas, perioral skin, back of legs, heels, perineum, lower abdomen, buttocks, thighs, and distal extremities. The eruption is characterized by spontaneous remissions or relapses without predisposing factors. It evolves in 1–4 weeks with erythematous macula, vesicles, eroded surface, and then crusts. This rash can be painful, itchy, and often superinfected. Central healing occurs which gives an aspect of arcuate, polycyclic serpiginous lesions with brown pigmented scars. Cutaneous lesions of different age are very common. It may be accompanied by alopecia, pubic and axillary hair removal, nail dystrophy, conjunctivitis, cheilitis, glossitis, or stomatitis (Fig. 9.1a, b).

The typical feature in skin biopsy is necrolysis of the upper epidermis with vacuolated keratinocytes (Fig. 9.1c). Psoriasiform epidermal hyperplasia, hypogranulosis, and thickened stratum corneum with parakeratosis as well as perivascular lymphohistiocytic infiltrate in the superficial dermis are characteristic histopathologic features [11, 14]. Similar lesions of the skin can occur in pseudoglucagonomas without pancreatic tumor, usually due to generalized malabsorption syndrome or specific nutritional deficiencies (i.e., zinc and essential fatty acids). Same aspects on skin biopsy can be found in other deficiency dermatoses, such as pellagra or acrodermatitis enteropathica [15]. Necrolytic

migratory erythema may be misinterpreted as other dermatoses (pemphigoid, mucocutaneous candidiasis, psoriasis, eczema, seborrheic or contact dermatitis) [15]. Due to nonspecific aspects of the cutaneous lesions and the rarity of this kind of tumor, skin involvement precedes the diagnosis of glucagonoma of 6–8 years on average [13].

Worsening or onset of diabetes mellitus is frequent (70–87 %) due to the plasmatic secretion of glucagon [9, 13]. It can be a glucose intolerance or a diabetes necessitating oral antidiabetics or insulin and can be cured with glucagon normalization. Weight loss is usually significant, higher than 20 kg and very evocative of the disease because, in general, it is not present in case of well-differentiated, slow-growing NET. It is secondary to the hypercatabolism of glucagon and is not a prognostic factor [13]. Venous thromboembolisms occur sometimes (25 %), and few cases of dilated heart disease with improvement of the cardiac function with the decrease of the plasmatic glucagon are described [16]. Diarrhea can be present (14 %) without malabsorption but conversely with villous hypertrophy. Finally, psychiatric disorders or deficiency encephalopathies have been observed [13].

Biologically, except diabetes, normochromic and normocytic anemia is characteristic and is related to the severity of the glucagonoma syndrome [9, 17]. Hypoaminoacidemia can occur in 40 % of the glucagonoma syndrome with frequent hypoalbuminemia [9, 13].

When the clinical diagnosis of glucagonoma syndrome is suggested, it should be confirmed by the dosage of the plasma glucagon. The excessive secretion is usually obvious [9, 13]. In basal conditions, plasma glucagon is continuously increased (N, 150 pg/ml), very often greater than 1,000 pg/ml. Hyperglucagonemia less than 500 pg/ml can be observed in other pathological conditions: diabetes mellitus (except those following pancreatectomy or pancreatitis), insufficiency of glucagon catabolism (renal failure, severe liver disease), serious diseases with hypercatabolism (infections, stress, burns), and

Fig. 9.1 Cutaneous manifestations of necrolytic migratory erythema. Glossitis (**a**) may be associated with the cutaneous lesions (**b**). The lesions are erythematous and polycyclic. The skin biopsy (**c**) shows a parakeratotic psoriasiform epidermis with superficial cleft, necrolysis in the upper epidermis, vacuolated keratinocytes, and mild perivascular lymphocytic infiltration

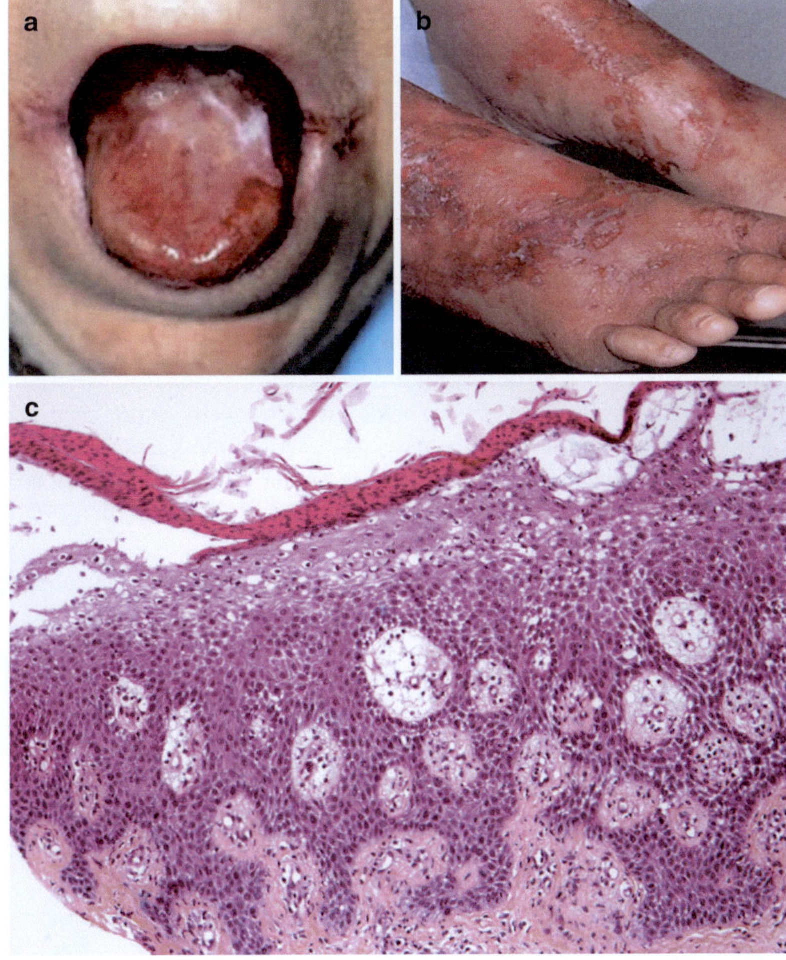

hyperglucagonemia family. However, usually, differential diagnoses in these conditions are not a problem [13, 17].

After the biological confirmation of the glucagonoma syndrome, morphological exams have to be done to localize the primary tumor, always located in the pancreas [8, 9], more often (53 %) in the tail [7, 9]. At diagnosis, the primary is usually large, greater than 3 cm in 60 % of cases and greater than 10 cm in 20 % of cases according to Guillausseau [5]. The disease is often malignant at diagnosis, mostly (80 %) with liver metastases [7–9]. For these reasons, CT scan with arterial and venous phases (Fig. 9.2a) or MRI (Fig. 9.2b) has a good diagnostic accuracy and shows a hyper-

vascularized tumor without necessity of EUS as in smaller tumor (insulinoma or gastrinoma). Due to the presence of somatostatin receptors, somatostatin receptor scintigraphy is usually positive and can be helpful for the confirmation of the neuroendocrine origin and the staging (Fig. 9.2c, d).

9.4 Morphology

9.4.1 Macroscopy

Glucagonomas are pancreatic, usually single large tumors. Their diameter is mainly comprised between 3 and 7 cm, but they vary in size from 2 to 25 cm. They frequently occur in the tail of the pancreas [18]. Like most other PanNETs, they are well demarcated from the adjacent pancreas, but in some cases, they can infiltrate the parenchyma (Fig. 9.3a, b). They can be cystic [19].

9.4.2 Histology

The histological features of glucagonomas are quite the same as those of other well-differentiated PanNETs (Fig. 9.4a). They show a predominance of a mixed trabecular-solid patterns [10]. No poorly differentiated functioning glucagonoma has been described.

9.4.3 Immunohistochemistry

As other PanNETs, glucagonomas express both synaptophysin (Fig. 9.4b) and chromogranin. They stain for glucagon (Fig. 9.4c). PP-positive cells can also be frequently identified in glucagonomas. Glucagonomas can also produce peptides derived from proglucagon (glycentin, glucagon-like peptides 1 and 2) [10].

PanNET can produce more than one type of hormone, including glucagon, especially in the context of MEN1 disease [20, 21]. Presence of cells expressing glucagon can be observed in non-glucagonoma PanNETs. In MEN1, the most frequent tumors are mainly glucagon positive, followed by PP, insulin, and somatostatin.

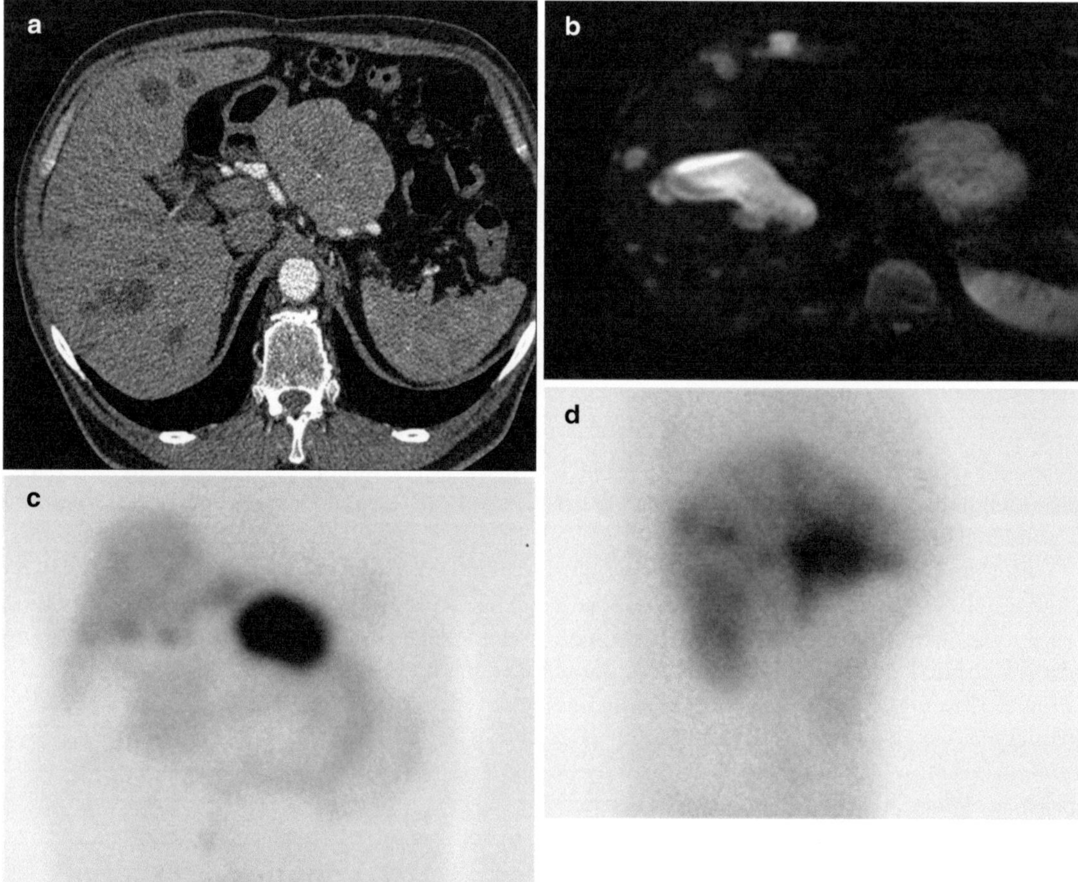

Fig. 9.2 Imaging of a pancreatic glucagonoma with liver metastasis. CT scan (**a**) shows a large tumor on the left of the pancreas without enhancement on the arterial phase and hypodense bilobar liver metastases. MRI (**b**) shows same lesions with very hyperintense liver metastases on T2 phase due to their cystic appearance which can explain a slight uptake on the Octreoscan ® of the liver in contrast to the important uptake of the pancreatic primary (**c, d**)

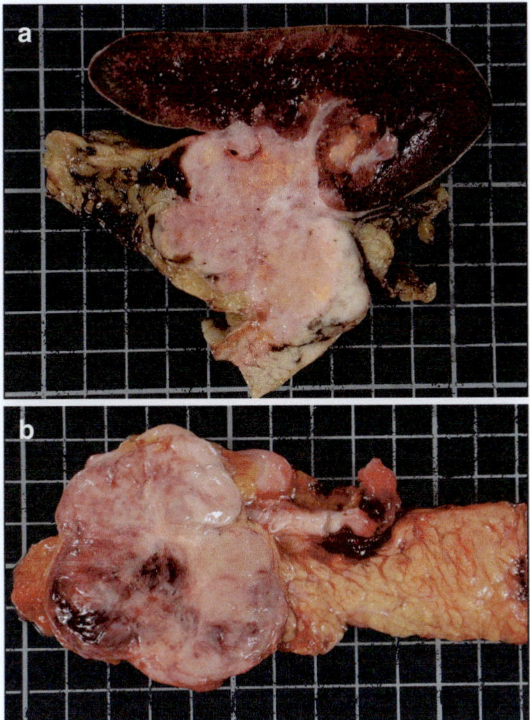

Fig. 9.3 Macroscopic appearance of glucagonomas. Two large, 6 cm-diameter glucagonomas of the caudal pancreas in two different patients, infiltrating the pancreas, peripancreatic adipose tissue, and spleen (**a**) or better limited (**b**). These tumors contain small areas of necrosis and hemorrhage

However, glucagon-positive NETs in the context of MEN1 are usually nonfunctioning [20]. The glucagonoma syndrome may be associated with or followed by another syndrome (insulinoma, VIPoma syndromes, etc.). A secretion of parathyroid hormone-related peptide (PTHrP) was described in a patient presenting a large pancreatic glucagonoma with hypercalcemia [22].

9.4.4 Grading and Predictive Factors

There are few data on grading in the literature (Fig. 9.4d). The retrospective series from Wermers et al. describing 21 cases in 1996 and from Vauleon in 2004 do not give any data on

proliferation [12, 18]. In Eldor's study, the Ki67 was available in only 2/6 cases, evaluated at 2 % and 4 % [23].

9.4.5 Spreading and Metastases

Glucagonomas spread by local invasion into the pancreas and the surrounding tissue. They metastasize frequently, as other PanNETs, into lymph nodes and liver. Patients with glucagonomas characteristically have advanced metastatic disease at the time of diagnosis [18]. In a recent study presenting a series of six patients diagnosed with glucagonoma, the authors found 6/6 metastatic patients; four patients presented with hepatic metastasis upon diagnosis, and in the two remaining patients, metastasis developed after 4 and 6 years from the time of diagnosis [23]. In a report of 21 glucagonomas, all patients had a metastatic disease at presentation, and metastatic disease was noted in the liver ($n=20$), lymph nodes ($n=10$), bone ($n=4$), kidney ($n=2$), mesentery ($n=1$), and adrenal gland ($n=1$) [12]. In another report of 23 glucagonoma, 78 % had metastatic disease to the liver at diagnosis [24]. Other sites of metastasis have been described, such as the ovary [25].

9.4.6 Glucagon Cell Adenomatosis

The glucagon cell adenomatosis (GCA) is a recently described neoplastic disease, also called Mahvash disease [26–28], not related to VHL or MEN1 diseases. It is characterized by multiple microadenomas and NETs composed of glucagon cells. The presence of microadenomas is preceded by glucagon cell hyperplasia of the islets. Clinically, the patients have elevated serum glucagon levels but usually do not present any glucagonoma syndrome. However, in a recent case, the GCA was functional, and the patient presented a necrotizing migratory erythema [29]. For further morphological and molecular features, see Chap. 19.

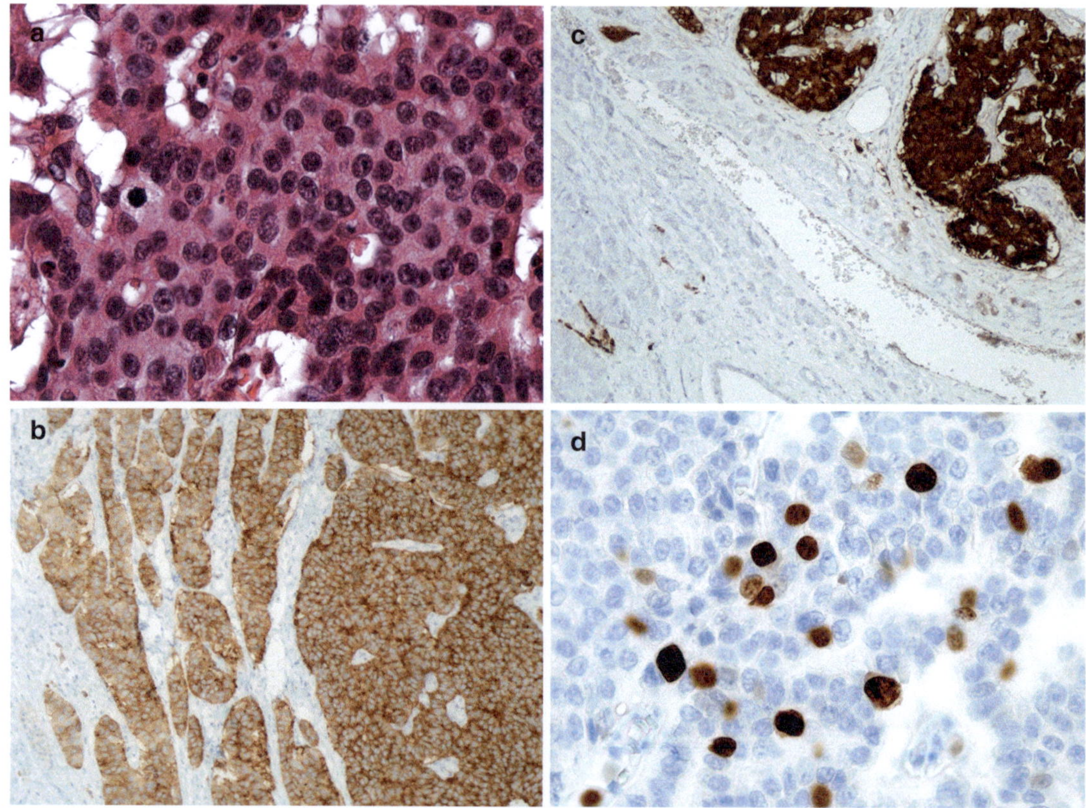

Fig. 9.4 Histologic appearance of glucagonomas. This glucagonoma is a well-differentiated neuroendocrine tumor, grade 2. Some mitoses are present. Tumor cells are regular, and anisonucleosis is mild (**a**; H&E staining × 40). Tumor cells diffusely express synaptophysin (**b**; immunohistochemistry × 20). Tumor cells (*top right*) strongly express glucagon; some cells are detected in adjacent islets in the surrounding parenchyma (**c**; immunohistochemistry × 20). Ki67 is expressed by 8 % of tumor cells in this grade 2 tumor according to WHO 2010 classification (**d**; immunohistochemistry; ×40)

9.4.7 Prognosis

As for other PanNETs, the prognosis depends on several factors such as differentiation, grade, and TNM classification [10]. Usually, glucagonomas are large pancreatic tumors with metastatic spread. In the SEER analysis of 1,310 PanNETs, the prognosis of glucagonomas does not differ from all the other PanNETs if accorded to the staging.

The median overall survival for all stages was 38 months and 124 months, 70 months and 23 months if tumor was localized, with regional or with distant metastases, respectively [7]. In a series of 425 PanNETs analyzed to confirm the validity of the AJCC TNM classification for the assessment of the prognosis, overall survival did not significantly differ between functioning (excluding insulinomas) and nonfunctioning tumors [30–32].

References

1. Becker SW, Kahn D, Rothman S (1942) Cutaneous manifestations of internal malignant tumours. Arch Derm Syphilol 45:1069–1080
2. McGavran MH, Unger RH, Recant L (1966) A glucagon-secreting alpha-cell carcinoma of the pancreas. N Engl J Med 274:1408–1413
3. Wilkinson DS (1973) Necrolytic migratory erythema with carcinoma of the pancreas. Trans St Johns Hosp Dermatol Soc 59:244–250
4. Mallison CN, Bloom SR, Warin AP et al (1974) A glucagonoma syndrome. Lancet 2:1–5
5. Guillausseau PJ, Guillausseau C, Villet R et al (1982) Glucagonomas. Clinical, biological, anatomopathological and therapeutic aspects (general review of 130 cases). Gastroenterol Clin Biol 6:1029–1041
6. Lombard-Bohas C, Mitry E, O'Toole D et al (2009) Thirteen-month registration of patients with gastroenteropancreatic endocrine tumours in France. Neuroendocrinology 89:217–222

7. Yao JC, Eisner MP, Leary C et al (2007) Population-based study of islet cell carcinoma. Ann Surg Oncol 14:3492–3500

8. Jensen RT, Cadiot G, Brandi ML et al (2012) ENETS consensus guidelines for the management of patients with digestive neuroendocrine neoplasms: functional pancreatic endocrine tumor syndromes. Neuroendocrinology 95:98–119

9. Soga J, Yakuwa Y (1998) Glucagonomas/diabetico-dermatogenic syndrome (DDS): a statistical evaluation of 407 reported cases. J Hepatobiliary Pancreat Surg 5:312–319

10. Klimstra DS, Arnold R, Capella C et al (2010) Neuro-endocrine neoplasms of the pancreas. In: Bosman FT, Carneiro F, Hruban RH, Theise ND (eds) WHO classification of tumours of the digestive system. IARC Press, Lyon, pp 322–326

11. Stavropoulos PG, Papafragkaki DK, Avgerinou G et al (2013) Necrolytic migratory erythema: a common cutaneous clue of uncommon syndromes. Cutis 92:1–4

12. Wermers RA, Fatourechi V, Wynne AG et al (1996) The glucagonoma syndrome. Clinical and pathologic features in 21 patients. Medicine (Baltimore) 2:53–63

13. Cadiot G, Mignon M (2005) Différents types de tumeurs endocrines fonctionnelles. In: Lévy P, Ruzsniewski P, Sauvanet A (eds) Traité de pancréatologie clinique. Médecine Sciences Flammarion, Paris, pp 317–320

14. Compton NL, Chien AJ (2013) A rare but revealing sign: necrolytic migratory erythema. Am J Med 126:387–3899

15. Lobo I, Carvalho A, Amaral C et al (2010) Glucagonoma syndrome and necrolytic migratory erythema. Int J Dermatol 49:24–29

16. De mestier L, Hammel P, Hentic O et al (2010) Dramatic efficacy of chemotherapy with 5-fluorouracil and dacarbazine in a patient with metastatic glucagonoma and cardiac insufficiency. Gastroenterol Clin Biol 34:106–110

17. Bloom SR, Polak JM (1987) Glucagonoma syndrome. Am J Med 82:25–36

18. Vauleon E, Egreteau J, Boucher E et al (2004) Glucagonoma: a recent series of 7 cases. Bull Cancer 91:637–640

19. Brown K, Kristopaitis T, Yong S et al (1998) Cystic glucagonoma: a rare variant of an uncommon neuro-endocrine pancreas tumor. J Gastrointest Surg 2:533–536

20. Anlauf M, Perren A, Klöppel G (2007) Endocrine precursor lesions and microadenomas of the duodenum and pancreas with and without MEN1: criteria, molecular concepts and clinical significance. Pathobiology 74:279–284

21. Varsavsky M, Reyes-García R, Alonso García G et al (2012) An unusual association of neuroendocrine tumors in MEN 1A. Pituitary 15:393–397

22. Shirai K, Inoue I, Kato J et al (2011) A case of a giant glucagonoma with parathyroid hormone-related peptide secretion showing an inconsistent postsurgical endocrine status. Intern Med 50:1689–1694

23. Eldor R, Glaser B, Fraenkel M et al (2011) Glucagonoma and the glucagonoma syndrome – cumulative experience with an elusive endocrine tumour. Clin Endocrinol (Oxf) 74:593–598

24. Kindmark H, Sundin A, Granberg D et al (2007) Endocrine pancreatic tumors with glucagon hypersecretion: a retrospective study of 23 cases during 20 years. Med Oncol 24:330–337

25. Watt DG, Pandanaboyana S, Herrington CS et al (2013) Pancreatic glucagonoma metastasising to the right ovary five years after initial surgery: a case report. JOP 14:510–514

26. Henopp T, Anlauf M, Schmitt A et al (2009) Glucagon cell adenomatosis: a newly recognized disease of the endocrine pancreas. J Clin Endocrinol Metab 94:213–217

27. Klöppel G, Anlauf M, Perren A et al (2014) Hyperplasia to neoplasia sequence of duodenal and pancreatic neuroendocrine diseases and pseudohyperplasia of the PP-cells in the pancreas. Endocr Pathol 25:181–185

28. Zhou C, Dhall D, Nissen NN et al (2009) Homozygous P86S mutation of the human glucagon receptor is associated with hyperglucagonemia, alpha cell hyperplasia, and islet cell tumor. Pancreas 38:941–946

29. Otto AI et al (2011) Glucagon cell adenomatosis: a new entity associated with necrolytic migratory erythema and glucagonoma syndrome. J Am Acad Dermatol 65:458–459

30. Strosberg JR, Cheema A, Weber J et al (2011) Prognostic validity of a novel American Joint Committee on cancer staging classification for pancreatic neuroendocrine tumors. J Clin Oncol 29:3044–3049

31. Sobin LH, Gospodarowicz MK, Wittekind C (eds) (2009) TNM classification of malignant tumours. Wiley & Blackwell, Chichester

32. Rindi G, Falconi M, Klersy C et al (2012) TNM staging of neoplasms of the endocrine pancreas: results from a large international cohort study. J Natl Cancer Inst 104:764–777

Paul Komminoth

Somatostatin-producing neuroendocrine tumors are neoplasms with evidence of D-cell differentiation, while the so-called somatostatinomas additionally show clinical symptoms associated with chronic inappropriate secretion of somatostatin (somatostatinoma syndrome). Pancreatic neuroendocrine tumors and extrapancreatic tumors such as those of the duodenum, lung, thyroid, ovaries, kidney, and paraganglia [1–7] composed either exclusively or predominantly of somatostatin immunoreactive cells but, without a proven somatostatinoma syndrome, should not be called "somatostatinomas" but designated as somatostatin-producing neuroendocrine tumors (or D-cell tumors) [8].

10.1 Historical Background

Somatostatin is a secretory inhibitory decapeptide, which was first isolated and characterized from the hypothalamus in 1973 [9]. Since then, it has been found also in cells of the gastrointestinal tract as well as the endocrine pancreas and could be localized to D cells [10–12].

In 1977, two tumors of the pancreas mainly containing somatostatin were described independently by two groups [13, 14]. Ganda et al. reported a 46-year-old woman with a long-standing diabetes mellitus and a pancreatic mass, which became apparent during cholecystectomy for cholelithiasis. The tumor ultrastructurally exhibited a distinctive endocrine morphology, resembling D cells and contained a large quantity of immunoreactive somatostatin. After complete resection of the tumor, the patient became normoglycemic [14].

The second case described by Larsson et al. was a 55-year-old woman with diarrhea and steatorrhea, abdominal pain, hypochlorhydria, and diabetic glucose tolerance. During cholecystectomy, a tumor located in the head of the pancreas with liver metastases was detected. Examination of biopsy specimens showed a neuroendocrine tumor with cells indistinguishable from islet D cells. Radioimmunoassay of blood samples obtained by tumor vein catheterization revealed very high levels of somatostatin [13].

Based on these findings together with the known pharmaceutical effects of somatostatin, a description of the somatostatin syndrome was published by Unger in 1977 [15]. The full biochemical, morphologic, and clinical syndrome was characterized by Krejs et al. in 1979 [16].

According to the WHO definition, the somatostatinoma syndrome includes (1) markedly elevated somatostatin levels in the plasma

P. Komminoth
Institute of Pathology, City Hospital Triemli,
Birmensdorferstrasse 497, CH-8063 Zürich,
Switzerland
e-mail: paul.komminoth@triemli.zuerich.ch,
http://www.triemli.ch/pathologie

S. La Rosa, F. Sessa (eds.), *Pancreatic Neuroendocrine Neoplasms: Practical Approach to Diagnosis,
Classification, and Therapy*, DOI 10.1007/978-3-319-17235-4_10,
© Springer International Publishing Switzerland 2015

and/or tumor, (2) diabetes of recent onset, (3) hypo- or achlorhydria, (4) gallbladder disease (cholelithiasis, suppression of gallbladder motility), (5) diarrhea and steatorrhea, and (6) anemia and weight loss [8].

All these symptoms are attributed to the effects of somatostatin, which is secreted by the tumor in excess, leading to hypersomatostatinemia. Since somatostatin physiologically exhibits mostly inhibitory effects on various neuroendocrine and non-neuroendocrine secretory cells, it is thought that hypersomatostatinemia leads to inhibition of insulin release resulting in diabetes mellitus, inhibition of cholecystokinin causing reduced gallbladder contractility and cholelithiasis, and inhibition of pancreatic enzyme, bicarbonate secretion, and intestinal absorption of lipids resulting in diarrhea and steatorrhea. Furthermore, decreased gastrin secretion due to its inhibition by somatostatin is the possible reason for gastric hypo- or achlorhydria.

It has been estimated that only about 10 % of reported patients with somatostatin-producing tumors presented with the syndrome at the time of diagnosis [17]. While this has been attributed by some to the level and molecular form of the secreted somatostatin and/or other hormones released by the tumors [18], others have questioned the existence of such a syndrome [19] on the ground that these features are nonspecific and very common in the older age group in which these tumors usually arise. Thus, in the overview by Tanaka et al. in 2000 [20] and the report by House et al. in 2002 [21], none of the patients exhibited any symptom of the somatostatinoma syndrome. In the series of Pipelees et al., three of five patients exhibited an incomplete somatostatinoma syndrome [22]. Furthermore, in a recently published series of 541 pancreatic neuroendocrine tumors of different centers, 21 (4 %) tumors expressed somatostatin predominantly or exclusively [23]. None of the 17 patients for whom appropriate clinical data were available met the criteria for the somatostatinoma syndrome according to their records. They presented with nonspecific symptoms such as abdominal pain, or the tumors were detected incidentally. Three patients exhibited cholelithiasis and one patient showed weight loss and another diarrhea [23],

but the full syndrome with at least three of six WHO criteria fulfilled could not be found.

While this failure to identify the somatostatinoma syndrome may be due to the retrospective nature of the study, it might also be explained by the very short biological half-life of somatostatin [24] and marked differences in the circulating levels of biologically active somatostatin [23]. From all these findings, it is reasonable to conclude that a somatostatinoma syndrome is possible but only in patients with large tumors and advanced tumor stages in which the neoplasm secretes enough somatostatin to induce the abovementioned symptoms.

Furthermore, it is likely that many of the published cases and series of so-called somatostatinomas were in fact neuroendocrine tumors expressing somatostatin by immunohistochemistry or biochemical assays (somatostatin-producing tumors) but with no proven somatostatinoma syndrome fulfilling all the criteria mentioned in the WHO book [18].

10.2 Epidemiology

Somatostatin-producing tumors of the pancreas are rare [25–39], and true functioning pancreatic somatostatinomas causing the somatostatinoma syndrome are even rarer. Thus, the knowledge about these neoplasms is based on single or small series of patients and reviews [7, 28, 39, 40]. The incidence is considered 1 in 40 million population [41, 42], and it is estimated that somatostatinomas encompass less than 1 % of functioning pancreatic neuroendocrine tumors [8, 43].

Pancreatic somatostatinomas occur more frequently in females and arise in middle-aged to older patients [7, 39, 43] with an average age at diagnosis of 55 years (30–74) [43]. In the recently published series of Garbrecht et al., the mean age of patients was 53 years (17–79 years) and the female to male ratio 1.3:1 [23].

A minority of patients with somatostatin-expressing pancreatic neuroendocrine tumors exhibit a MEN1 syndrome [7, 23]. A few patients with the von Hippel-Lindau disease (VHL) [32] or neurofibromatosis type 1 (NF1) [44] have been described.

10.3 Morphology

Most of the reported somatostatinomas occurred in the head of the pancreas followed by the tail [23, 39, 43], but they may arise anywhere in the gland [28, 39]. The tumors are usually single, well circumscribed (but not encapsulated), soft, gray white to yellow tan in color, and large in size (average diameter 5–6 cm) [7, 43]. In the series of Garbrecht et al., the mean size of tumors was 4.25 cm [23].

The majority (approx. two-third) of pancreatic somatostatinomas are reported to be malignant as evidenced by metastases or invasive growth. Metastases are most frequently seen in lymph nodes and the liver and are present in 35 and 69 % of patients, respectively, at the time of diagnosis [28]. In the reported series of Garbrecht et al., 41 % of patients presented with metastases [23].

The majority of reported somatostatinomas of the pancreas are histologically well- or moderately differentiated neoplasms and rarely poorly differentiated [23]. Tumor cells generally exhibit mild atypia and few mitoses. Extensive necrosis is usually absent, but perineural invasion and angio-invasion are often found [43]. Amyloid deposits are rare and, unlike those of insulinomas, do not react with anti-amylin antibodies [29].

In contrast to duodenal somatostatin-producing neuroendocrine neoplasms, which frequently exhibit a pseudoglandular pattern and typical psammomatous calcifications [45, 46], pancreatic somatostatinomas exhibit no distinct morphology. Most show the usual histological features observed in all pancreatic neuroendocrine neoplasms such as solid, acinar, or trabecular growth patterns [43]. As reported by Garbrecht et al., most tumors reveal a trabecular pattern (Fig. 10.1), and in 22 %, an additional

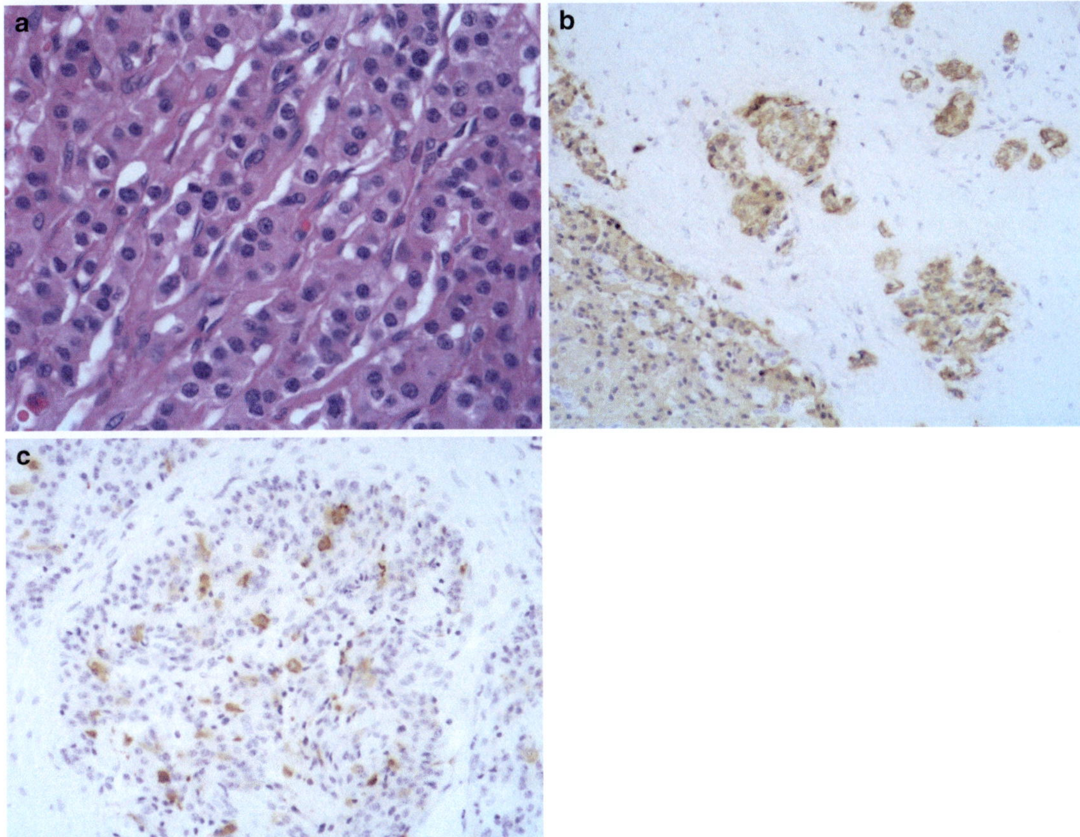

Fig. 10.1 Functioning somatostatinoma characterized by a trabecular architecture (**a**) and showing somatostatin (**b**) and calcitonin (**c**) immunoreactivity (H original magnification ×400; immunohistochemistry original magnification ×200)

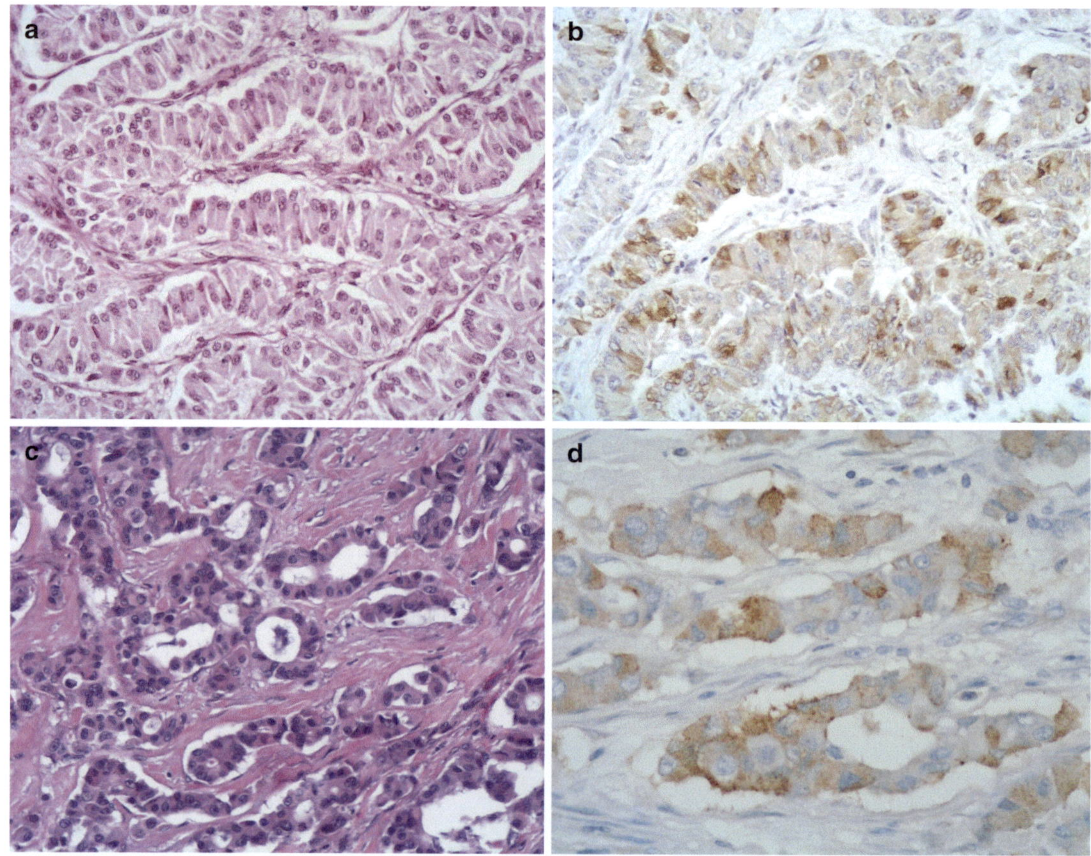

Fig. 10.2 Nonfunctioning somatostatin-producing pancreatic neuroendocrine tumor with a trabecular structure (**a**) (H&E, original magnification ×400) and showing somatostatin immunoreactivity (**b**) (immunohistochemistry original magnification; ×400). (**c**) Example of a nonfunctioning somatostatin-producing pancreatic neuroendocrine tumor positive for somatostatin (**d**) showing an acinar structure resembling that of duodenal somatostatin-producing neuroendocrine tumors (H&E and immunohistochemistry; original magnification ×400)

pseudoglandular component (Fig. 10.2) may be encountered. Few tumors may also have a paraganglioma-like appearance [23]. Psammomatous calcifications – similar to those seen in duodenal tumors – may also be found in a subset of pancreatic tumors and have been reported in 37 % of the cases described by Garbrecht et al. [23]. In that series, they were found in sporadic and in MEN1-associated tumors and in gangliocytic paragangliomas but not in poorly differentiated somatostatin-producing neuroendocrine neoplasms [23].

By special stains, tumor cells are uniformly non-argentaffin and show argyrophilia only with the Hellerstrom-Hellman technique which is selective for somatostatin-producing cells [8].

Immunohistochemically, tumor cells are strongly positive for synaptophysin and with varying degree of immunoreactivity for somatostatin [43] (Figs. 10.1 and 10.2). Immunolabeling for chromogranin A, however, may be negative [23]. More than half of the tumors additionally exhibit scattered cells with immunoreactivity for other peptides such as pancreatic polypeptide (PP), insulin, glucagon, gastrin, adrenocorticotropin, and calcitonin [23, 43, 47]. As in other types of pancreatic neuroendocrine tumors, the transcription factor islet 1 gene product (ISL1) is also expressed in somatostatin-producing tumors [48]. In the series of Garbrecht et al., tumors with a gangliocytic appearance typically showed

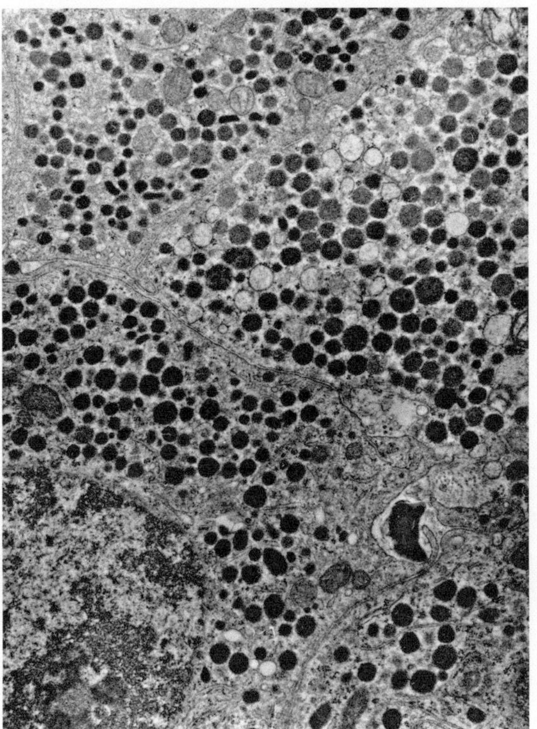

Fig. 10.3 Ultrastructural features of the functioning somatostatinoma showed in Fig. 10.1 containing numerous large, round, and moderately electron-dense membrane-bound secretory granules (original magnification ×10,000)

immunohistochemical positivity for somatostatin, VIP, and PP [23].

By electron microscopy, tumor cells contain two distinct populations of intracytoplasmic membrane-bound neurosecretory granules (Fig. 10.3). The majority of the secretory granules are large (range of diameter 250–450 nm), round, and moderately electron dense, resembling those of normal D cells. The second subset consists of smaller granules (range of diameter 150–300 nm), with dense cores surrounded by a thin peripheral halo [43].

Because of the rarity of these tumors, there are only very few molecular data on somatostatinomas available in the literature. Recently, somatic and germline mutations in the HIF2A gene of patients with pheochromocytomas/paragangliomas associated with polycythemia, and in some of them also with somatostatinomas were described [49].

10.4 Clinical Diagnosis

The clinical features of the somatostatinoma syndrome include the classical triad of diabetes mellitus, gallstones, and steatorrhea [13, 25, 50]. Additional symptoms consist of hypochlorhydria, weight loss, and anemia [13, 16, 19, 22, 51].

The diagnosis of a "somatostatinoma" is confirmed by documentation of elevated plasma concentrations of somatostatin and the presence of the abovementioned somatostatinoma syndrome.

The normal plasma level of somatostatin is less than 100 pg/ml. Patients with a functioning somatostatinoma usually have very high levels of somatostatin. A mean of 15.5 ng/ml (range, 0.16–107 ng/ml) has been reported [52]. Mild elevations of somatostatin, however, may also occur in other endocrine disorders. The value of provocation tests, such as with tolbutamide, calcium, secretin, etc., has been debated but can be useful in some cases [53].

Tumor localization is usually accomplished by computed tomography (CT) or magnetic resonance imaging (MRI). Endoscopic ultrasound (EUS) is a very sensitive method which may be combined with endoscopic ultrasound-guided fine-needle aspiration (EUS-FNA) allowing preoperative diagnosis [54]. Somatostatin receptor scintigraphy (SRS) using radiolabeled octreotide may also be useful in somatostatin-producing tumors [55] and may be helpful to identify clinically unsuspected extra-abdominal metastases. FDG-PET imaging has also been reported to be useful in detecting somatostatin-producing tumors, although its place in the diagnostic evaluation is uncertain [56].

10.5 Prognosis

The largest experience with these uncommon endocrine tumors estimates a 75.2 % 5-year overall survival, with 59.9 % of the patients with metastases and 100 % of the patients without metastases [7].

Acknowledgments I thank Prof. S. La Rosa for providing the histological and EM pictures.

References

1. Chamberlain RS, Blumgart LH (1999) Carcinoid tumors of the extrahepatic bile duct. A rare cause of malignant biliary obstruction. Cancer 86(10): 1959–1965
2. Gregersen G, Holst JJ, Trankjaer A, Stadil F, Mogensen AM (2002) Case report: somatostatin producing teratoma, causing rapidly alternating extreme hyperglycemia and hypoglycemia, and ovarian somatostatinoma. Metabolism 51(9):1180–1183
3. Hamid QA, Bishop AE, Rode J, Dhillon AP, Rosenberg BF, Reed RJ, Sibley RK, Polak JM (1986) Duodenal gangliocytic paragangliomas: a study of 10 cases with immunocytochemical neuroendocrine markers. Hum Pathol 17(11):1151–1157
4. Tomic S, Warner T (1996) Pancreatic somatostatin-secreting gangliocytic paraganglioma with lymph node metastases. Am J Gastroenterol 91(3): 607–608
5. Ghose RR, Gupta SK (1981) Oat cell carcinoma of bronchus presenting with somatostatinoma syndrome. Thorax 36(7):550–551
6. Walsh IK, Kernohan RM, Johnston CF, Keane PF (1996) Somatostatinoma in a horseshoe kidney. Br J Urol 78(6):958–959
7. Soga J, Yakuwa Y (1999) Somatostatinoma/inhibitory syndrome: a statistical evaluation of 173 reported cases as compared to other pancreatic endocrinomas. J Exp Clin Cancer Res 18(1):13–22
8. Dayal Y, Oberg K, Perren A, Komminoth P (2004) Somatostatinoma. In: DeLellis RA, Lloyd RV, Heitz PU, Eng C (eds) World Health Organization classification of tumors. Pathology and genetics of tumors of endocrine organs. IARC Press, Lyon, pp 189–190
9. Brazeau P, Vale W, Burgus R, Ling N, Butcher M, Rivier J, Guillemin R (1973) Hypothalamic polypeptide that inhibits the secretion of immunoreactive pituitary growth hormone. Science 179(4068):77–79
10. Luft R, Efendic S, Hokfelt T, Johansson O, Arimura A (1974) Immunohistochemical evidence for the localization of somatostatin–like immunoreactivity in a cell population of the pancreatic islets. Med Biol 52(6):428–430
11. Arimura A, Sato H, Dupont A, Nishi N, Schally AV (1975) Somatostatin: abundance of immunoreactive hormone in rat stomach and pancreas. Science 189(4207):1007–1009
12. Polak JM, Pearse AG, Grimelius L, Bloom SR (1975) Growth-hormone release-inhibiting hormone in gastrointestinal and pancreatic D cells. Lancet 1(7918):1220–1222
13. Larsson LI, Hirsch MA, Holst JJ, Ingemansson S, Kuhl C, Jensen SL, Lundqvist G, Rehfeld JF, Schwartz TW (1977) Pancreatic somatostatinoma. Clinical features and physiological implications. Lancet 1(8013):666–668
14. Ganda OP, Weir GC, Soeldner JS, Legg MA, Chick WL, Patel YC, Ebeid AM, Gabbay KH, Reichlin S (1977) "Somatostatinoma": a somatostatin-containing tumor of the endocrine pancreas. N Engl J Med 296(17):963–967
15. Unger RH (1977) Somatostatinoma. N Engl J Med 296(17):998–1000
16. Krejs GJ, Orci L, Conlon JM, Ravazzola M, Davis GR, Raskin P, Collins SM, McCarthy DM, Baetens D, Rubenstein A, Aldor TA, Unger RH (1979) Somatostatinoma syndrome. Biochemical, morphologic and clinical features. N Engl J Med 301(6):285–292
17. Jensen RT, Norton JA (1995) Endocrine neoplasms of the pancreas. In: Yamada T (ed) Textbook of gastroenterology. Lippincott, Philadelphia, p 2131
18. Dayal Y, Ganda OP (1991) Somatostatin-producing tumors. In: Dayal Y (ed) Endocrine pathology of the gut and pancreas. CRC Press, Boca Raton, p 241
19. Stacpoole PW, Kasselberg AG, Berelowitz M, Chey WY (1983) Somatostatinoma syndrome: does a clinical entity exist? Acta Endocrinol (Copenh) 102(1):80–87
20. Tanaka S, Yamasaki S, Matsushita H, Ozawa Y, Kurosaki A, Takeuchi K, Hoshihara Y, Doi T, Watanabe G, Kawaminami K (2000) Duodenal somatostatinoma: a case report and review of 31 cases with special reference to the relationship between tumor size and metastasis. Pathol Int 50(2):146–152
21. House MG, Yeo CJ, Schulick RD (2002) Periampullary pancreatic somatostatinoma. Ann Surg Oncol 9(9):869–874
22. Pipeleers D, Couturier E, Gepts W, Reynders J, Somers G (1983) Five cases of somatostatinoma: clinical heterogeneity and diagnostic usefulness of basal and tolbutamide-induced hypersomatostatinemia. J Clin Endocrinol Metab 56(6):1236–1242
23. Garbrecht N, Anlauf M, Schmitt A, Henopp T, Sipos B, Raffel A, Eisenberger CF, Knoefel WT, Pavel M, Fottner C, Musholt TJ, Rinke A, Arnold R, Berndt U, Plockinger U, Wiedenmann B, Moch H, Heitz PU, Komminoth P, Perren A, Kloppel G (2008) Somatostatin-producing neuroendocrine tumors of the duodenum and pancreas: incidence, types, biological behavior, association with inherited syndromes, and functional activity. Endocr Relat Cancer 15(1):229–241
24. Pless J (2005) The history of somatostatin analogs. J Endocrinol Invest 28(11 Suppl International):1–4
25. Jackson JA, Raju BU, Fachnie JD, Mellinger RC, Janakiraman N, Lloyd RV, Vinik AI (1987) Malignant somatostatinoma presenting with diabetic ketoacidosis. Clin Endocrinol (Oxf) 26(5):609–621
26. Harris GJ, Tio F, Cruz AB Jr (1987) Somatostatinoma: a case report and review of the literature. J Surg Oncol 36(1):8–16
27. Levi S, Bjarnason I, Swinson CM, Polak JM, Murray W, Levi AJ (1988) Malignant pancreatic somatostatinoma in a patient with dermatitis herpetiformis and coeliac disease. Digestion 39(1):1–6
28. Konomi K, Chijiiwa K, Katsuta T, Yamaguchi K (1990) Pancreatic somatostatinoma: a case report and review of the literature. J Surg Oncol 43(4): 259–265
29. Ohsawa H, Kanatsuka A, Tokuyama Y, Yamaguchi T, Makino H, Yoshida S, Horie H, Mikata A, Kohen Y

(1991) Amyloid protein in somatostatinoma differs from human islet amyloid polypeptide. Acta Endocrinol (Copenh) 124(1):45–53

30. Stavri GT, Pritchard GA, Williams EJ, Stamatakis JD (1992) Somatostatinoma of the pancreas with hypercalcaemia. A case report. Eur J Surg Oncol 18(3):298–300

31. Dominioni L, Dionigi R, Benevento A, Capella C, La Rosa S, Roncari G, Garancini S (1995) Very late recurrence of a somatostatin cell tumor of the head of the pancreas. Pancreas 10(4):417–419

32. Maki M, Kaneko Y, Ohta Y, Nakamura T, Machinami R, Kurokawa K (1995) Somatostatinoma of the pancreas associated with von Hippel-Lindau disease. Intern Med 34(7):661–665

33. Anene C, Thompson JS, Saigh J, Badakhsh S, Ecklund RE (1995) Somatostatinoma: atypical presentation of a rare pancreatic tumor. Am J Gastroenterol 90(5):819–821

34. Barbato A, Roviello F, De Stefano A, Marrelli D, Messano A, Guarnieri A, Pinto E (1996) A case of pancreatic somatostatinoma. Minerva Chir 51(6):475–479

35. Roy J, Pompilio M, Samama G (1996) Pancreatic somatostatinoma and MEN 1. Apropos of a case. Review of the literature. Ann Endocrinol (Paris) 57(1):71–76

36. Roy J, Pompilio M, Yvin JL (1993) Pancreatic somatostatinoma. A new case. Presse Med 22(21):1012

37. Sessa F, Arcidiaco M, Valenti L, Solcia M, Di Maggio E, Solcia E (1997) Metastatic psammomatous somatostatinoma of the pancreas causing severe keto-acidotic diabetes cured by surgery. Endocr Pathol 8(4):327–333

38. Moayedoddin B, Booya F, Wermers RA, Lloyd RV, Rubin J, Thompson GB, Fatourechi V (2006) Spectrum of malignant somatostatin-producing neuroendocrine tumors. Endocr Pract 12(4):394–400

39. Vinik AI, Strodel WE, Eckhauser FE, Moattari AR, Lloyd R (1987) Somatostatinomas, PPomas, neurotensinomas. Semin Oncol 14:263–281

40. Theodoraki A, Khoo B, Hamda A, Grillo F, Meyer T, Bouloux PM (2010) Malignant somatostatinoma presenting with diabetic ketoacidosis and inhibitory syndrome: pathophysiologic considerations. Endocr Pract 16(5):835–837

41. Hammond PJ, Gilbey SG, Wynick D, Bloom SR (1993) Glucagonoma, vipoma, somatostatinoma, other hormones and nonfunctional tumors. In: Mazzaferri EL, Samaan NA (eds) Endocrine tumors. Blackwell Scientific Publications, Boston, pp 457–483

42. Mozell E, Stenzel P, Woltering EA, Rosch J, O'Dorisio TM (1990) Functional endocrine tumors of the pancreas: clinical presentation, diagnosis, and treatment. Curr Probl Surg 27(6):301–386

43. La Rosa S, Furlan D, Sessa F, Capella C (2010) The endocrine pancreas. In: Lloyd RV (ed) Endocrine pathology. Differential diagnosis and molecular advances. Springer, New York, pp 367–413

44. Thannberger P, Wilhelm JM, Derragui A, Saraceni O, Kieffer P (2001) Von Recklinghausen's disease associated with pancreatic somatostatinoma. Presse Med 30(35):1741–1743

45. Taccagni GL, Carlucci M, Sironi M, Cantaboni A, Di Carlo V (1986) Duodenal somatostatinoma with psammoma bodies: an immunohistochemical and ultrastructural study. Am J Gastroenterol 81(1):33–37

46. Dayal Y, Tallberg KA, Nunnemacher G, DeLellis RA, Wolfe HJ (1986) Duodenal carcinoids in patients with and without neurofibromatosis. A comparative study. Am J Surg Pathol 10(5):348–357

47. Sugimoto F, Sekiya T, Saito M, Iiai T, Suda K, Nozawa A, Nakazawa T, Ishizaki T, Ikarashi T (1998) Calcitonin-producing pancreatic somatostatinoma: report of a case. Surg Today 28(12):1279–1282

48. Hermann G, Konukiewitz B, Schmitt A, Perren A, Kloppel G (2011) Hormonally defined pancreatic and duodenal neuroendocrine tumors differ in their transcription factor signatures: expression of ISL1, PDX1, NGN3, and CDX2. Virchows Arch 459(2):147–154

49. Jochmanova I, Zelinka T, Widimsky J Jr, Pacak K (2014) HIF signaling pathway in pheochromocytoma and other neuroendocrine tumors. Physiol Res 63(Suppl 2):S251–S262

50. Willcox PA, Immelman EJ, Barron JL, Klaff LJ, Harries-Jones EP, Hainsworth M, Millar RP (1988) Pancreatic somatostatinoma: presentation with recurrent episodes of severe hyperglycaemia and ketoacidosis. Q J Med 68(255):559–571

51. Galmiche JP, Chayvialle JA, Dubois PM, David L, Descos F, Paulin C, Ducastelle T, Colin R, Geffroy Y (1980) Calcitonin-producing pancreatic somatostatinoma. Gastroenterology 78(6):1577–1583

52. Boden G, Shimoyama R (1985) Somatostatinoma. In: Cohen S, Soloway RD (eds) Hormone-producing tumors of the gastrointestinal tract. Churchill Livingstone, New York, p 85

53. Economopoulos P, Christopoulos C (2001) Somatostatinoma syndrome. Ann Gastroenterol 14:252–260

54. Mori Y, Sato N, Taniguchi R, Tamura T, Minagawa N, Shibao K, Higure A, Nakamoto M, Taguchi M, Yamaguchi K (2014) Pancreatic somatostatinoma diagnosed preoperatively: report of a case. J Periodontol 15(1):66–71

55. Angeletti S, Corleto VD, Schillaci O, Marignani M, Annibale B, Moretti A, Silecchia G, Scopinaro F, Basso N, Bordi C, Delle Fave G (1998) Use of the somatostatin analogue octreotide to localise and manage somatostatin-producing tumours. Gut 42(6):792–794

56. Suzuki H, Kuwano H, Masuda N, Hashimoto S, Kanoh K, Nomoto K, Shimura T, Katoh H (2008) Diagnostic usefulness of FDG-PET for malignant somatostatinoma of the pancreas. Hepatogastroenterology 55(85):1242–1245

VIPoma

Carlo Capella and Stefano La Rosa

11.1 Historical Background

11.1.1 Definition

A VIPoma is a functionally active and commonly malignant neuroendocrine tumor predominantly arising in the pancreas, which produces the WDHA (watery diarrhea, hypokalemia, achlorhydria) syndrome through ectopic secretion of vasoactive intestinal peptide (VIP), peptide histidine methionine (PHM), and other hormone-like substances. The majority of VIPomas are in the pancreas and are represented by epithelial neoplasms. However, VIP-producing neurogenic tumors are occasionally observed in the sympathetic chain and adrenal glands, particularly in children.

11.1.2 Synonyms

VIPomas have also been named "diarrheagenic tumors of the pancreas" or "islet cell tumors of the pancreas with watery diarrhea" [1]. The syndrome associated with VIPomas, firstly known as Verner–Morrison syndrome due to their original description in 1958 [2], has also been denominated pancreatic cholera [3] and WDHA syndrome [4].

11.2 Epidemiology

11.2.1 Incidence

Pancreatic VIPomas are rare neoplasms. The incidence of new cases/10^6 population/year is 0.05–0.2 [5]. Based on a large pathological series, they constitute 6 % of functioning and 1.7 % of all neuroendocrine tumors in the pancreas [6], although they represent 80 % of diarrheagenic neoplasms. About 56 % of pancreatic VIPomas are malignant (with metastases) when first diagnosed [7]. Males are affected less frequently than females with a M/F ratio of 0.9 [7], and the average age of patients is 50.5 years with a range of 15–82 years [7]. On the contrary, neurogenic VIPomas mostly (about two thirds) affect pediatric patients at an average age of 7.3 years with a range of 1–61 years [7]. A family history is usually absent, but an association with the MEN 1 has been reported in some cases of pancreatic VIPomas [8, 9]. Association with von Hippel–Lindau syndrome or neurofibromatosis has not been reported for epithelial VIPomas, while at least one case of a VIP-producing composite

C. Capella (✉)
Department of Surgical and Morphological Sciences,
University of Insubria,
Via O. Rossi 9, 21100 Varese, Italy
e-mail: carlo.capella@uninsubria.it

S. La Rosa
Department of Pathology, Ospedale di Circolo,
Varese, Italy

S. La Rosa, F. Sessa (eds.), *Pancreatic Neuroendocrine Neoplasms: Practical Approach to Diagnosis, Classification, and Therapy*, DOI 10.1007/978-3-319-17235-4_11,
© Springer International Publishing Switzerland 2015

pheochromocytoma in a patient with neurofibromatosis 1 (NF1) has been described [10].

11.2.2 Etiology

Apart from rare cases associated with MEN1 or NF1, no causative factors are known for VIPomas.

11.2.3 Tumor Sites

VIPomas are located in the pancreas in about 75 % of cases. Approximately 20 % are represented by neurogenic neoplasms, including pheochromocytomas, ganglioneuromas, ganglioneuroblastomas, and neuroblastomas located in adrenal glands, retroperitoneum, and mediastinum. The remaining 5 % of cases are represented by extrapancreatic epithelial neoplasms located in the small intestine/duodenum, esophagus, lung, large bowel, and kidney [1, 7].

11.3 Diagnosis

11.3.1 Clinical Features

The WDHA syndrome is the distinctive feature of VIPomas and comprises watery diarrhea, hypokalemia, and achlorhydria (or hypochlorhydria) [2, 4]. Additional features include alkalosis, hypercalcemia, hyperglycemia, flushing, and dilated gallbladder. Diarrhea is always the most prominent symptom at presentation. The volume of stool is usually 700 ml or more daily and may reach several liters per day with severe loss of potassium and bicarbonate, resulting in metabolic acidosis and dehydration. Stools characteristically resemble diluted tea. Most patients have significant weight loss, and some patients report flushing of the face and chest, but this is not associated with the excretion of serotonin and its metabolites. Tetany is rare; it is thought to be due to hypomagnesemia and may occur in presence of hypercalcemia. The evidence for VIP as a major mediator of the WDHA syndrome is as follows: (1) high concentrations of VIP have been detected in tumors associated with the WDHA syndrome [11]; (2) many of the symptoms in the WDHA syndrome can be explained by the biologic action of VIP recorded in experimental animals [12]; (3) patients with high circulating levels of VIP before tumor resection demonstrated normal VIP levels after surgery, with disappearance of the diarrhea [13]. The syndrome can be mimicked in healthy humans by prolonged VIP infusion [13]. VIPomas have been shown to cosecrete a peptide (P) with an amino terminal histidine (H) and a carboxyl terminal methionine (M). PHM shares a common precursor (prepro-VIP) with VIP as well as some biologic actions [14]. Levels of pancreatic polypeptide (PP) can be elevated in about 75 % of patients with VIPomas [15]; however, PP does not show a secretagogue effect on the intestine of experimental animals [16].

11.3.2 Clinical Diagnosis

In patients with characteristic symptoms, the diagnosis of VIPoma is established with a plasma VIP assay indicating a level above 200 pg/mL [17]. The standard imaging procedures for VIPomas include contrast-enhanced helical CT or MRI of the abdomen for both the primary tumor and the detection of metastases, combined with octreotide scintigraphy and PET scans [18].

11.4 Morphology and Genetics

11.4.1 Gross Findings

A careful review of 179 pancreatic VIPomas, reported in the literature up to 1998 [7], in which the exact tumor site was known, indicates that the tumor is usually solitary (95 % of cases) and most often located in the pancreatic tail (42.4 %), followed by the head (28 %), the body and tail together (17.1 %), the body (8.2 %), and the head and body together (1.3 %). Pancreatic VIPomas range in size from 1.5 to 20 cm, with an average diameter of 5.9 cm [7] which is much larger than that of insulinomas (1.5–2 cm) and similar to the size of glucagonomas and gastrinomas. They appear as circumscribed but unencapsulated red-tan or yellow solid masses, sometimes displaying fibrous septa, calcification, or focal cystic change.

11.4.2 Microscopic Findings

Pancreatic tumors display three main structural patterns: solid, broad trabecular, and tubuloacinar, in order of decreasing frequency. The solid pattern in about half of the cases is characteristically interrupted by irregular cystic spaces filled with weakly eosinophilic fluid (Fig. 11.1). Tumor cells have modest amount of faintly granular eosinophilic or clear cytoplasm. The nuclei are bland, without prominent nucleoli in the majority of the cases. The mitotic count is usually low (<2 per mm^2) including in tumors with metastases; in a few cases, frequent and often atypical mitoses are observed. Vascular and perineural invasion at the periphery of the tumor are detected in about 50 % of cases, most of which are associated with lymph node or liver metastases. As with other pancreatic neuroendocrine tumors, focal or extensive oncocytic change and/or clear cell change can be observed (Fig. 11.1).

11.4.3 Immunohistochemical Findings

In 28 pancreatic tumors studied by one of the authors up to 1988 [19] and in three cases examined in the subsequent 24 years, immunohisto-

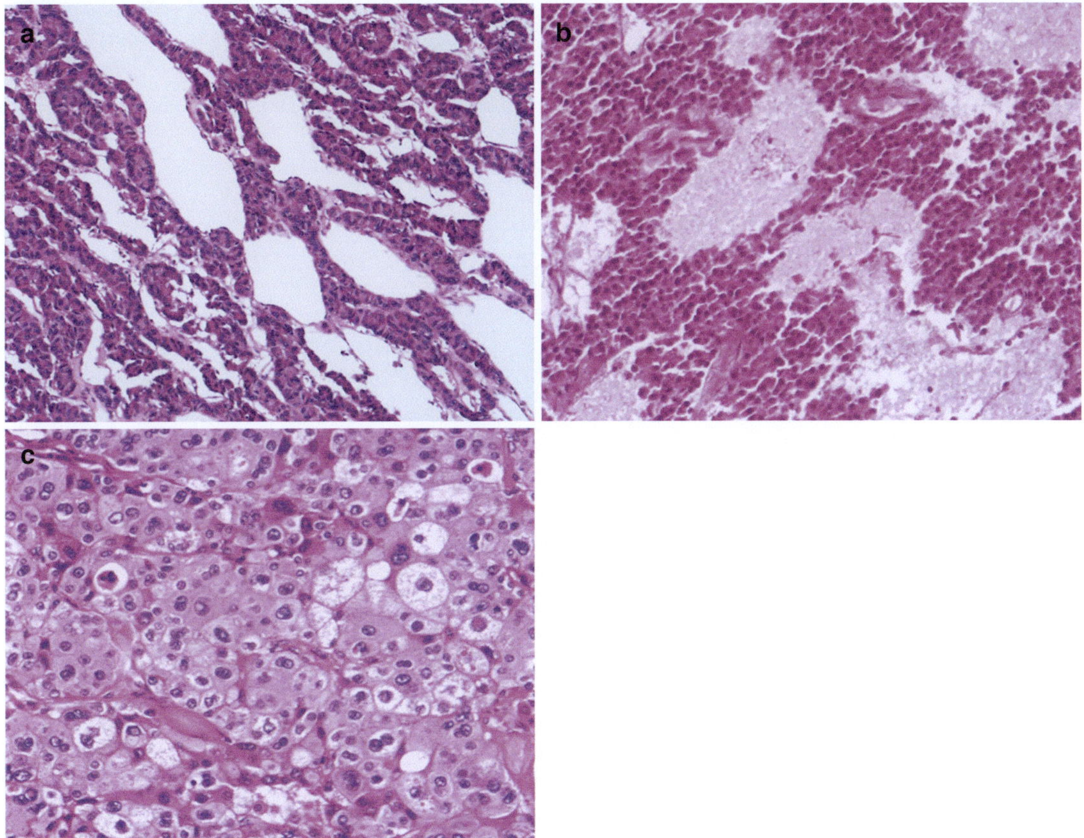

Fig. 11.1 Histologic features of VIPoma: (**a**) trabecular pattern, (**b**) diffuse pattern interrupted by cystic spaces containing pale serum-like material, (**c**) oncocytic area of a VIPoma with some lipid-rich foam cells

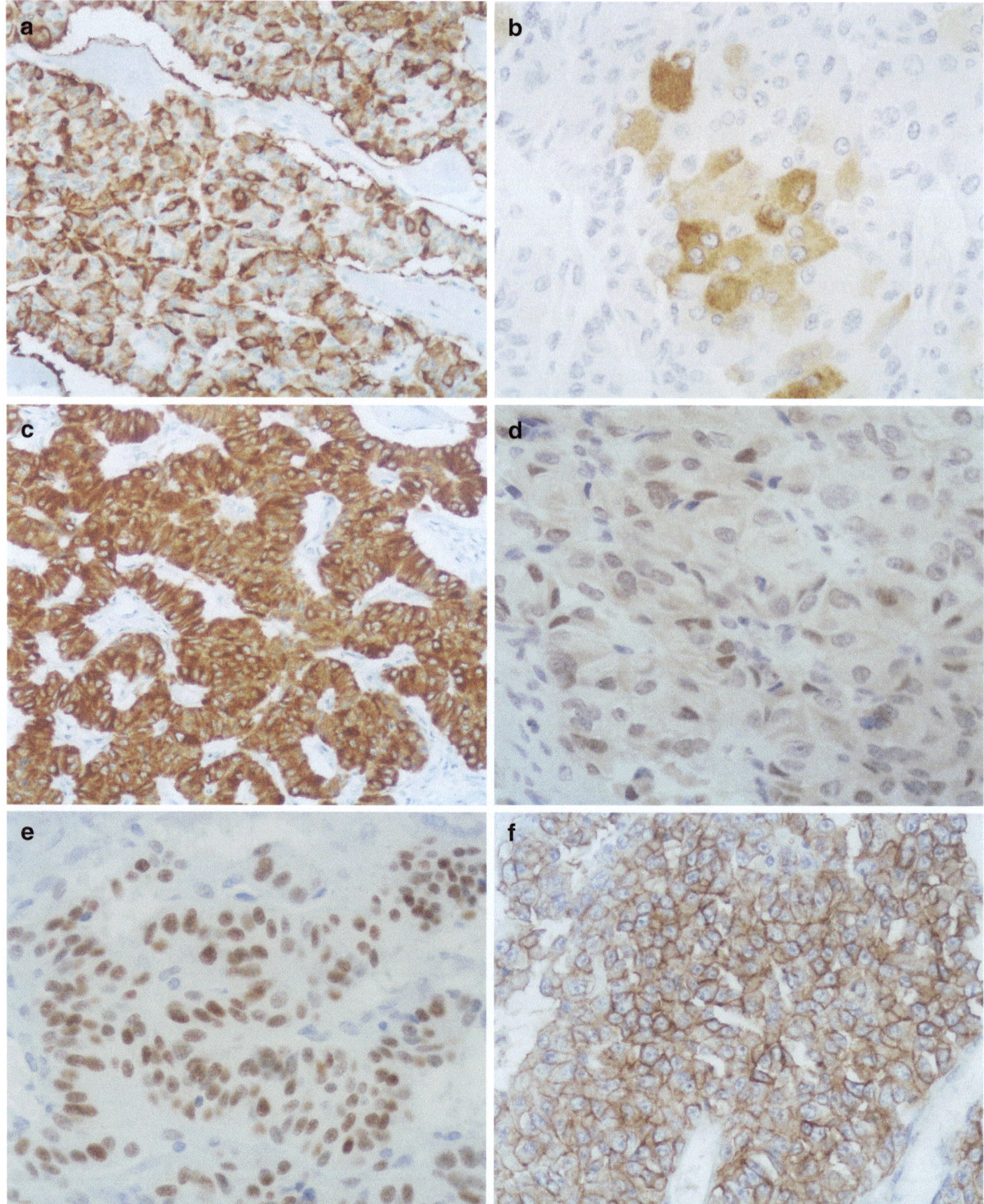

Fig. 11.2 Immunohistochemical immunoreactions of VIPomas: (**a**) chromogranin A, (**b**) VIP, (**c**) cytokeratin 8/18, (**d**) PDX1, (**e**) progesterone receptor, (**f**) somatostatin receptor 2A

chemical stainings showed positivity for the following markers of epithelial neuroendocrine cells: neuron-specific enolase (95 % of cases), synaptophysin (93 %), chromogranin A (83 %), cytokeratin (CK) AE1/AE3 (61 %), CK 8–18 (100 %), and CK19 (100 %) (Fig. 11.2). In some cases, low molecular weight CK is expressed as paranuclear dots (Fig. 11.3). Neural markers

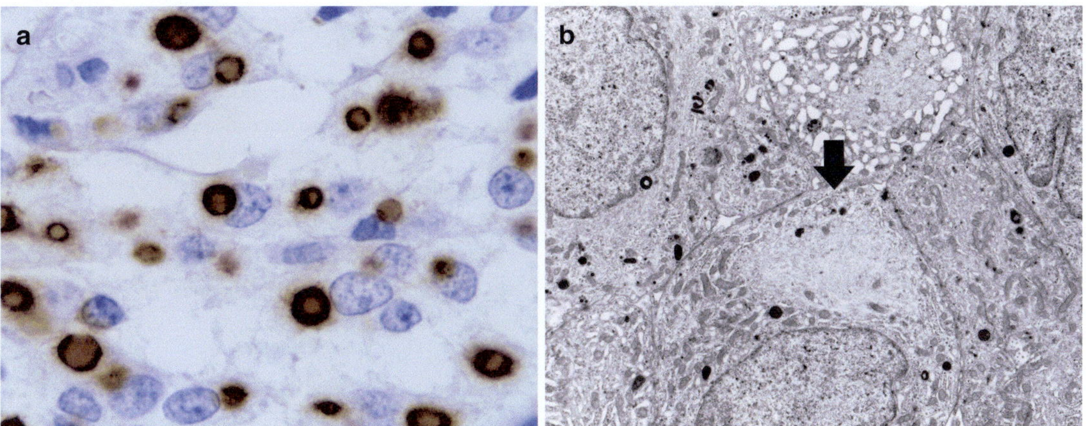

Fig. 11.3 Fibrous bodies in VIPoma: (**a**) CK8/18 immunoreactivity; (**b**) electron microscopic image showing balls of cytokeratin filaments (*arrow*)

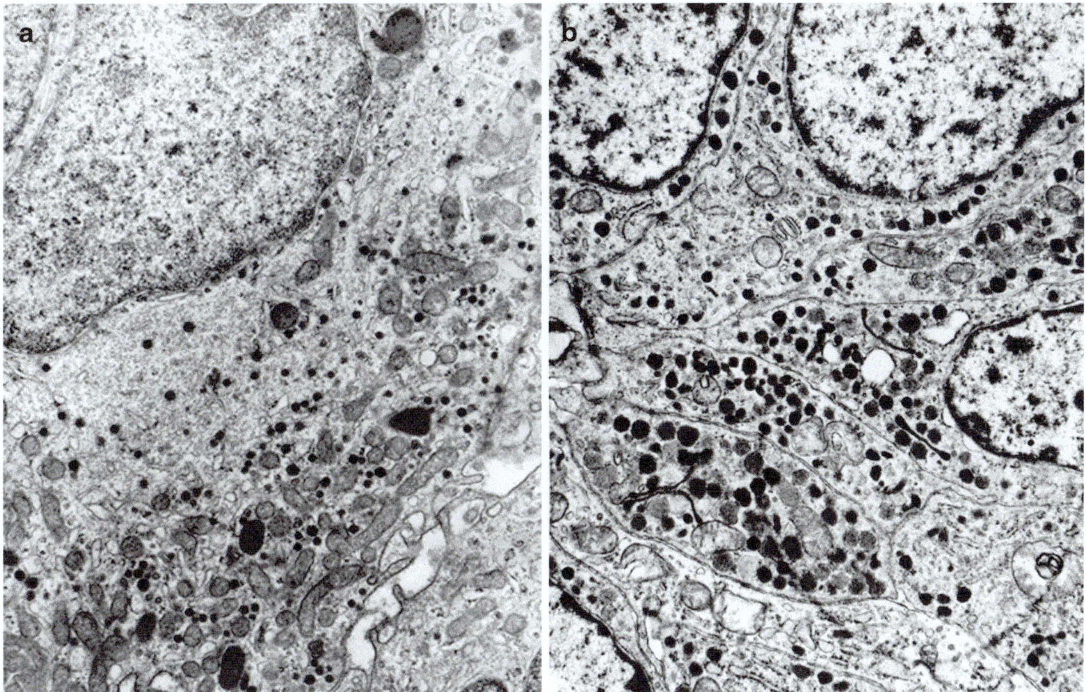

Fig. 11.4 Electron microscopy of pancreatic VIPoma. (**a**) Tumor cells containing small thin-haloed secretory granules. (**b**) Tumor cells containing F-type granules similar to those of PP cells

such as neurofilament protein, microtubule-associated protein (MAP2), and S-100 protein have never been detected. In contrast, neuroendocrine peptide VIP (90 % of the cases), PHM (60 %), growth hormone-releasing hormone (GHRH; 50 %), PP (53 %), alpha chain of human chorionic gonadotropin (alpha-hCG; 50 %), insulin (17 %), ghrelin (20 %), neurotensin (18 %), glucagon (10 %), and met-enkephalin (8 %) were detected. In the majority of pancreatic VIPomas, only a modest number of VIP-immunoreactive cells were present (Fig. 11.2), in agreement with the sparsely granulated ultrastructural pattern of the majority of tumor cells (Fig. 11.4) [11]. Both findings point to a defective storage mechanism with rapid release of the synthesized hormone into the blood. Production of VIP and PHM, which are normally present in neuroectodermal cells [20], may be tentatively explained by the increased plasticity in differentiation shown by the tumor cells. The frequent occurrence of PP cells in pancreatic VIPomas and the expression of both PP and VIP in the same neoplastic cells favor the interpretation that a cell line somewhat related to dorsal pancreas PP cells might be involved in the histogenesis of VIPomas [19]. Eighty percent of pancreatic VIPomas that we examined expressed the lineage marker PDX1 (Fig. 11.2), a transcription factor involved in pancreatic differentiation, which is also represented in the majority of functioning and non-functioning pancreatic neuroendocrine tumors [21]. Eighty percent of VIPomas show strong membranous labeling for somatostatin receptor 2A (Fig. 11.2).

The Ki67 proliferation index of VIPomas has rarely been reported. The average Ki67 index of six of our cases and of three reported cases [22–24] was 3.99 % (range 0.55–7 %) with five tumors having a Ki67 index around 2 %, corresponding to grade 1 (G1) and four tumors having a Ki67 index more than 3 % corresponding to grade 2 of the 2010 WHO classification [25].

11.4.4 Electron Microscopy

Most tumors are formed by sparsely granulated or agranular cells with a well-developed endoplasmic reticulum and Golgi complex. Secretory granules are generally round and small (120–190 nm). Two types of secretory granules can be indentified: (1) small (120–160 nm), thin-haloed granules containing a moderately dense core, which react with VIP antibodies in electron immunocytochemical tests and (2) slightly larger (140–190 nm), in part irregularly shaped, more solid granules which react with anti-PP antibodies and reproduce the characteristics of those of PP cells of PP-rich islets of the human normal pancreas (Fig. 11.4) [26].

11.4.5 Somatic Genetics

Frequent chromosomal gains and losses involving several chromosomes have been detected in eight out of nine VIPomas examined with comparative genomic hybridization (CGH). Similar loci were involved in both VIPomas and different types of malignant neuroendocrine neoplasms. Nevertheless, a higher frequency of corresponding allelic imbalances was detected in VIPomas with LOH analysis [27–29]. In genome and gene expression analysis of a pancreatic VIPoma metastatic to the liver, defects in mismatch repair gene MSH2 and strong overexpression of the chemokine CXCR4, involved in metastasis development, have been reported [30]. Mutations of the *MEN1* gene have been detected in four of nine sporadic VIPomas investigated [31, 32].

11.5　Prognosis

Most VIPomas have been classified as well-differentiated endocrine tumors (WDETs) or well-differentiated endocrine carcinomas (WDECs) according to the 2000 WHO classification [33] or as grade 1 (G1) and G2 neuroendocrine tumors (NETs) according to the 2010 WHO criteria [25]. High-grade poorly differentiated endocrine carcinomas (PDECs, WHO 2000) or neuroendocrine carcinomas (NECs, WHO 2010) have rarely been reported in association with the WDHA syndrome [34]. The average rate of metastases for patients with pancreatic VIPomas is 56.4 % [7]. Metastases are more frequently detected in the liver than in lymph nodes [7, 11, 35]. The staging systems for VIPomas are those proposed by the European Neuroendocrine Tumor Society (ENETS) [36] and by the 2010 WHO [25]. According to both systems, about one half of the cases of pancreatic VIPomas present at stage IV.

In a statistical evaluation of 179 cases of pancreatic VIPomas, Soga and Yakuwa reported 59.6 % 5-year survival for patients with metastases and 94.4 % for patients without metastasis [7]. Similar survival rates were found in our review of pancreatic VIPomas reported in the

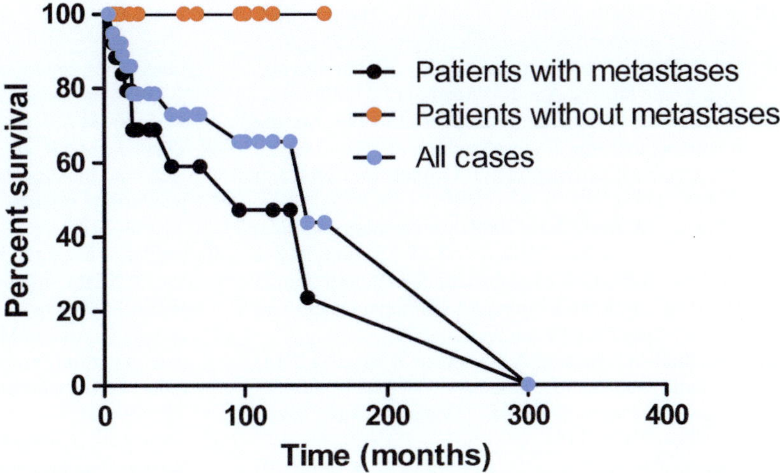

Fig. 11.5 Treatment outcome in patients with pancreatic VIPomas, reported in the literature from 1999 to September 2014, as calculated by the Kaplan–Meyer methods

literature from 1999 to 2013 with 100 % 5-year survival for patients without metastases and 59 % for patients with metastases (Fig. 11.5).

References

1. Solcia E, Capella C, Kloppel G (1997) Tumors of the pancreas, 3rd edn. Armed Forces Institute of Pathology, Washington, DC
2. Verner JV, Morrison AB (1958) Islet cell tumor and a syndrome of refractory watery diarrhea and hypokalemia. Am J Med 25:374–380
3. Matsumoto KK, Peter JB, Schultze RE et al (1966) Watery diarrhea and hypokalemia associated with pancreatic islet cell adenoma. Gastroenterology 50:231–242
4. Marks IN, Bank S, Louw JH (1967) Islet cell tumor of the pancreas with reversible watery diarrhea and achlorhydria. Gastroenterology 52:695–708
5. Jensen RT, Cadiot G, Brandi ML et al (2012) ENETS consensus guidelines for the management of patients with digestive neuroendocrine neoplasms: functional pancreatic endocrine tumor syndromes. Neuroendocrinology 95:98–119
6. Rindi G, Falconi M, Klersy C et al (2012) TNM staging of neoplasms of the endocrine pancreas: results from a large international cohort study. J Natl Cancer Inst 104:764–777
7. Soga J, Yakuwa Y (1998) Vipoma/diarrheagenic syndrome: a statistical evaluation of 241 reported cases. J Exp Clin Cancer Res 17:389–400
8. Hutcheon DF, Bayless TM, Cameron JL et al (1979) Hormone-mediated watery diarrhea in a family with multiple endocrine neoplasms. Ann Intern Med 90:932–934
9. Ooi A, Kameya T, Tsumuraya M et al (1985) Pancreatic endocrine tumours associated with WDHA syndrome. An immunohistochemical and electron microscopic study. Virchows Arch A Pathol Anat Histopathol 405:311–323
10. Onozawa M, Fukuhara T, Minoguchi M et al (2005) Hypokalemic rhabdomyolysis due to WDHA syndrome caused by VIP-producing composite pheochromocytoma: a case in neurofibromatosis type. Jpn J Clin Oncol 35:559–563
11. Capella C, Polak JM, Buffa R et al (1983) Morphologic patterns and diagnostic criteria of VIP-producing endocrine tumors. A histologic. histochemical, ultrastructural and biochemical study of 32 cases. Cancer 52:1860–1874
12. Said SI (1981) VIP overview. In: Bloom SA, Polak JM (eds) Gut hormones, 2nd edn. Churchill Livingstone, Edinburgh, pp 379–384
13. Kreis GJ (1987) VIPoma syndrome. Am J Med 82:37–48
14. Yiangau Y, Williams SJ, Bishop AE et al (1987) Peptide histidine-methionine immunoreactivity in plasma and tissue from patients with vasoactive intestinal peptide-secreting tumors and watery diarrhea syndrome. J Clin Endocrinol Metab 64: 131–139
15. Polak JM, Bloom SR, Adrian TE et al (1976) Pancreatic polypeptide in insulinomas, gastrinomas, vipomas, and glucagonomas. Lancet 1: 328–330
16. Wu ZC, O'Dorisio TM, Cataland S et al (1979) Effects of pancreatic polypeptide and vasoactive intestinal polypeptide on rat ileal and colonic water and electrolyte transport in vivo. J Dig Dis Sci 24:625–630
17. Boushey RP, Drucker DJ (2002) Gastrointestinal hormones and gut endocrine tumors. In: Larsen PR (ed) Williams textbook of endocrinology. Saunders, Philadelphia, pp 1773–1796
18. O'Toole D, Salazar R, Falconi M et al (2006) Rare functioning pancreatic endocrine tumors. Neuroendocrinology 84:189–195

19. Solcia E, Capella C, Riva C et al (1988) The morphology and neuroendocrine profile of pancreatic epithelial VIPomas and extrapancreatic, VIP-producing, neurogenic tumors. Ann NY Acad Sci 527:508–517

20. Larsson LI, Polak JM, Buffa R et al (1979) On the immunocytochemical localization of the vasoactive intestinal polypeptide. J Histochem Cytochem 27:936–938

21. Srivastava A, Hornick JL (2009) Immunohistochemical staining for CDX-2, PDX-1, NESP-55, and TTF-1 can help distinguish gastrointestinal carcinoid tumors from pancreatic endocrine and pulmonary carcinoid tumors. Am J Surg Pathol 33:626–632

22. Abu-Zaid A, Azzam A, Abudan Z et al (2014) Sporadic pancreatic vasoactive intestinal peptide-producing tumor (VIPoma). Hematol Oncol Stem Cell Ther 7:109–115

23. Urdangarin A, Iniquez G, Benavides C et al (2010) Pancreatic VIPoma. Report of one case. Rev Med Chile 138:841–846

24. Moug SJ, Leen E, Horgan PG et al (2006) Radiofrequency ablation has a valuable therapeutic role in metastatic VIPoma. Pancreatology 6:155–159

25. Rindi G, Arnold R, Bosman FT et al (2010) Nomenclature and classification of neuroendocrine neoplasms of the digestive system. In: Bosman FT, Carneiro F, Hruban RH, Theise ND (eds) WHO classification of tumours of the digestive system. IARC Press, Lyon, pp 13–14

26. Fiocca R, Sessa F, Tenti P et al (1983) Pancreatic polypeptide (PP) cells in the PP-rich lobe of the human pancreas are identified ultrastructurally and immunocytochemically as F cells. Histochemistry 77:511–523

27. Speel EJ, Richter J, Moch H et al (1999) Genetic differences in endocrine pancreatic tumor subtypes detected by comparative genomic hybridization. Am J Pathol 155:1787–1794

28. Speel EJ, Zhao J et al (2001) Genetic evidence for early divergence of small functioning and nonfunctioning endocrine pancreatic tumors: gain of 9Q34 is an early event in insulinomas. Cancer Res 61:5186–5192

29. Zhao J, Moch H, Scheidweiler AF et al (2001) Genomic imbalances in the progression of endocrine pancreatic tumors. Genes Chromosomes Cancer 32:364–372

30. Muller S, Kupka S, Königsrainer I et al (2012) MSH2 and CXCR4 involvement in malignant VIPoma. World J Surg Oncol 10:264

31. Asteria C, Anagni M, Fugazzola L et al (2002) MEN1 gene mutations are a rare event in patients with sporadic neuroendocrine tumors. Eur J Intern Med 13:319–323

32. Shan L, Nakamura Y, Nakamura M et al (1998) Somatic mutations of multiple endocrine neoplasia type 1 gene in the sporadic endocrine tumors. Lab Invest 78:471–475

33. Solcia E, Klöppel G, Sobin LH (eds) (2000) Histological typing of endocrine tumours. WHO international histological classification of tumours, 2nd edn. Springer, Berlin

34. Nikou GC, Toubanakis C, Nikolaou P et al (2005) VIPomas: an update in diagnosis and management in a series of 11 patients. Hepatogastroenterology 52:1259–1265

35. Smith S, Branton SA, Avino AJ et al (1998) Vasoactive intestinal polypeptide secreting islet cell tumors: a 15-year experience and review of the literature. Surgery 124:1050–1055

36. Rindi G, Klöppel G, Alhman H et al (2006) TNM staging of foregut (neuro)endocrine tumors: a consensus proposal including a grading system. Virchows Arch 449:395–491

Gastrinoma

12

Anja M. Schmitt, Annika Blank, and Aurel Perren

12.1 Definition

Gastrinomas are neuroendocrine tumors which occur most frequently in the duodenum (70 %), followed by the pancreas (25 %), and are found only rarely in other abdominal or extra-abdominal sites (5 %) [1–4]. Clinically, gastrinomas are characterized by the secretion of gastrin, resulting in gastric acid hypersecretion and eventually in peptic ulcer disease and gastroesophageal reflux disease [1, 5, 6]. This syndrome is named Zollinger-Ellison syndrome (ZES) after the surgeons Robert Milton Zollinger and Edwin Homer Ellison who first described in 1955 the association between peptic ulcer disease and pancreatic neuroendocrine tumors [7]. Gastrinomas have to be separated from functionally inactive neuroendocrine tumors expressing gastrin which are not associated with ZES and seem to have a different biology [2].

12.2 Epidemiology

Among functioning pancreatic neuroendocrine tumors, gastrinomas represent the most common malignant subtype with an incidence of

0.5–2/million/year [1, 5, 8, 9]. Gastrinomas differ concerning their site of origin and their genetic background. Sporadic gastrinomas are slightly more often found in men (54–56 %), and the mean age of patients at diagnosis is between 48 and 55 years. They arise either in the duodenum (50–88 %) or in the pancreas. In contrast, gastrinomas in the hereditary setting of MEN1 develop in younger patients with a mean age of 32–35 years [10, 11]. In these cases, ZES will be due to multiple and small gastrinomas in the duodenal wall in 80–100 % of the cases. Of note, the pancreatic tumors in MEN1 syndrome usually represent nonfunctioning tumors [2, 4, 11].

12.3 Clinical Presentation and Diagnosis

Independent from the site of origin of the primary tumor, patients invariably will present with symptoms related to gastric acid hypersecretion ranging from gastroesophageal reflux disease with heartburn, nausea and vomiting, diarrhea, and weight loss over peptic (most often duodenal) ulcer up to ulcer complications [1, 5, 6, 10, 12–16]. If in a patient, a peptic ulcer is not due to *H. pylori* infection or NSAID intake; if it is recurrent or treatment resistant; if it presents with either complications or in combination with severe gastroesophageal reflux, diarrhea, or

A.M. Schmitt (✉) • A. Blank • A. Perren
Institute of Pathology, University of Bern,
Murtenstrasse 31, 3010 Bern, Switzerland
e-mail: anja.schmitt@pathology.unibe.ch;
annika.blank@pathology.unibe.ch;
aurel.perren@pathology.unibe.ch

S. La Rosa, F. Sessa (eds.), *Pancreatic Neuroendocrine Neoplasms: Practical Approach to Diagnosis, Classification, and Therapy*, DOI 10.1007/978-3-319-17235-4_12,
© Springer International Publishing Switzerland 2015

endocrinopathies; and if there is a family history of peptic ulcer disease, ZES should be suspected [1, 6, 15–19]. The confirmation of the clinically suspected diagnosis of ZES requires the demonstration of hypergastrinemia in the presence of hyperchlorhydria or an acidic pH [1, 9, 14, 15, 17–19]. It is important to note that PPIs interfere with and thus can lead to a delay of the diagnosis of ZES in a twofold manner: firstly, they can mask the symptoms [12, 14–17, 20], and, secondly, they can induce elevated gastrin levels in patients without ZES and lead to false-positive secretin tests [21]. Therefore, it is recommended to stop PPIs at least 1 week before performing the laboratory tests (see Chap. 4). The proof of ZES especially against the background of a family or personal history of endocrinopathies or recurrent peptic ulcer, symptoms of hyperparathyroidism such as renal colics or nephrolithiasis, or the presence of other tumors associated with MEN1 should lead to further laboratory and possibly genetic testing for MEN1, as in 25 % of MEN1 patients there will be no obvious MEN1 family history. On the other hand, as 20–30 % of MEN1 patients develop ZES and ZES can precede the symptoms of hyperparathyroidism, it should be looked for specifically in these patients.

a less aggressive behavior than sporadic tumors. Histologically, gastrinomas do not exhibit any specific features but are mostly well-differentiated neuroendocrine tumors with a trabecular and pseudoglandular growth pattern. In most instances, immunohistochemically they stain positive for gastrin (Fig. 12.1). Usually, they correspond to NET G1 or G2 according to WHO 2010, their proliferation index ranging between 2 % and 10 % [1, 4]. The presence of liver metastases at the time of diagnosis is the most important prognostic factor (10–20 % 10-year survival vs. 90–100 % without liver metastases) [1, 5, 22, 23]. Further poor prognostic factors in addition to those histological features generally admitted for pancreatic neuroendocrine tumors (i.e., angioinvasion, perineural invasion, >2 mitoses/10 HPF, proliferation index >2, poor differentiation) include pancreatic site of origin, lymph node metastases, bone metastases, large primary tumor (1–3 cm), advanced TNM stage, female gender, inadequate control of gastric acid hypersecretion, markedly increased fasting gastrin levels, short history from onset of symptoms to diagnosis, ectopic Cushing's syndrome, and molecular features like overexpression of HER2/neu, 1q LOH, and overexpression of EGFR or IGF1R [1, 3, 5, 22–29].

12.4 Clinicopathological and Prognostic Features

Gastrinomas differ in their clinicopathological features and their biological behavior according to their site of origin and their genetic background. Sporadic duodenal gastrinomas arise in the first and the second part of the duodenum, are usually small (77 % of cases <1 cm), and are associated with liver metastases in 5–10 % at the time of diagnosis. In contrast, sporadic pancreatic gastrinomas arise in any part of the pancreas, although the majority are found in the pancreatic head [1, 3, 4]. With a mean diameter of 3.8 cm, usually they are large tumors and are associated with liver metastases at the time of diagnosis in 20–25 % of the cases [1, 5, 22, 23]. Duodenal gastrinomas in the setting of MEN1 will present as multiple small tumors and are associated with

12.5 Determination of the Site of Origin and Therapy

Surgery is the only curative treatment for sporadic gastrinomas and has been shown to decrease the rate of development of liver metastases, to increase disease-free survival and to result in a long-term cure in 20–45 % of patients. However, as gastrinomas can arise in different sites, their site of origin unavoidably has to be determined to plan the correct surgical procedure. Somatostatin receptor scintigraphy has been shown to be the most sensitive and widely available method for localizing the primary tumor, nevertheless >50 % of the tumors <1 cm are missed. As these tumors almost certainly will be duodenal gastrinomas, the routine use of duodenotomy with intraoperative ultrasound and transillumination

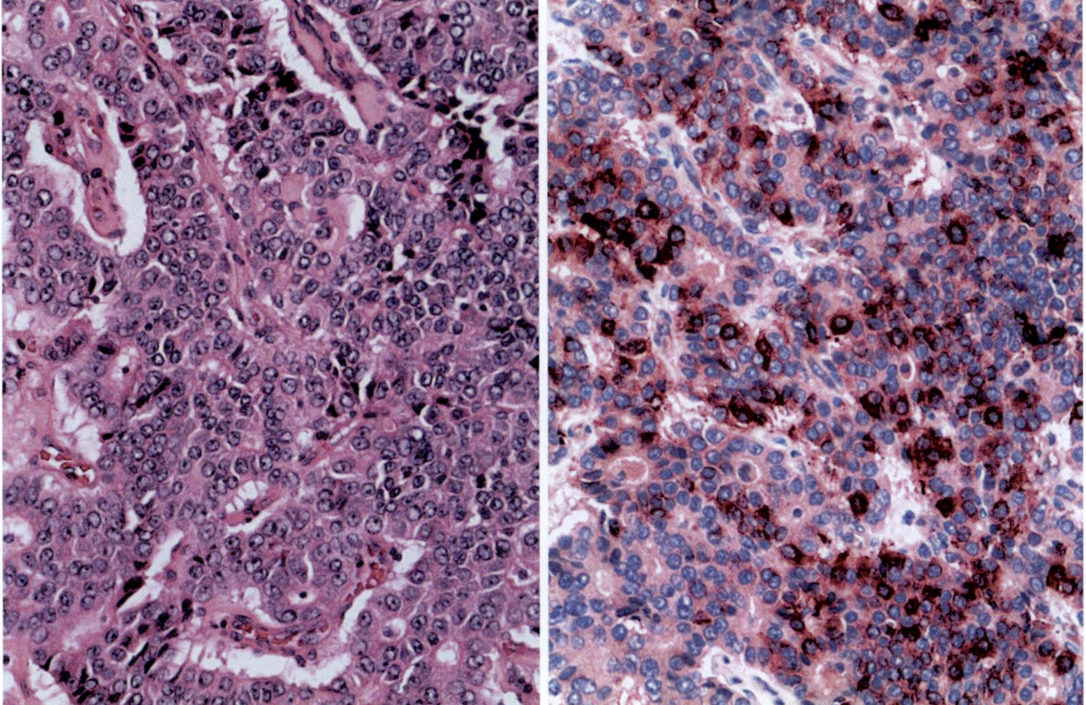

Fig. 12.1 Histology of a gastrinoma. *Left*: H&E, 20×. *Right*: Immunohistochemical staining for gastrin, 20×

of the duodenum should be performed. Pancreaticoduodenectomy should only be discussed in cases with tumor localization in the pancreatic head or in case of a persistent or recurrent tumor after previous resection [1, 28, 30–32]. In the setting of MEN1, the presence of only small (<2 cm) or no tumors in imaging studies is associated with a favorable outcome. Thus, the general recommendation to prevent malignant transformation in MEN1 patient is to confine surgery to pancreatic tumors >2 cm.

References

1. Jensen RT, Niederle B, Mitry E et al (2006) Gastrinoma (duodenal and pancreatic). Neuroendocrinology 84(3):173–182
2. Anlauf M, Garbrecht N, Henopp T et al (2006) Sporadic versus hereditary gastrinomas of the duodenum and pancreas: distinct clinico-pathological and epidemiological features. World J Gastroenterol 12(34):5440–5446
3. Gibril F, Jensen RT (2005) Advances in evaluation and management of gastrinoma in patients with Zollinger-Ellison syndrome. Curr Gastroenterol Rep 7(2):114–121
4. Kloppel G, Anlauf M (2007) Gastrinoma – morphological aspects. Wien Klin Wochenschr 119(19–20):579–584
5. Ellison EC, Johnson JA (2009) The Zollinger-Ellison syndrome: a comprehensive review of historical, scientific, and clinical considerations. Curr Probl Surg 46(1):13–106
6. Roy PK, Venzon DJ, Shojamanesh H et al (2000) Zollinger-Ellison syndrome. Clinical presentation in 261 patients. Medicine (Baltimore) 79(6): 379–411
7. Zollinger EH, Ellison RM (1955) Primary peptic ulcerations of the jejunum associated with islet cell tumors of the pancreas. Ann Surg 142(4):709–723; discussion 724–748
8. Oberg K (2010) Pancreatic endocrine tumors. Semin Oncol 37(6):594–618
9. Metz DC, Jensen RT (2008) Gastrointestinal neuroendocrine tumors: pancreatic endocrine tumors. Gastroenterology 135(5):1469–1492
10. Gibril F, Schumann M, Pace A et al (2004) Multiple endocrine neoplasia type 1 and Zollinger-Ellison syndrome: a prospective study of 107 cases and comparison with 1009 cases from the literature. Medicine (Baltimore) 83(1):43–83
11. Jensen RT, Berna MJ, Bingham DB et al (2008) Inherited pancreatic endocrine tumor syndromes:

advances in molecular pathogenesis, diagnosis, management, and controversies. Cancer 113(7 Suppl):1807–1843

12. Corleto VD, Annibale B, Gibril F et al (2001) Does the widespread use of proton pump inhibitors mask, complicate and/or delay the diagnosis of Zollinger-Ellison syndrome? Aliment Pharmacol Ther 15(10):1555–1561

13. Berna MJ, Hoffmann KM, Serrano J et al (2006) Serum gastrin in Zollinger-Ellison syndrome: I. Prospective study of fasting serum gastrin in 309 patients from the National Institutes of Health and comparison with 2229 cases from the literature. Medicine (Baltimore) 85(6):295–330

14. Banasch M, Schmitz F (2007) Diagnosis and treatment of gastrinoma in the era of proton pump inhibitors. Wien Klin Wochenschr 119(19–20):573–578

15. Osefo N, Ito T, Jensen RT (2009) Gastric acid hypersecretory states: recent insights and advances. Curr Gastroenterol Rep 11(6):433–441

16. Kulke MH, Anthony LB, Bushnell DL et al (2010) NANETS treatment guidelines: well-differentiated neuroendocrine tumors of the stomach and pancreas. Pancreas 39(6):735–752

17. Arnold R (2007) Diagnosis and differential diagnosis of hypergastrinemia. Wien Klin Wochenschr 119(19–20):564–569

18. Vinik AI, Woltering EA, Warner RR et al (2010) NANETS consensus guidelines for the diagnosis of neuroendocrine tumor. Pancreas 39(6):713–734

19. O'Toole D, Grossman A, Gross D et al (2009) ENETS consensus guidelines for the standards of care in neuroendocrine tumors: biochemical markers. Neuroendocrinology 90(2):194–202

20. Niederle B (2007) Hypergastrinemia – diagnosis and treatment. Wien Klin Wochenschr 119(19–20): 561–563

21. Goldman JA, Blanton WP, Hay DW et al (2009) False-positive secretin stimulation test for gastrinoma associated with the use of proton pump inhibitor therapy. Clin Gastroenterol Hepatol 7(5):600–602

22. Weber HC, Venzon DJ, Lin JT et al (1995) Determinants of metastatic rate and survival in patients with Zollinger-Ellison syndrome: a prospective long-term study. Gastroenterology 108(6): 1637–1649

23. Yu F, Venzon DJ, Serrano J et al (1999) Prospective study of the clinical course, prognostic factors, causes of death, and survival in patients with long-standing Zollinger-Ellison syndrome. J Clin Oncol 17(2):615–630

24. Pape UF, Jann H, Muller-Nordhorn J et al (2008) Prognostic relevance of a novel TNM classification system for upper gastroenteropancreatic neuroendocrine tumors. Cancer 113(2):256–265

25. Gibril F, Venzon DJ, Ojeaburu JV et al (2001) Prospective study of the natural history of gastrinoma in patients with MEN1: definition of an aggressive and a nonaggressive form. J Clin Endocrinol Metab 86(11):5282–5293

26. Maton PN, Gardner JD, Jensen RT (1986) Cushing's syndrome in patients with the Zollinger-Ellison syndrome. N Engl J Med 315(1):1–5

27. Cadiot G, Vuagnat A, Doukhan I et al (1999) Prognostic factors in patients with Zollinger-Ellison syndrome and multiple endocrine neoplasia type 1. Groupe d'Etude des Neoplasies Endocriniennes Multiples (GENEM and groupe de Recherche et d'Etude du Syndrome de Zollinger-Ellison (GRESZE). Gastroenterology 116(2):286–293

28. Norton JA, Jensen RT (2004) Resolved and unresolved controversies in the surgical management of patients with Zollinger-Ellison syndrome. Ann Surg 240(5):757–773

29. Goh BK, Chow PK, Tan YM et al (2011) Validation of five contemporary prognostication systems for primary pancreatic endocrine neoplasms: results from a single institution experience with 61 surgically treated cases. ANZ J Surg 81(1–2):79–85

30. Fendrich V, Waldmann J, Bartsch DK et al (2009) Surgical management of pancreatic endocrine tumors. Nat Rev Clin Oncol 6(7):419–428

31. Tonelli F, Fratini G, Nesi G et al (2006) Pancreatectomy in multiple endocrine neoplasia type 1-related gastrinomas and pancreatic endocrine neoplasias. Ann Surg 244(1):61–70

32. Grobmyer SR, Vogel SB, McGuigan JE et al (2009) Reoperative surgery in sporadic Zollinger-Ellison Syndrome: longterm results. J Am Coll Surg 208(5):718–722; discussion 722–724

ACTH-Producing Tumor

13

Silvia Uccella, Roberta Maragliano,
and Francesca Magnoli

13.1 Historical Background

Adrenocorticotropic hormone (*ACTH*) is physiologically secreted by basophil cells of the anterior pituitary gland as a cleavage product of pro-opiomelanocortin (POMC), together with other POMC-related hormonal products. It plays a key role in the regulation of the hypothalamic-pituitary-adrenal axis, stimulating adrenal cortical cells to produce and release corticosteroid hormones. An excess of circulating ACTH, due to ACTH-producing tumors, results in chronically increased circulating levels of corticosteroids and is responsible for ACTH-dependent *Cushing's syndrome* (CS). The hyperproduction of ACTH is most frequently related to a corticotroph pituitary adenoma; however, ACTH can be ectopically secreted by malignant tumors of extrapituitary sites, creating the physiopathological basis of the ectopic Cushing's syndrome (ECS). ECS accounts for about one third of all ACTH-dependent Cushing's syndromes. According to an extensive literature review, the four most common causes of ectopic ACTH syndrome are small cell carcinomas of the lung (27 %), bronchial carcinoids (21 %), neuroendocrine tumors of the pancreas (16 %), and thymic carcinoids (10 %) [1].

The first association between CS and ectopic ACTH production by pancreatic tumors was described in 1946 by Arthur Carleton Crooke, who reviewed four cases of acinar or ductal pancreatic adenocarcinomas associated with adrenocortical hyperfunction [2]. Four years later, Del Castillo and coworkers reported the first islet cell carcinoma of the pancreas causing hypercortisolism [3]. Since then, a total of 134 cases of ACTH-producing *pancreatic neuroendocrine tumors* (PanNETs) have been described, in 89 different papers published in the English literature, mostly including single case reports or small series [4–91]. Very recently, all of these tumors and ten additional cases have been reviewed by Maragliano and colleagues [92].

It is also worth noting that other pancreatic neoplasms, namely, acinar cell carcinoma and pancreatoblastoma, can cause an ECS, especially in pediatric age.

13.2 Epidemiology

ECS-associated PanNETs occur most frequently in females (M:F ratio = 1:2). The patients are frequently young or middle aged, with more than two thirds being less than 50 years old and a non-negligible proportion of cases occurring in pediatric age.

S. Uccella (✉) • R. Maragliano • F. Magnoli
Department of Surgical and Morphological Sciences,
University of Insubria, Via O. Rossi, 9,
Varese 21100, Italy
e-mail: silvia.uccella@uninsubria.it;
roberta.maragliano@gmail.com;
magnoli.francesca@gmail.com

S. La Rosa, F. Sessa (eds.), *Pancreatic Neuroendocrine Neoplasms: Practical Approach to Diagnosis, Classification, and Therapy*, DOI 10.1007/978-3-319-17235-4_13,
© Springer International Publishing Switzerland 2015

The signs and symptoms of CS are almost invariably present, with high circulating levels of ACTH and cortisol. The presence of another endocrine syndrome in the same patient is a common event, reported in about 40 % of the patients. *Zollinger-Ellison syndrome* (ZES), with gastrin overproduction by the same tumor, is the most frequent accompanying syndrome. A few patients present with an *insulinoma syndrome* associated to ECS, while *carcinoid syndrome* is anecdotally reported [10]. The signs and symptoms related to hypergastrinemia or hyperinsulinemia may be synchronous with those of CS, but in the majority of the reported cases, they occur after or, even more frequently, before the ACTH hypersecretion becomes evident. The latency between the onsets of the different syndromes is possibly related to the differently evident biological activities of ACTH and other hormones. Alternatively, the acquisition of ACTH secretion may be looked at as a part of the malignant progression, as plurisyndromic tumors seem to have a worse prognosis.

Of all reported ECS-associated PanNETs, only two cases were related to a genetically transmitted syndrome. One patient had multiple endocrine neoplasia type 1 syndrome (MEN-1) [61], and the other one had von Hippel-Lindau (VHL) syndrome [92].

13.3 Diagnosis

The signs and symptoms of ACTH-producing PanNETs encompass all of the possible manifestations of Cushing's syndrome and are related to chronically elevated cortisol concentrations. Clinical features are wide ranging and include weight gain, central obesity, moon face, violaceous striae, and easy bruising. The usual presentations in children are obesity and growth retardation. Hypertension is a frequent finding, as well as insulin resistance, glucose hypersensitivity, and overt diabetes mellitus. Severe hypokalemia, life-threatening infections, psychiatric disorders, osteoporosis, and fractures are seen more frequently in ECS than in Cushing's disease related to pituitary ACTH hypersecretion.

Cutaneous hyperpigmentation can be present in patients with high levels of circulating ACTH or other melanotropin hormones. In addition to endocrine manifestations, mass symptoms can be evident, in particular when the tumor is located in the head of the pancreas.

The laboratory workup of Cushing's syndrome includes the measurement of urinary cortisol levels, the dexamethasone suppression test, and the determination of plasma ACTH concentration. Once the syndrome has been determined to be ACTH dependent, the high-dose dexamethasone suppression test and the metyrapone test are useful to discriminate between a pituitary and an ectopic source of ACTH. In addition, it has been reported that the levels of ACTH precursors present in the circulation of patients with ectopic tumors are greater than those found in the circulation of patients with pituitary tumors indicating a less efficient processing of pro-opiomelanocortin (POMC) in tumors outside the pituitary. Overall, the reported data indicate that patients with ectopic tumors have ACTH precursor levels greater than 100 pmol/l [93].

The identification of the extrapituitary site of ACTH production is then accomplished by radiological imaging, that should include a complete chest and abdomen computed tomography (CT) scan or nuclear magnetic resonance (NMR). As the majority of ACTH-producing pancreatic tumors present with distant metastasis, a spiral CT and an Octreoscan may also be helpful for staging the tumor.

13.4 Morphology

ACTH-producing PanNETs may arise in any pancreatic portion; however, these neoplasms are more frequently found in the head, followed by the tail and, more rarely, the body of the pancreas. Macroscopically, tumor masses are generally large, with a mean diameter of the described cases of 4.8 cm (range: 2.5–15 cm) [92]. They are generally well circumscribed but non-encapsulated, and the cut surface is gray to pink and usually homogeneous.

Microscopically, these neoplasms have the morphological features of *well-differentiated*

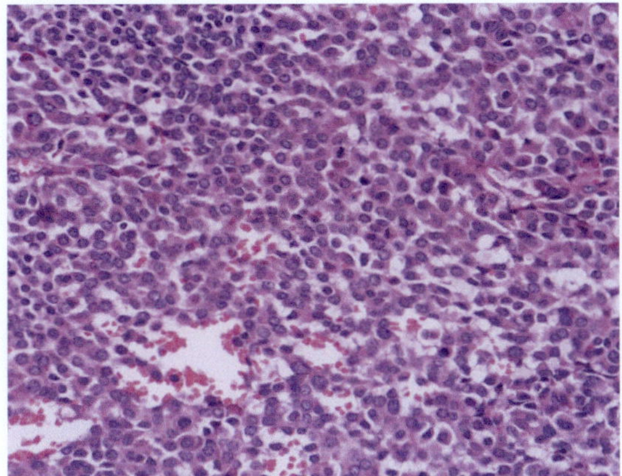

Fig. 13.1 ACTH-producing PanNET. The tumor cells grow in solid sheets (H&E, ×200)

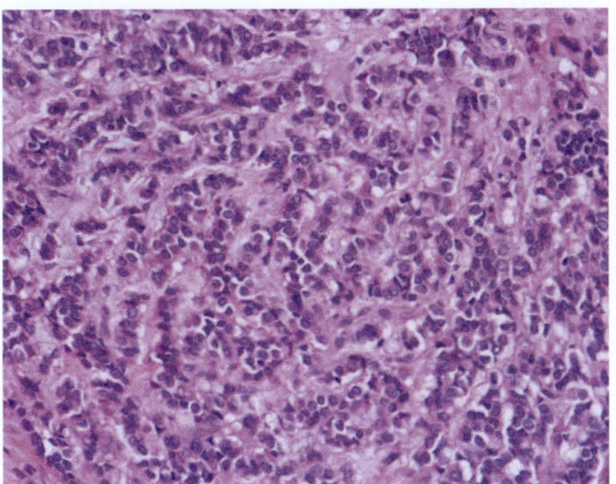

Fig. 13.2 ACTH-producing PanNET with a trabecular pattern of growth and moderate stromal fibrosis (H&E, ×200)

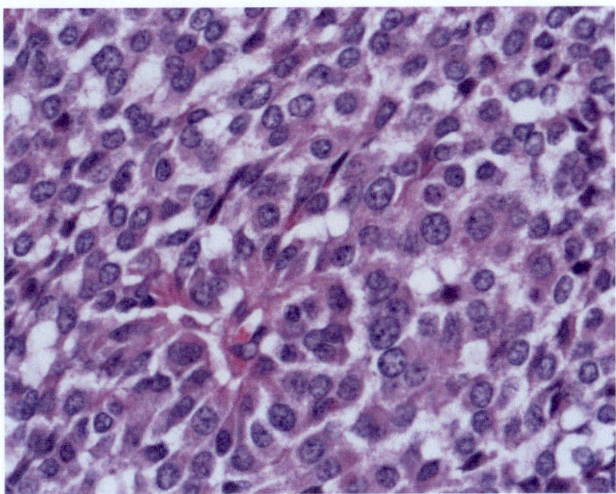

Fig. 13.3 ACTH-producing PanNET. Tumor cells show moderately abundant, eosinophilic, granular cytoplasms and round to oval nuclei with regular contours, evident nuclear membrane, "salt and pepper" chromatin, and small nucleoli (H&E, ×400)

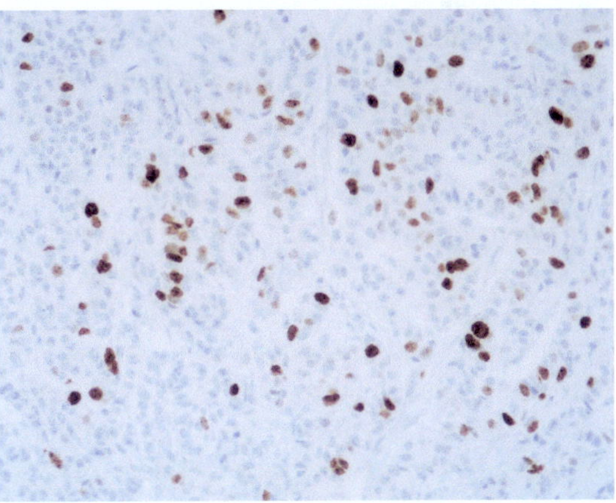

Fig. 13.4 Ki67 immunoreactivity in an ACTH-producing PanNET G2 reveals a proliferative index higher than 3 % (immunoperoxidase and hematoxylin, ×200)

PanNETs, as they are defined by the 2000 WHO classification [94]. The neoplastic population is composed of relatively uniform cuboidal cells with centrally located nuclei and eosinophilic or amphophilic granular cytoplasm arranged in nests, trabeculae, pseudoglands, or solid sheets, being undistinguishable from other well-differentiated neuroendocrine tumors of the pancreas (Figs. 13.1, 13.2, and 13.3). A spindle-cell, ACTH-secreting neuroendocrine tumor of the pancreas has also been reported [72], albeit this peculiar aspect seems not to recur in these neoplasms. Mitotic count and proliferative index have been inconstantly reported in these tumors, making it difficult to assess whether

ACTH-producing PanNETs were NET G1 or G2. However, in our series of ten well-characterized tumors, we observed that most cases were NET G2 [92] (Fig. 13.4). In addition, histological features of aggressiveness (invasion of lymphatic and blood vessels and perineural invasion), which are features of NET G2, were observed in the majority of tumors [92], mirroring the aggressive behavior of these neoplasms. Focal necrosis is not a frequent finding. Cytoplasmic basophilia and Crooke's hyalinization, which are features of ACTH-producing

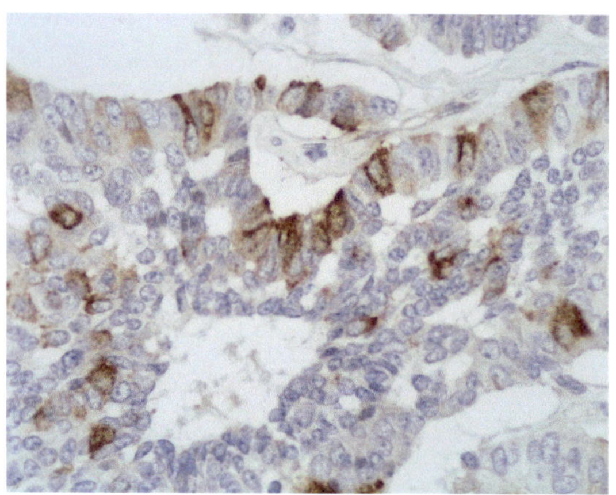

Fig. 13.5 ACTH immunoreactivity is observed in a fraction of neoplastic cells in a Cushing's syndrome-associated PanNET (immunoperoxidase and hematoxylin, ×400)

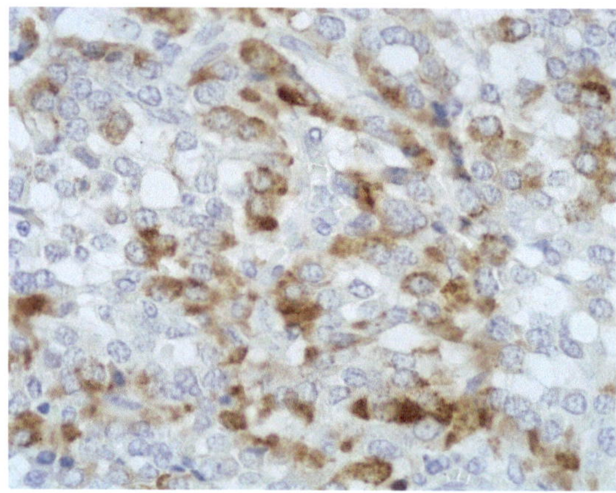

Fig. 13.6 This ACTH-producing PanNET is also immunoreactive for β-endorphin (immunoperoxidase and hematoxylin, ×400)

pituitary adenomas, are not usually found in these pancreatic tumors [92].

Immunohistochemically, all ACTH-producing pancreatic neuroendocrine tumors react with general neuroendocrine markers (synaptophysin, neuron-specific enolase, chromogranin A, CD56). These tumors are also immunoreactive for ACTH and/or other ACTH-related peptide hormones, such as pro-opiomelanocortin (POMC), melanotropin (MSH), β-endorphin, and met-enkephalin, all identifiable using specific antibodies in at least a fraction of tumor cells [93] (Figs. 13.5 and 13.6). Intriguingly, several neuroendocrine tumors of the pancreas have been reported to show ACTH expression and clinical features of CS only in recurrences or in metastatic localization, while the primary neoplasm was ACTH negative [63, 74]. As it is also clinically evident, plurihormonality is not an infrequent feature of CS-associated PanNETs. Interestingly, a few of these neoplasms have been found to be immunoreactive also for *corticotropin-releasing hormone* (CRH), including malignant plurihormonal neuroendocrine tumors associated with ZES [74]. In addition, a case of CRH-immunoreactive PanNET associated with ECS, with no expression of ACTH or other hormones, has also been described [69]. All ZES-associated tumors show positive immunostaining for gastrin (Fig. 13.7), whereas insulin was detected in tumors associ-

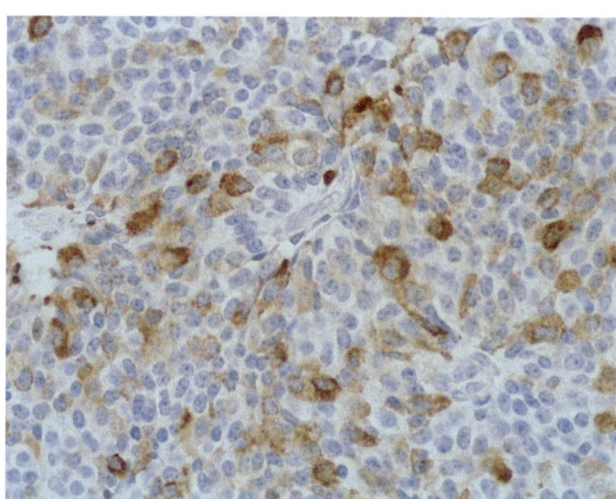

Fig. 13.7 Gastrin immunoreactivity in an ACTH-producing PanNET associated with Cushing's syndrome and Zollinger-Ellison syndrome (immunoperoxidase and hematoxylin, ×400)

ated with insulinoma syndrome. It has been recently reported that ACTH-producing neuroendocrine tumors of the pancreas can be immunoreactive for CD117 and galectin-3, although the meaning of the expression of these molecules is still unclear [92]. Finally, ACTH-secreting PanNETs show a weak expression of SSRT2A, possibly due to the downregulation of the SSTR by high levels of glucocorticoids, as reported in ACTH-secreting pituitary adenomas [95–97]. However, octreotide therapy has been shown to suppress ACTH and cortisol secretion in several patients with ectopic ACTH production from

PanNETs, bronchial carcinoids, and medullary carcinoma of the thyroid [1].

ACTH-producing PanNETs have a high metastatic rate, with 79 % of all cases presenting with systemic disease or developing distant metastases during the history of the disease [91]. As a consequence, the majority of these tumors have a high stage at diagnosis, according to the ENETS system [98]. The liver is the most frequent site of hematogenous localization, and it is almost invariably involved in metastatic disease. Less frequently, distant metastases may occur in the lung, in the bones, and in pelvic organs, i.e., ovaries [91].

13.5   Prognosis

ACTH-producing PanNETs are aggressive tumors, with a median overall survival (OS) of 30 months and a 5-year OS of 25 % [91]. These figures are significantly worse than that of other PanNET subtypes (5-year survival of 97 % for insulinomas, 72 % for gastrinomas, 75 % for somatostatinomas, and 80 % for nonfunctioning PanNETs [see specific chapters in this book]). The association of an ECS and a ZES due to a PanNET in the same patient significantly worsens the patients' outcome. If this group of patients is excluded from the general ACTH-producing PanNETs population, the median and the 5-year OS rise to 50 months and to 35 %, respectively. By contrast, the association with insulinoma syndrome, as well as the detection of the production of other hormones, does not seem to produce a different prognosis.

References

1. Beuschlein F, Hammer GD (2002) Ectopic pro-opiomelanocortin syndrome. Endocrinol Metab Clin N Am 31:191–234
2. Crooke AC (1946) Basophilism and carcinoma of the pancreas. J Pathol Bacteriol 58:667–673
3. Del Castillo EB, Trucco E, Manzuoli J (1950) Maladie de Cushing et cancer du pancréas. Presse Med 58:783
4. Rosenberg AA (1956) Fulminating adrenocortical hyperfunction associated with islet-cell carcinoma of the pancreas; case report. J Clin Endocrinol Metab 16:1364–1373
5. Balls KF, Nicholson JT, Goodman HL et al (1959) Functioning islet-cell carcinoma of the pancreas with Cushing's syndrome. J Clin Endocrinol Metab 19:1134–1143
6. Meador CK, Liddle GW, Island DP et al (1962) Cause of Cushing's syndrome in patients with tumors arising from "nonendocrine" tissue. J Clin Endocrinol Metab 22:693–703
7. Liddle GW, Island DP, Ney RL et al (1963) Nonpituitary neoplasms and Cushing's syndrome. Ectopic "adrenocorticotropin" produced by nonpituitary neoplasms as a cause of Cushing's syndrome. Arch Intern Med 111:471–475
8. Hallwright GP, North KA, Reid JD (1964) Pigmentation and Cushing's syndrome due to malignant tumor of the pancreas. J Clin Endocrinol Metab 24:496–500
9. Marks V, Samols E, Bolton R (1965) Hyperinsulinism and Cushing's syndrome. Br Med J 1:1419–1420
10. Sayle BA, Lang PA, Green WO Jr et al (1965) Cushing's syndrome due to islet cell carcinoma of the pancreas. Report of two cases: one with elevated hydroxyindole acetic acid and complicated by aspergillosis. Ann Intern Med 63:58–68
11. Geokas MC, Chun JY, Dinan JJ et al (1965) Islet-cell carcinoma (Zollinger-Ellison syndrome) with fulminating adrenocortical hyperfunction and hypokalemia. Can Med Assoc J 93:137–1343
12. Law DH, Liddle GW, Scott HW Jr et al (1965) Ectopic production of multiple hormones (ACTH, MSH and gastrin) by a single malignant tumor. N Engl J Med 273:292–296
13. Burkinshaw JH, O'Brien D, Pendower JE (1967) Cushing's syndrome associated with an islet-cell tumour of the pancreas in a boy aged 2 years. Arch Dis Child 42:525–531
14. Uei Y, Kim U, Itatsu Y (1968) An autopsy case of islet-cell carcinoma with Cushing's syndrome. Acta Pathol Jpn 18:333–343
15. O'Neal LW, Kipnis DM, Luse SA et al (1968) Secretion of various endocrine substances by ACTH-secreting tumors – gastrin, melanotropin, norepinephrine, serotonin, parathormone, vasopressin, glucagon. Cancer 21:1219–1232
16. Vieweg WV, Graber AL, Cerchio GM (1969) Pancreatic islet cell carcinoma with hyperinsulinism and probable, ectopic ACTH-MSH secretion. Arch Intern Med 124:731–735
17. Frederick WC, Gross L (1972) Surgical correction of functioning islet cell carcinoma of the pancreas associated with hyperadrenocorticism. Am J Gastroenterol 57:146–151
18. Rawlinson DG (1973) Electron microscopy of an ACTH-secreting islet cell carcinoma. Cancer 31:1015–1019
19. Corrin B, Gilby ED, Jones NF et al (1973) Oat cell carcinoma of the pancreas with ectopic ACTH secretion. Cancer 31:1523–1527

20. Belchetz PE, Brown CL, Makin HL et al (1973) ACTH, glucagon and gastrin production by a pancreatic islet cell carcinoma and its treatment. Clin Endocrinol 2:307–316

21. Walter RM, Ensinck JW, Ricketts H et al (1973) Insulin and ACTH production by a streptozotocin responsive islet cell carcinoma. Am J Med 55:667–670

22. Sadoff L, Gordon J, Goldman S (1975) Amelioration of hypoglycemia in a patient with malignant insulinoma during the development of the ectopic ACTH syndrome. Diabetes 24:600–603

23. Craig ID, Nelson PG (1975) Pancreatic islet-cell tumour associated with Cushing's syndrome. Report of a case with estimation of tumour ACTH content. Ulster Med J 44:68–70

24. Imura H, Matsukura S, Yamamoto H et al (1975) Studies on ectopic ACTH-producing tumors. II. Clinical and biochemical features of 30 cases. Cancer 35:1430–1437

25. Kovacs K, Horvath E, Ezrin C et al (1977) Immunoreactive somatostatin in pancreatic islet-cell carcinoma accompanied by ectopic A.C.T.H. syndrome. Lancet 1:1365–1366

26. Kawaoi A, Okano T, Uchida T (1977) Immunohistological study on the ACTH producing islet cell carcinoma of the pancreas. Acta Pathol Jpn 27:265–273

27. Joffe SN, Elias E, Rehfeld JF et al (1978) Clinically silent gross hypergastrinaemia from a multiple hormone-secreting pancreatic apudoma. Br J Surg 65:277–280

28. Kyriakides GK, Silvis SE, Ahmed M et al (1979) Gastrinoma associated with common bile duct obstruction and the ectopic production of ACTH. Am J Surg 137:800–802

29. Asa SL, Kovacs K, Killinger DW et al (1980) Pancreatic islet cell carcinoma producing gastrin, ACTH, alpha-endorphin, somatostatin and calcitonin. Am J Gastroenterol 74:30–35

30. Daniels GH (1981) Case records of the Massachusetts General Hospital. Weekly clinicopathological exercises. Case 10. N Engl J Med 304:591–599

31. Heitz PU, Klöppel G, Polak JM et al (1981) Ectopic hormone production by endocrine tumors: localization of hormones at the cellular level by immunocytochemistry. Cancer 48:2029–2037

32. Kitchens CS, Alexander RW (1981) Cushing's syndrome secondary to a neuroendocrine tumor: relapse after bilateral adrenalectomy. Cancer 48:1873–1876

33. Davies CJ, Joplin GF, Welbourn RB (1982) Surgical management of the ectopic ACTH syndrome. Ann Surg 196:246–258

34. Drury PL, Ratter S, Tomlin S et al (1982) Experience with selective venous sampling in diagnosis of ACTH-dependent Cushing's syndrome. Br Med J (Clin Res Ed) 284:9–12

35. Santelices R, Bobadilla E, Pineda G et al (1983) Cushing's syndrome due to ectopic ACTH production by a carcinoid tumor not producing serotonin. N Engl J Med 308:463

36. Styne DM, Isaac R, Miller WL et al (1983) Endocrine, histological, and biochemical studies of adrenocorticotropin-producing islet cell carcinoma of the pancreas in childhood with characterization of proopiomelanocortin. J Clin Endocrinol Metab 57:723–731

37. Lyons DF, Eisen BR, Clark MR et al (1984) Concurrent Cushing's and Zollinger-Ellison syndromes in a patient with islet cell carcinoma. Case report and review of the literature. Am J Med 76:729–733

38. Clark ES, Carney JA (1984) Pancreatic islet cell tumor associated with Cushing's syndrome. Am J Surg Pathol 8:917–924

39. Allison MC, Renfrew CC, Webb WJ et al (1985) Neuroendocrine islet cell tumour producing gastrin and ACTH in a patient with calcifying chronic pancreatitis. Gut 26:426–428

40. Jex RK, van Heerden JA, Carpenter PC et al (1985) Ectopic ACTH syndrome. Diagnostic and therapeutic aspects. Am J Surg 149:276–282

41. Howlett TA, Drury PL, Perry L et al (1986) Diagnosis and management of ACTH-dependent Cushing's syndrome: comparison of the features in ectopic and pituitary ACTH production. Clin Endocrinol 24:699–713

42. Maton PN, Gardner JD, Jensen RT (1986) Cushing's syndrome in patients with the Zollinger-Ellison syndrome. N Engl J Med 315:1–5

43. Findling JW, Tyrrell JB (1986) Occult ectopic secretion of corticotropin. Arch Intern Med 146:929–933

44. Long SI (1987) ACTH-producing apudoma metastatic to the liver. J Natl Med Assoc 79:122–123

45. Souquet JC, Sassolas G, Forichon J et al (1987) Clinical and hormonal effects of a long-acting somatostatin analogue in pancreatic endocrine tumors and in carcinoid syndrome. Cancer 59:1654–1660

46. Melmed S, Yamashita S, Kovacs K et al (1987) Cushing's syndrome due to ectopic proopiomelanocortin gene expression by islet cell carcinoma of the pancreas. Cancer 59:772–778

47. Lokich J, Bothe A, O'Hara C et al (1987) Metastatic islet cell tumor with ACTH, gastrin, and glucagon secretion. Clinical and pathologic studies with multiple therapies. Cancer 59:2053–2058

48. Ruszniewski P, Girard F, Benamouzig R et al (1988) Long acting somatostatin treatment of paraneoplastic Cushing's syndrome in a case of Zollinger-Ellison syndrome. Gut 29:838–842

49. Garg SK, Vashist R, Pathak IC et al (1988) Ectopic ACTH syndrome due to islet cell carcinoma in a 12-year old child. Indian J Pediatr 55:155–160

50. Lamberts SW, Tilanus HW, Klooswijk AI et al (1988) Successful treatment with SMS 201-995 of Cushing's syndrome caused by ectopic adrenocorticotropin secretion from a metastatic gastrin-secreting pancreatic islet cell carcinoma. J Clin Endocrinol Metab 67:1080–1083

51. Torriani F, Uske A, Temler E et al (1989) Pancreatic insulinoma causing Cushing's syndrome. J Endocrinol Invest 12:313–319

52. Bertagna X, Favrod-Coune C, Escourolle H et al (1989) Suppression of ectopic adrenocorticotropin secretion by the long-acting somatostatin analog octreotide. J Clin Endocrinol Metab 68:988–991

53. Doppman JL, Nieman L, Miller DL et al (1989) Ectopic adrenocorticotropic hormone syndrome: localization studies in 28 patients. Radiology 172:115–124

54. van Coevorden A, Laurent E, Rickaert F et al (1990) Cushing's syndrome with intermittent ectopic ACTH production. J Endocrinol Invest 13:317–326

55. Gullo L, De Giorgio R, D'Errico A et al (1992) Pancreatic exocrine carcinoma producing adrenocorticotropic hormone. Pancreas 7:172–176

56. Doppman JL, Nieman LK, Cutler GB Jr et al (1994) Adrenocorticotropic hormone–secreting islet cell tumors: are they always malignant? Radiology 190:59–64

57. Ishido H, Yamashita N, Kitaoka M et al (1994) A case of ectopic ACTH syndrome associated with Zollinger-Ellison syndrome: long-term survival with chemical adrenalectomy. Endocr J 41:171–176

58. Amikura K, Alexander HR, Norton JA et al (1995) Role of surgery in management of adrenocorticotropic hormone-producing islet cell tumors of the pancreas. Surgery 118:1125–1130

59. Kelekis NL, Semelka RC, Molina PL et al (1995) ACTH-secreting islet cell tumor: appearances on dynamic gadolinium-enhanced MRI. Magn Reson Imaging 13:641–644

60. Zhu L, Domenico DR, Howard JM (1996) Metastatic pancreatic neuroendocrine carcinoma causing Cushing's syndrome. ACTH secretion by metastases 3 years after resection of nonfunctioning primary cancer. Int J Pancreatol 19:205–208

61. Sundaram V, Schuster DP, Falko JM (1998) Unusual manifestations of Cushing's syndrome in a multiple endocrine neoplasia type I kindred. Endocr Pract 4:190–194

62. Young J, Deneux C, Grino M et al (1998) Pitfall of petrosal sinus sampling in a Cushing's syndrome secondary to ectopic adrenocorticotropin-corticotropin releasing hormone (ACTH-CRH) secretion. J Clin Endocrinol Metab 83:305–308

63. Raddatz D, Horstmann O, Basenau D et al (1998) Cushing's syndrome due to ectopic adrenocorticotropic hormone production by a non-metastatic gastrinoma after long-term conservative treatment of Zollinger-Ellison syndrome. Ital J Gastroenterol Hepatol 30:636–640

64. Grobholz R, Back W, Porner T et al (1999) Fatal Aspergillus fumigatus septicemia in a patient with an ectopic ACTH-producing neuroendocrine pancreatic tumor. Endocr Pathol 10:181–185

65. Hinnie J, Gray CE, McNicol AM et al (2000) Cushing's syndrome in a 16 year old girl due to ectopic ACTH precursor production from a pancreatic tumour. Clin Endocrinol 53:539–540

66. Brandt L (2000) Case records of the Massachusetts General Hospital. Weekly clinicopathological exercises. Case 4-2000. A 64-year-old man with Cushing's syndrome and a pancreatic mass. N Engl J Med 342:414–420

67. Kasperlik-Zaluska AA, Jeske W, Cichocki A (2001) Cushing's syndrome in a 16-year-old girl due to ectopic ACTH precursor production from a pancreatic tumour. Clin Endocrinol 55:558–559

68. Oberg KC, Wells K, Seraj IM et al (2002) ACTH-secreting islet cell tumor of the pancreas presenting as bilateral ovarian tumors and Cushing's syndrome. Int J Gynecol Pathol 21:276–280

69. Babu AR, Dwarakanathan AA (2003) Cushing's syndrome from ectopic production of corticotropin by a metastatic gastrinoma. Endocr Pract 9:229–232

70. Lee T, Karl M, Solorzano CC (2004) Adrenocorticotropic hormone-secreting pancreatic islet cell carcinoma. J Am Coll Surg 199:336–337

71. Miehle K, Tannapfel A, Lamesch P et al (2004) Pancreatic neuroendocrine tumor with ectopic adrenocorticotropin production upon second recurrence. J Clin Endocrinol Metab 89:3731–3736

72. Chetty R, Serra S (2005) Spindle cell pancreatic endocrine tumor associated with Cushing's syndrome. Endocr Pathol 16:145–151

73. Pivonello R, Ferone D, de Herder WW et al (2007) Dopamine receptor expression and function in corticotroph ectopic tumors. J Clin Endocrinol Metab 92:65–69

74. Park SY, Rhee Y, Youn JC et al (2007) Ectopic Cushing's syndrome due to concurrent corticotropin-releasing hormone (CRH) and adrenocorticotropic hormone (ACTH) secreted by malignant gastrinoma. Exp Clin Endocrinol Diabetes 115:13–16

75. Benitez Velazco A, Pacheco Capote C, Latre Romero JM (2008) Ectopic Cushing's syndrome caused by a functioning pancreatic neuroendocrine tumour in a patient with von Hippel-Lindau disease. Rev Esp Med Nucl 27:29–33

76. Said R, O'Reilly EM, Blumgart L et al (2010) Pancreatic islet cell carcinoma presenting with concurrent Cushing's and Zollinger-Ellison syndromes: case series and literature review. Eur J Gastroenterol Hepatol 22:246–252

77. Kondo T, Matsuyama R, Ashihara H et al (2010) A case of ectopic adrenocorticotropic hormone-producing pancreatic neuroendocrine tumor with multiple liver metastases. Endocr J 57:229–236

78. Doi M, Sugiyama T, Izumiyama H et al (2010) Clinical features and management of ectopic ACTH syndrome at a single institute in Japan. Endocr J 57:1061–1069

79. Filippella M, Davi MV, Doveri G et al (2011) Hyperinsulinemic hypoglycemia associated with ectopic Cushing's syndrome due to a pancreatic endocrine tumor in a Type 2 diabetes mellitus patient:

clinical implications of a rare association. J Endocrinol Invest 34:175–179

80. Chowdry RP, Bhimani C, Delgado MA et al (2012) Unusual suspects: pulmonary opportunistic infections masquerading as tumor metastasis in a patient with adrenocorticotropic hormone-producing pancreatic neuroendocrine cancer. Ther Adv Med Oncol 4:295–300

81. Wu H, Wang C, Liu S et al (2012) Adrenocorticotropic hormone-secreting tumor in the pancreas identified by PET/CT. Clin Nucl Med 37:296–297

82. Patel FB, Khagi S, Daly KP et al (2013) Pancreatic neuroendocrine tumor with ectopic adrenocorticotropin production: a case report and review of literature. Anticancer Res 33:4001–4005

83. Chertman M, Chertman L (2013) Ectopic ACTH secretion by islet cell neuroendocrine carcinoma: case report and review of the literature. World J Med Surg Case Rep 3:56–63

84. Treglia G, Salomone E, Petrone G et al (2013) A rare case of ectopic adrenocorticotropic hormone syndrome caused by a metastatic neuroendocrine tumor of the pancreas detected by 68Ga-DOTANOC and 18F-FDG PET/CT. Clin Nucl Med 38:e306–e308

85. Sauer N, Zur Wiesch CS, Flitsch J et al (2014) Cushing's syndrome due to a CRH and ACTH-producing neuroendocrine pancreatic tumor. Endocr Pract 20:e53–e57

86. Surace A, Ferrarese A, Benvenga R et al (2014) ACTH-secreting neuroendocrine pancreatic tumor: a case report. Int J Surg. pii: S1743-9191(14)00134-4

87. La Rosa S, Marando A, Ghezzi F et al (2011) Cushing's syndrome due to a pancreatic neuroendocrine tumor metastatic to the ovaries: a clinicopathological description of a case. Endocr Pathol 22:118–124

88. Passmore SJ, Berry PJ, Oakhill A (1988) Recurrent pancreatoblastoma with inappropriate adrenocorticotrophic hormone secretion. Arch Dis Child 63: 1494–1496

89. Matarazzo P, Tuli G, Tessaris D et al (2011) Cushing syndrome due to ectopic adrenocorticotropic hormone secretion in a 3-year-old child. J Pediatr Endocrinol Metab 24:219–222

90. Kletter GB, Sweetser DA, Wallace SF et al (2007) Adrenocorticotropin-secreting pancreatoblastoma. J Pediatr Endocrinol Metab 20:639–642

91. Illyes G, Luczay A, Benyo G et al (2007) Cushing's syndrome in a child with pancreatic acinar cell carcinoma. Endocr Pathol 18:95–102

92. Maragliano R, Vanoli A, Albarello L et al (2015) ACTH-secreting pancreatic neoplasms associated with Cushing syndrome: clinicopathologic study of 11 cases and review of the literature. Am J Surg Pathol 39:374–382

93. Oliver RL, Davis JRE, White A (2003) Characterization of ACTH related peptides in ectopic Cushing's syndrome. Pituitary 6:119–126

94. Solcia E, Klöppel G, Sobin LH et al (2000) Histological typing of endocrine tumours. WHO international histological classification of tumours, 2nd edn. Springer, Berlin

95. Celio MR, Pasi A, Bürgisser E, Buetti G, Höllt V, Gramsch C (1980) 'Proopiocortin fragments' in normal human adult pituitary. Distribution and ultrastructural characterization of immunoreactive cells. Acta Endocrinol 95:27–40

96. de Herder WW, Lamberts SW (1999) Octapeptide somatostatin-analogue therapy of Cushing's syndrome. Postgrad Med J 75:65–66

97. Cingolani N, Shaco-Levy R, Farruggio A et al (2000) Alpha-fetoprotein production by pancreatic tumors exhibiting acinar cell differentiation: study of five cases, one arising in a mediastinal teratoma. Hum Pathol 31:938–944

98. Sanchez-Franco F, Patel YC, Reichlin S (1981) Immunoreactive adrenocorticotropin in the gastrointestinal tract and pancreatic islets of the rat. Endocrinology 108:2235–2238

Serotonin-Producing Tumor

14

Stefano La Rosa, Nora Sahnane, and Laura Cimetti

14.1 Historical Background

The first tumor showing the typical morphological features of neoplasms producing serotonin was reported in 1907 by Siegfried Oberndorfer who used the term "carcinoid" ("Karzinoide") to describe a set of ileal tumors composed of monomorphic cells forming nests and/or trabeculae rather than true glands that behaved better than carcinomas [1]. Since then, this terminology has largely been used to identify a wide spectrum of neuroendocrine neoplasms arising in the digestive system, including the pancreas, but originating from several different neuroendocrine cell types. However, although this term has become very popular among pathologists and clinicians and has been widely used, it has failed to adequately convey the variety of such tumors which show different morphological, biological, clinical, and molecular features, in part related to their site of origin along the digestive system. For this reason, the use of the term "carcinoid" has been discouraged in diagnostic practice in favor of "neuroendocrine tumor (NET)," maintaining the

term carcinoid solely in the context of the "carcinoid syndrome" [2–4].

The term "carcinoid" has also historically been used to identify rare pancreatic neuroendocrine tumors (PanNETs) composed of serotonin-producing EC cells that, for the reasons mentioned above, would be better named "serotonin-producing PanNETs" [5]. The first well-documented case of a serotonin-producing PanNET, which included serotonin demonstration in tumor tissue, was described by Peart et al. in 1963 [6], and since then, 88 cases have been reported in the medical literature, either associated with the carcinoid syndrome (17 cases) or clinically nonfunctioning (71 cases) [6–46].

14.2 Epidemiology

Due to the confusing use of the term "carcinoid" in previous years as aforesaid, it is difficult to determine the real incidence and prevalence of serotonin-producing PanNETs. In epidemiological studies including large series of digestive neuroendocrine neoplasms defined as carcinoids, pancreatic tumors, which probably correspond to serotonin-producing neoplasms, accounted for 0.58–1.4 % of the entire series and represented about 1 % of all PanNETs [47–49]. However, it is probable that the actual incidence and prevalence of pancreatic serotonin-producing tumors have been underestimated because

S. La Rosa (✉)
Department of Pathology, Ospedale di Circolo,
Viale Borri 57, 21100 Varese, Italy
e-mail: stefano.larosa@ospedale.varese.it

N. Sahnane • L. Cimetti
Department of Surgical and Morphological Sciences,
University of Insubria, Varese, Italy

S. La Rosa, F. Sessa (eds.), *Pancreatic Neuroendocrine Neoplasms: Practical Approach to Diagnosis,*
Classification, and Therapy, DOI 10.1007/978-3-319-17235-4_14,
© Springer International Publishing Switzerland 2015

serotonin production is not generally routinely investigated and the clinical picture of the carcinoid syndrome is very rare. Indeed, in our series of 362 functioning and nonfunctioning PanNETs systematically investigated for serotonin expression with immunohistochemistry, serotonin-producing PanNETs represented 4 % of cases, and all of them were nonfunctioning [42]. In a recent published series including 1,072 patients who underwent pancreatic surgery for PanNETs, functioning serotonin-producing PanNETs associated with the carcinoid syndrome represented 1.4 % [50].

Females seem to be slightly more frequently affected by this tumor type, and functioning tumors arise in younger patients (mean age, 41 years) compared to nonfunctioning neoplasms (mean age, 54 years) [42].

14.3 Diagnosis

Since most of serotonin-producing PanNETs are nonfunctioning, they are often incidentally found during ultrasound examination performed for other reasons. Patients can show unspecific symptoms related to tumor growth including abdominal pain, jaundice, or weight loss. In these cases, the final diagnosis relies on the immunohistochemical demonstration of serotonin in tumor cells.

Conversely, patients with functioning serotonin-producing PanNETs show symptoms of the carcinoid syndrome which has a clinical spectrum including hypotension or hypertension, facial flushing, diarrhea, wheezing, colicky abdominal pain, edema, and carcinoid heart disease. Since serotonin is secreted by such tumors, the most common diagnostic test is the 24-h urinary 5-hydroxyindoleacetic acid (5-HIAA) assay, which monitors the metabolite of serotonin. Normal levels of 5-HIAA are less than 10 mg in a 24-h urine sample. Levels greater than 25 mg per 24 h have been considered diagnostic for carcinoid tumor. However, it is worth noting that up to 20 % of carcinoid patients have normal urinary 5-HIAA levels. During this test, patients must avoid serotonin-rich foods such as bananas, avo-cadoes, plums, tomatoes, pineapples, kiwis, eggplant, plantain, and walnuts [51]. In most reported patients with functioning serotonin-producing PanNETs, increased levels of 5-HIAA have been demonstrated.

14.4 Morphology

Macroscopically, the mean tumor diameter for reported cases is 3.4 cm, ranging from 0.5 to 9 cm. Some tumors have been described to originate closely to the main pancreatic duct, and they tended to be smaller than tumors arising in the pancreatic parenchyma. However, specific macroscopic features peculiar of serotonin-producing PanNETs have not yet been described.

Histologically, most reported neoplasms were well differentiated, while poorly differentiated neuroendocrine carcinomas account for only a few cases [7, 9, 13, 42]. Tumors can show different architectural features according to the scheme proposed by Soga and Tazawa [52] and include trabecular (type B), solid nest (type A), or acinar (type C) patterns of growths, while a diffuse architecture (type D) with or without necrosis has only been observed in large malignant tumors (Fig. 14.1). Histological signs of malignancy including vascular and perineural invasion as well as infiltration of peripancreatic tissues have been observed in some tumors and were associated with tumor aggressiveness. Interestingly, serotonin expression did not correlate per se with specific signs of aggressive behavior [42, 45]. In other words, these tumors showed all the different macroscopic and microscopic features that can be observed in the other neuroendocrine pancreatic tumor types.

Tumors arising within the main pancreatic duct were reported as well differentiated and small ranging from 5 to 15 mm in size. They resulted in a localized stricture or stenosis of the duct, which, in turn, determined an upstream dilatation of the ducts associated with chronic obstructive pancreatitis [41, 43–46].

McCall and coworkers have reported that serotonin-producing PanNETs were more

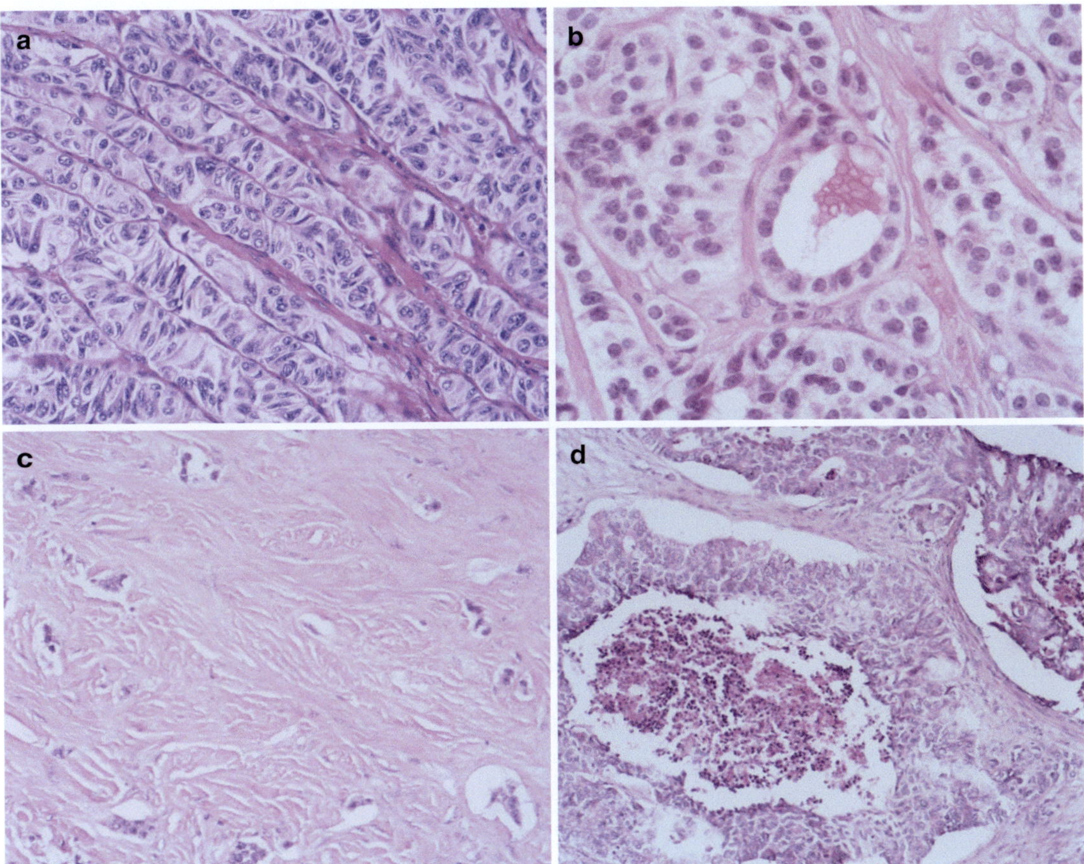

Fig. 14.1 Serotonin-producing PanNETs show different architectural features including trabecular (**a**) or acinar (**b**) patterns of growths, and some cases can present marked stromal fibrosis (**c**). Although serotonin-producing PanNETs are generally well differentiated, some cases can show poorly differentiated morphology including cell atypia with focal necrosis (**d**)

frequently associated with fibrosis than other PanNET types [45]. It is worth noting that serotonin-producing NETs arising in the small intestine produce several growth factors that stimulate fibroblast proliferation and function, resulting in marked stromal fibrosis [53–56]. However, it has been recently demonstrated that, conversely to ileal serotonin-producing NETs, serotonin-producing PanNETs do not express acidic fibroblast growth factor (aFGF) and express connective tissue growth factor (CTGF) at a low level [42]. These are well-known growth factors involved in tumor fibrosis development, and these findings suggest that stromal fibrosis observed in several serotonin-producing PanNETs may be due to different factors that have to be identified.

Most of reported serotonin-producing pancreatic neuroendocrine neoplasms were morphologically well differentiated, so they have to be considered as neuroendocrine tumors (NETs) according to the 2010 WHO classification [57]. However, since mitotic count and Ki67 index were not reported in several cases, the tumor grade of all published cases is not known. Among the 36 reported PanNETs for which the proliferative assessment was available, 25 (69.4 %) were G1 (grade 1) showing less than 2 mitoses × 10 HPF and less than 3 % of Ki67 proliferative index [42–46].

Immunohistochemical analyses have demonstrated that serotonin-producing PanNETs express general neuroendocrine markers, serotonin, and somatostatin receptor 2A (Fig. 14.2),

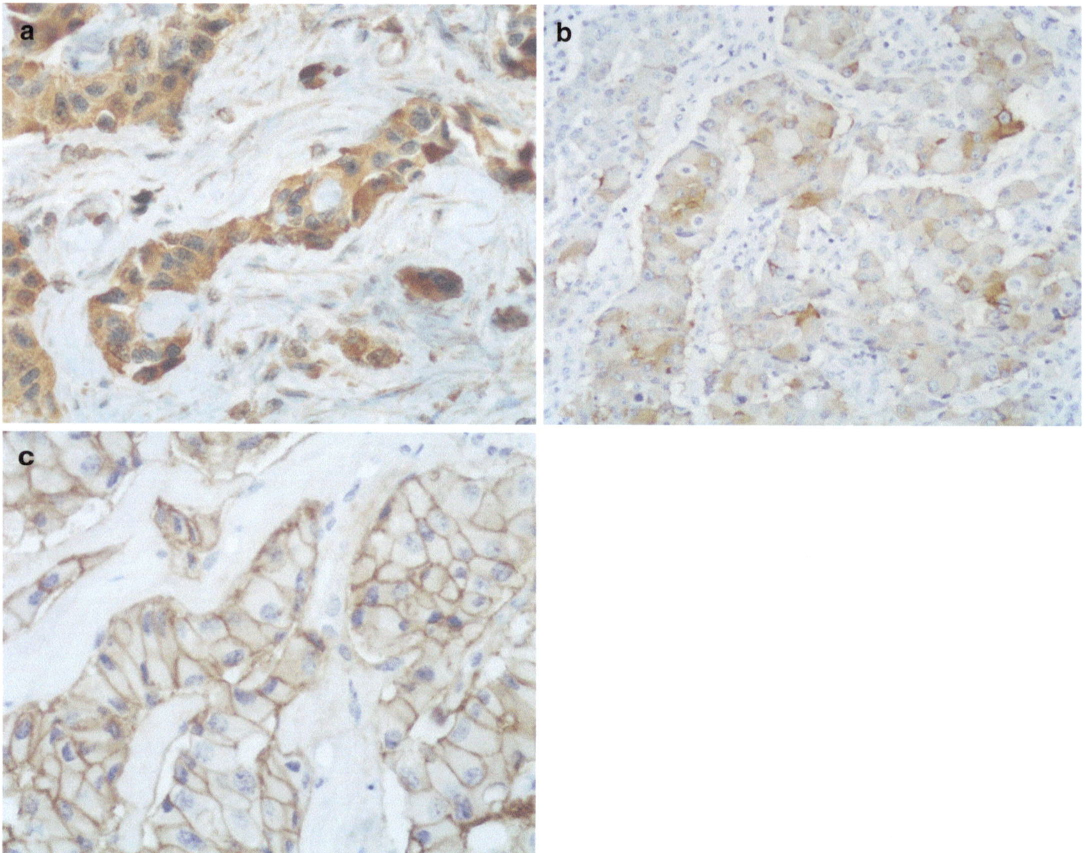

Fig. 14.2 Serotonin-producing PanNETs are strongly and diffusely positive for serotonin (**a**), vesicular monoamine transporter 2 (VMAT2, **b**), and somatostatin receptor 2A (**c**)

while they generally lack the expression of pancreatic hormones (insulin, glucagon, somatostatin, and pancreatic polypeptide) and gastrin. Interestingly, additional immunohistochemical investigations demonstrated that serotonin-producing PanNETs show a different immunophenotype with respect to intestinal serotonin-producing NETs. These differences include the lack of substance P and aFGF immunoreactivity; the lack of S100-positive sustentacular cells; the low expression of CDX2, prostate acid phosphatase, CTGF, and vesicular monoamine transporter 1 (VMAT1); and a strong expression of VMAT2 [42, 45]. These different immunohistochemical features suggest that serotonin-producing PanNETs are different from their intestinal counterparts, and this has also been demonstrated at the ultrastructural level.

Indeed, tumor cells show ultrastructural features resembling those of the so-called "gastric-type" EC cells which differ from "intestinal-type" EC cells (Fig. 14.3) [42].

Despite the various differences described above, a similar cytogenetic pattern of chromosome 18 has been demonstrated in both serotonin-producing pancreatic and ileal NETs [42]. Chromosome 18 deletions have been frequently found in ileal NETs and have also been described, although less frequently, in pancreatic neuroendocrine neoplasms [58–60]. Although the molecular mechanisms underlying the pathogenesis and progression of serotonin-producing PanNETs are largely unknown, this finding suggests that there is at least a common molecular alteration between pancreatic and ileal serotonin-producing NETs.

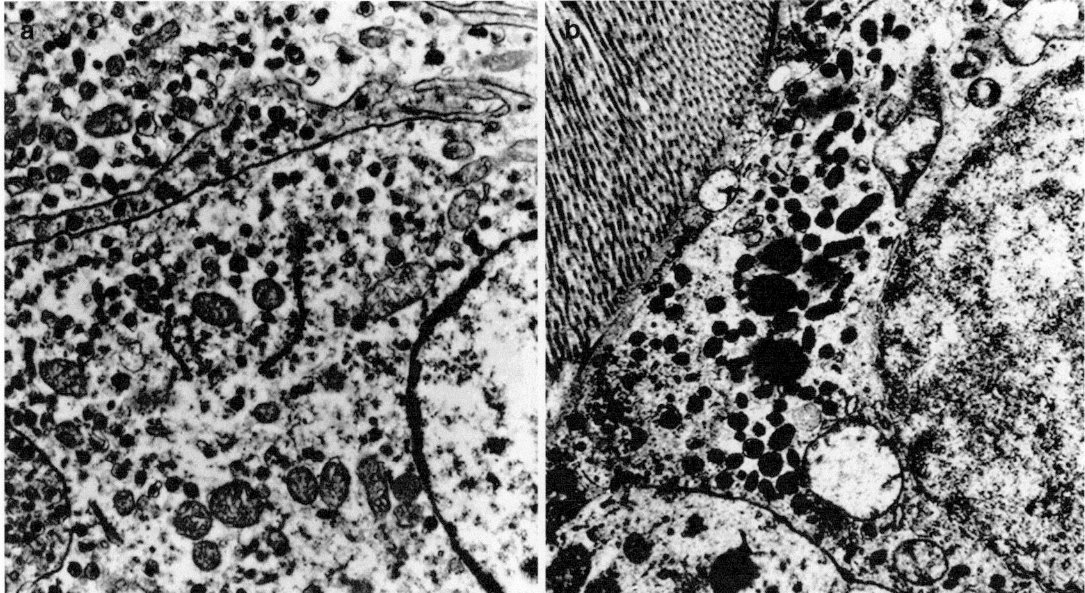

Fig. 14.3 At the ultrastructural examination, serotonin-producing PanNETs are well granulated and show small (mean size of 170×120 nm) pleomorphic round-ovoid secretory granules (**a**). EC cells of ileal neoplasms are very densely granulated showing larger (mean size of 380×140 nm) pleomorphic rodlike or biconcave secretory granules (**b**) (original magnification ×10,000)

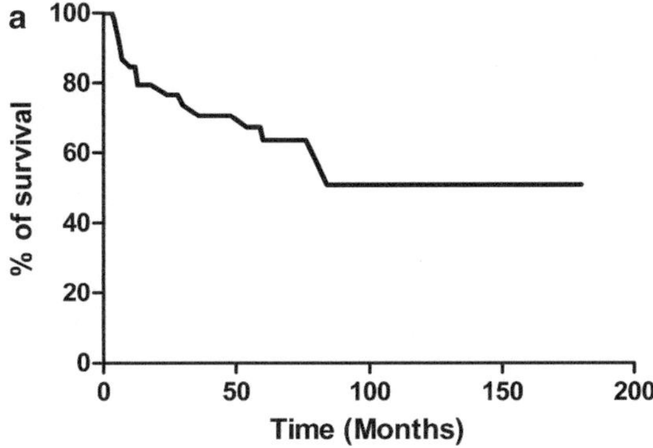

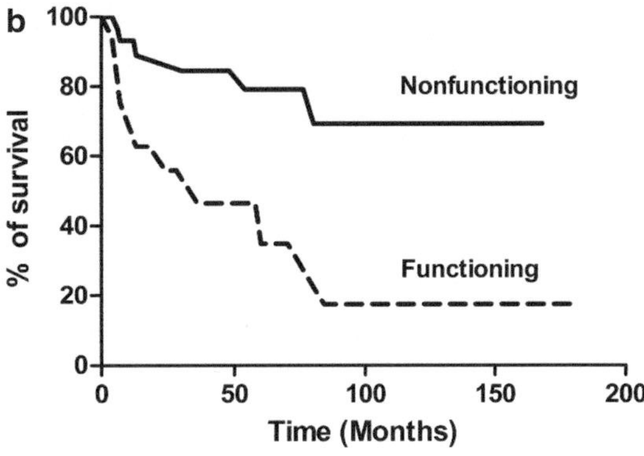

Fig. 14.4 (**a**) Overall survival of patients with serotonin-producing PanNETs. (**b**) Patients with nonfunctioning neoplasms (*black line*) show a statistically significant better survival rate (*p*, 0.0029) than patients with functioning tumors (*dotted line*) associated with the carcinoid syndrome

14.5 Prognosis

The overall survival of patients with serotonin-producing PanNETs is shown in Fig. 14.4a. The survival analysis of all cases reported in the medical literature shows that 60.5 % and 50.8 % of patients were alive 5 and 10 years after diagnosis, respectively. Patients with nonfunctioning neoplasms show a statistically significant better survival rate (*p*, 0.0029) than patients with functioning tumors associated with the carcinoid syndrome (Fig. 14.4b). In particular, 79.1 % and 69.3 % of patients with nonfunctioning serotonin-producing PanNETs were alive at 5 and 10 years after the diagnosis, respectively, showing a survival rate similar to patients with nonfunctioning neoplasms which accounts for 80 % at 5 years and 67 % at 10 years after diagnosis [50]. 34.9 %

of patients with functioning serotonin-producing PanNETs were alive 5 years after diagnosis as compared to 35 % of patients with functioning ACTH-secreting PanNETs [61], 97 % with insulinomas [62], 72 % with gastrinomas [63], and 75.2 % with somatostatinomas [64]. 17.4 % of patients with functioning serotonin-producing PanNETs were alive 10 years after diagnosis as compared to 16.2 % of patients with ACTH-secreting PanNETs [61], 86 % with insulinomas [62], and 59 % with gastrinomas [63].

From these prognostic evaluations, it appears that nonfunctioning serotonin-producing PanNETs have a survival rate similar to that of nonfunctioning PanNETs, while functioning serotonin-producing PanNETs are aggressive neoplasms with a survival rate similar to that of other aggressive functioning neuroendocrine pancreatic neoplasms like ACTH-secreting PanNETs associated with Cushing's syndrome.

References

1. Oberdorfer S (1907) Karzinoid tumoren des dünndarms. Frankfurt Z Pathol 1:426–429
2. Solcia E, Klöppel G, Sobin LH (eds) (2000) Histological typing of endocrine tumours. WHO International Histological Classification of Tumours, 2nd ed. Springer, Berlin
3. DeLellis RA (2001) The neuroendocrine system and its tumors: an overview. Am J Clin Pathol 115(suppl):S5–S16
4. Chetty R (2008) Requiem for the term "carcinoid tumour" in the gastrointestinal tract? Can J Gastroenterol 22:357–358
5. Osamura RY, Oberg K, Speel EJM et al (2004) Serotonin-secreting tumours. In: DeLellis RA, Lloyd RV, Heitz PU, Eng C (eds) World Health Organization classification of tumours. Pathology and genetics of tumours of endocrine organs. IARC Press, Lyon, p 198
6. Peart WS, Porter KA (1963) Carcinoid syndrome due to pancreatic-duct neoplasm secreting 5-hydroxytryotophan and 5-hydroxytryptamine. Lancet 1:239–243
7. van Der Sluys Veer J, Choufoer JC, Querido A et al (1964) Metastasising islet-cell tumour of the pancreas associated with hypoglycaemia and carcinoid syndrome. Lancet 1:1416–1419
8. Gloor VF, Pletscher A, Hardmeier T (1965) Metastasierendes inselzelladenom des pancreas mit 5-hydroxytryptamin und insulinproduktion. Schwaiz Med Wonchenschr 94:1476–1480
9. Dollinger MR, Ratner LH, Shamoian CA et al (1967) Carcinoid syndrome associated with pancreatic tumors. Arch Intern Med 120:575–580
10. Gordon DL, Chang M, Schwartz MA (1970) Carcinoid of the pancreas. Am J Med 51:412–415
11. Appleyard TN, Losowsky MS (1970) A pancreatic tumour with carcinoid syndrome and hypoglycaemia. Postgrad Med J 46:159–162
12. Persaud V, Walrond ER, Jamaica K (1971) Carcinoid tumor and cystadenoma of the pancreas. Arch Pathol 92:28–30
13. Patchefsky AS, Solit R, Phillips LD et al (1972) Hydroxyindole-producing tumors of the pancreas-carcinoid islet cell tumor and oat cell carcinoma. Ann Intern Med 77:53–61
14. Patchefsky AS, Gordon G, Harrer W et al (1974) Carcinoid tumor of the pancreas. Ultrastructural observations of a lymph node metastasis and comparison with bronchial carcinoid. Cancer 33:1349–1354
15. Greene JF, Doyle WF (1974) Pancreatic islet cell carcinoid: a highly malignant form of carcinoid tumor. J Surg Oncol 6:183–190
16. Pedinielli L, Quilichini R, Futsch D (1975) Les tumeurs pancréatiques à double composante endocrine et esocrine avec sindrome carcinoide. A propos de deux observations. Chirurgie 101:42–51
17. Wilander E, El-Salhy M, Willen R et al (1981) Immunocytochemistry and electron microscopy of an argentaffin endocrine tumour of the pancreas. Virchows Arch A 392:263–269
18. Prinz RA, Bermes EW, Chejfec G et al (1983) A serotonin and βHCG-producing islet cell carcinoma associated with focal nodular hyperplasia of the liver. J Surg Oncol 24:30–32
19. King MD, Young DG, Hann IM et al (1985) Carcinoid syndrome: an unusual cause of diarrhoea. Arch Dis Child 60:269–271
20. Ordonez NG, Manning JT, Raymond K (1985) Argentaffin endocrine carcinoma (carcinoid) of the pancreas with concomitant breast metastasis: an immunohistochemical and electron microscopic study. Hum Pathol 16:746–751
21. Lee CH, Ching KN, Lui WY et al (1986) Carcinoid tumor of the pancreas causing the diarrheogenic syndrome: report of a case combined with multiple endocrine neoplasia, type I. Surgery 99:123–129
22. Khorsand J, Katz RL, Savaraj N (1987) Malignant carcinoid of the pancreas: a cytologic, ultrastructural, and immunocytochemical study of a case diagnosed by fine-needle aspiration of a supraclavicular node metastasis. Diagn Cytopathol 3:222–227
23. Wilson RW, Gal AA, Cohen C et al (1987) Serotonin immunoreactivity in pancreatic endocrine neoplasms (carcinoid tumors). Mod Pathol 4:727–732
24. Carstens PHB, Cressman FK (1989) Malignant oncocytic carcinoid of the pancreas. Ultrastruct Pathol 13:69–75
25. Kanavaros P, Hoang C, Le Bodic MF et al (1990) Serotonin-producing pancreatic endocrine tumour.

Histological, ultrastructural and immunohistochemical study of a case. Histol Histopathol 5:325–328

26. Deixonne B, Duchene D, Eledjam JJ et al (1991) Carcinome endocrine pancréatique à cellules EC (carcinoide) responsable d'une diarrhée chronique. J Chir 128:415–418

27. Haq AU, Yook CR, Hiremath V et al (1992) Carcinoid syndrome in the absence of liver metastasis: a case report and review of the literature. Med Pediatr Oncol 20:221–223

28. Nagai E, Yamaguchi K, Hashimoto H et al (1992) Carcinoid tumor of the pancreas with obstructive pancreatitis. Am J Gastroenterol 87:361–364

29. Taidi C, Soyer P, Barge J et al (1993) Tumeur carcinoide primitive du pancréas. Aspect tomodensitométriques et écho-endoscopiques. J Radiol 74:347–350

30. Villanueva A, Pérez C, Llauger J et al (1994) Carcinoid tumors of the pancreas: CT findings. Abdom Imaging 19:221–224

31. Maurer CA, Glaser C, Reubi JC et al (1997) Carcinoid of the pancreas. Digestion 58:410–414

32. Mao C, El Attar A, Domenico DR et al (1998) Carcinoid tumors of the pancreas. Status report based on two cases and review of the world's literature. Int J Pancreatol 23:153–164

33. Hiller N, Berlowitz D, Fisher D et al (1998) Primary carcinoid tumor of the pancreas. Abdom Imaging 23:188–190

34. Migliori M, Tomassetti P, Lalli S et al (2002) Carcinoid of the pancreas. Pancreatology 2:163–166

35. Gunji N, Miyamoto H, Orii K et al (2003) Pancreatic carcinoid: transcatheter arterial chemoembolization of liver metastases. Hepatogastroenterology 50:2166–2168

36. Saint-Marc O, Cogliandolo A, Pozzo A et al (2004) A primary pancreatic carcinoid tumour with unusual clinical complaints: a case report. World J Surg Oncol 2:3

37. Outtas O, Barthet M, De Troyer J et al (2004) Panniculite nodulaire et tumeur carcinoide intracanalaire d'un pancreas divisum. Ann Dermatol Venereol 131:466–469

38. Kim HC, Park SI, Park SJ et al (2005) Pancreatic carcinoid tumor with obstructive pancreatitis: multislice helical CT appearance. Abdom Imaging 30:601–604

39. Bamba T, Kosugi SI, Kanda T et al (2007) Multiple carcinoids in the duodenum, pancreas and stomach accompanied with type A gastritis: a case report. World J Gastroenterol 13:2247–2249

40. Hamada Y, Nakayama Y, Maeshiro K et al (2009) Two cases of primary carcinoid tumor of the pancreas associated with marked stenosis of the main pancreatic duct. Pancreas 38:834–835

41. Shi C, Siegelman SS, Kawamoto S et al (2010) Pancreatic duct stenosis secondary to small endocrine neoplasms: a manifestation of serotonin production? Radiology 257:107–114

42. La Rosa S, Franzi F, Albarello L et al (2011) Serotonin-producing enterochromaffin cell tumors of the pancreas: clinicopathologic study of 15 cases and comparison with intestinal enterochromaffin cell tumors. Pancreas 40:883–895

43. Walter T, Hervieu V, Adham M et al (2011) Primary neuroendocrine tumors of the main pancreatic duct: a rare entity. Virchows Arch 458:537–546

44. Kawamoto S, Shi C, Hruban RH et al (2011) Small serotonin-producing neuroendocrine tumor of the pancreas associated with pancreatic duct obstruction. AJR Am J Roentgenol 197:W482–W888

45. McCall CM, Shi C, Klein AP et al (2012) Serotonin expression in pancreatic neuroendocrine tumors correlates with a trabecular histologic pattern and large duct involvement. Hum Pathol 43:1169–1176

46. Ogawa M, Kawaguchi Y, Maruno A et al (2012) Small serotonin-positive pancreatic endocrine tumors caused obstruction of the main pancreatic duct. World J Gastroenterol 18:6669–6673

47. Modlin IM, Lye KD, Kidd M (2003) A 5-decade analysis of 13,715 carcinoid tumors. Cancer 97:934–959

48. Modlin IM, Shapiro MD, Kidd M (2005) An analysis of rare carcinoid tumors: clarifying these clinical conundrums. World J Surg 29:92–101

49. Soga J (2005) Carcinoids of the pancreas. An analysis of 156 cases. Cancer 104:1180–1187

50. Rindi G, Falconi M, Klersy C et al (2012) TNM staging of neoplasms of the endocrine pancreas: results from a large international cohort study. J Natl Cancer Inst 104:764–777

51. Mancuso K, Kaye AD, Boudreaux JP et al (2011) Carcinoid syndrome and perioperative anesthetic considerations. J Clin Anesth 23:329–341

52. Soga J, Tazawa K (1971) Pathologic analysis of carcinoids. Histologic reevaluation of 62 cases. Cancer 28:990–998

53. La Rosa S, Chiaravalli AM, Capella C et al (1997) Immunohistochemical localization of acidic fibroblast growth factor in normal human enterochromaffin cells and related gastrointestinal tumours. Virchows Arch 430:117–124

54. La Rosa S, Uccella S, Capella C et al (1998) Localization of acidic fibroblast growth factor, fibroblast growth factor receptor-4, transforming growth factor-α, and epidermal growth factor receptor in human endocrine cells of the gut and related tumors: an immunohistochemical study. Appl Immunohistochem 6:199–208

55. La Rosa S, Uccella S, Capella C et al (2000) Localization of hepatocyte growth factor and its receptor met in endocrine cells and related tumors of the gut and pancreas: an immunohistochemical study. Endocr Pathol 11:315–329

56. Kidd M, Modlin I, Shapiro M et al (2007) CTGF, intestinal stellate cells and carcinoid fibrogenesis. World J Gastroenterol 13:5208–5216

57. Rindi G, Arnold R, Bosman FT et al (2010) Nomenclature and classification of neuroendocrine neoplasms of the digestive system. In: Bosman FT, Carneiro F, Hruban RH, Theise ND (eds) WHO classification of tumours of the digestive system. IARC Press, Lyon, pp 13–14

58. Löllgen RM, Hessman O, Szabo E et al (2001) Chromosome 18 deletions are common events in classical midgut carcinoid tumors. Int J Cancer 92:812–815
59. Kytola S, Hoog A, Norc B et al (2001) Comparative genomic hybridization identifies loss of 18q22-qte as an early and specific event in tumorigenesis of midgut carcinoids. Am J Pathol 158:1803–1808
60. Wang G, Yao JC, Worah S et al (2005) Comparison of genetic alterations in neuroendocrine tumors: frequent loss of chromosome 18 in ileal carcinoid tumors. Mod Pathol 18:1079–1087
61. Maragliano R, Vanoli A, Albarello L et al (2015) ACTH-secreting pancreatic neoplasms associated with Cushing's syndrome. Clinico-pathologic study of 11 cases and review of the literature. Am J Surg Pathol 39:374–382
62. Nikfarjam M, Warshaw AL, Axelrod L et al (2008) Improved contemporary surgical management of insulinomas: a 25-year experience at the Massachusetts General Hospital. Ann Surg 247:165–172
63. Weber HC, Venzon DJ, Lin JT et al (1995) Determinants of metastatic rate and survival in patients with Zollinger-Ellison syndrome: a prospective long-term study. Gastroenterology 108:1637–1649
64. Soga J, Yakuwa Y (1999) Somatostatinoma/inhibitory syndrome: a statistical evaluation of 173 reported cases as compared to other pancreatic endocrinomas. J Exp Clin Cancer Res 18:13–22

Pancreatic Neuroendocrine Tumors Producing GHRH, GH, Ghrelin, PTH, or PTHrP

Kai Duan, Shereen Ezzat, Sylvia L. Asa, and Ozgur Mete

15.1 Introduction

Pancreatic neuroendocrine tumors (PanNETs) encompass a heterogeneous group of neoplasms with distinct clinical, morphologic, and molecular features [1–5]. Approximately 9 % of these tumors give rise to specific functional syndromes, due to their ability to produce biologically active substances [6, 7]. With the exception of insulin- and gastrin-producing neuroendocrine tumors, the remainder of functioning pancreatic neuroendocrine neoplasms are currently termed "rare functioning pancreatic endocrine tumors," which include glucagon-, somatostatin-, vasoactive intestinal polypeptide-, corticotropin (ACTH)-, serotonin-, growth hormone-releasing hormone (GHRH)-, growth hormone (GH)-, ghrelin-, parathyroid hormone-related peptide (PTHrP)-, and parathyroid hormone (PTH)-producing tumors [3, 4]. Recognition of these rare neoplasms and their associated paraneoplastic syndromes carries

tremendous clinical importance, because they typically present with metastatic disease and are associated with poor patient outcome when the diagnosis is delayed [1–5, 8]. Over the last 2 years, some of the largest series of functioning GHRH- and PTHrP-producing tumors have been reported in the literature, providing much needed insight into the diagnostic and prognostic features of these exceptionally rare tumors [9, 10]. This chapter provides an update on the current knowledge of GHRH-, GH-, ghrelin-, PTHrP-, and PTH-producing pancreatic neuroendocrine tumors.

15.2 Historical Background

While the first case of functioning growth hormone-releasing hormone (*GHRH*)-*producing neuroendocrine tumor* may have been described as early as 1959 by Altmann and Schutz in an acromegalic patient who did not respond to pituitary irradiation but improved after resection of a bronchial neuroendocrine tumor, it was not until 1982 that two teams simultaneously isolated a peptide, known as growth hormone-releasing factor (GRF) or growth hormone-releasing hormone (GHRH), from pancreatic neuroendocrine tumors (Table 15.1) [9, 11–14]. The first team studied a 55-year-old French male, who had acromegaly without evidence of pituitary adenoma and a pancreatic tumor of 25 cm

K. Duan • S.L. Asa • O. Mete, MD (✉)
Department of Pathology, University Health Network, Toronto, ON, Canada

Department of Laboratory Medicine and Pathobiology, University of Toronto, 200 Elizabeth Street, 11th Floor, Toronto, ON M5G 2C4, Canada
e-mail: Ozgur.Mete2@uhn.ca

S. Ezzat
Department of Medicine, University Health Network and University of Toronto, Toronto, ON, Canada

S. La Rosa, F. Sessa (eds.), *Pancreatic Neuroendocrine Neoplasms: Practical Approach to Diagnosis, Classification, and Therapy*, DOI 10.1007/978-3-319-17235-4_15,
© Springer International Publishing Switzerland 2015

diameter, from which three peptides were identified: a main form of 44 amino acids (GHRH 1–44) and two reduced forms of 37 and 40 amino acids (GHRH 1–37 and GHRH 1–40) [12]. At the same time, a second team successfully isolated GHRH 1–40 from another pancreatic tumor in a 21-year-old acromegalic woman in the United States [13]. Both pancreatic GHRH 1–40 and GHRH 1–44 were subsequently found to be structurally similar to human hypothalamic GHRH. GHRH interacts with pituitary somatotroph cells via a G-protein-coupled receptor (GHRH-R) to regulate the release of growth hormone. The action of growth hormone is subsequently mediated by growth hormone receptors, which are expressed mainly in the liver but also in the cartilage, in the muscle, and ubiquitously throughout the body and induce the synthesis of peripheral insulin-like growth factor 1 (IGF-1) [15, 16]. While GHRH-producing tumors causing acromegaly are now well described in the literature, functioning *growth hormone (GH)-producing pancreatic neuroendocrine tumor* is exceptionally rare, with only a single case reported in 1985 by Melmed and colleagues [15–19].

In contrast to GH and GHRH, ghrelin is a more recent discovery in 1999 by Kojima et al. (Table 15.1) while searching for an endogenous ligand for the growth hormone secretagogue receptor (GHS-R) [20, 21]. Although initial studies localized this 28-amino acid peptide to the stomach, it was subsequently found in a wide range of normal and neoplastic tissues in the pancreas, small intestine, hypothalamus, pituitary, heart, lung, thyroid, adrenal, testis, prostate, and breast [22, 23]. In normal physiology, ghrelin is synthesized mainly in the gastrointestinal tract in response to the availability of nutrients; it exists in two forms, acylated and non-acylated, and acylation is mediated by the ghrelin O-acyltransferase (GOAT) enzyme discovered in 2008 [16, 22–24]. Acylated ghrelin has been shown to stimulate growth hormone release by binding growth hormone secretagogue receptor-1a (GHSR1a), which is widely expressed in the hypothalamic and pituitary regions [22–24]. Recent findings have also suggested that hypo-

thalamic mTOR signaling is responsible for the orexigenic effects of ghrelin [24]. In the context of pancreatic neuroendocrine tumors, the existence of a putative ghrelin syndrome has been proposed by Wang et al. in 2007 on the basis of body mass index preservation despite widely disseminated disease due to the orexigenic effect of extremely high levels of circulating ghrelin [5, 22–25]. However, this remains controversial, and only two cases of functioning *ghrelin-producing neuroendocrine tumors* ("ghrelinoma") have been reported (1 pancreatic ghrelinoma in 2003 and 1 gastric ghrelinoma in 2004; Tables 15.1 and 15.2) [22, 26–28].

While the existence of a parathyroid hormone (PTH)-like factor causing hypercalcemia may have been proposed as early as 1941 by Albright in a patient with renal cell carcinoma, this hypothesis was not clarified until 1987,

Table 15.1 Historical background of functioning GHRH-, GH-, ghrelin-, PTHrP-, and PTH-producing PanNETs

Year	Research	Investigators
1924	Isolation of PTH	Collip
1944	Isolation of GH	Li et al.
1982	Isolation of GHRH	Guillemin et al./ Rivier et al.[a]
	First report of functioning GHRH-producing PanNET	Guillemin et al./ Rivier et al.[a]
1985	First report of functioning GH-producing PanNET	Melmed et al.
1987	Isolation of PTHrP	Suva et al./Strewler et al./Burtis et al.[a]
1989	First report of functioning PTHrP-producing PanNET	Drucker et al.
1999	Isolation of ghrelin	Kojima et al.
2003	First report of functioning ghrelin-producing PanNET	Corbetta et al.
2006	First report of functioning PTH-producing PanNET	VanHouten et al.

Abbreviations: *GHRH* growth hormone-releasing hormone, *GH* growth hormone, *PTHrP* parathyroid hormone-related peptide, *PTH* parathyroid hormone, *PanNET* pancreatic neuroendocrine tumor
[a]Indicates simultaneous discovery

Table 15.2 Epidemiology of functioning GHRH-, GH-, ghrelin-, PTHrP-, and PTH-producing NETs

NET type	GHRH	GH	Ghrelin	PTHrP	PTH
Number of cases	~100	2	2	~40	<10
Tumor location	Pancreas (34), Lung (51), GI (7)	Pancreas (1)	Pancreas (1)	Pancreas (30), GI (3)	Pancreas (3)[a], Lung (3),
	Adrenal (2), Thymus (2), Pit (1)	Lung (1)	Stomach (1)	Thymus (1), Adrenal (2)	H&N (1), GI (1)
	Mediastinum (1), Unknown (1)	–	–	Lung (1), Cervix[b]	Ovary (1), Thyroid (1)
Age	Mean ~40 (range 14–77) years	Not defined[a]	Not defined[a]	50–60 years	Not defined[a]
Sex	60–65 % female	Not defined[a]	Not defined[a]	Male predominance[a]	Not defined[a]

Abbreviations: *GHRH* growth hormone-releasing hormone, *GH* growth hormone, *PTHrP* parathyroid hormone-related peptide, *PTH* parathyroid hormone, *NET* neuroendocrine tumor, H&N head and neck, *GI* gastrointestinal *Pit* pituitary
[a]Indicates scarce or conflicting data
[b]Indicates unclear incidence

when several investigators simultaneously isolated parathyroid hormone-related peptide (PTHrP) from cancer cells (Suva et al.; Strewler et al.; Burtis et al.; Table 15.1) [29–36]. PTHrP is now known to cause 80 % of cases of hypercalcemia associated with cancer (humoral hypercalcemia of malignancy) [37]. PTHrP is a polypeptide that has a significant structural homology with the amino terminus of parathyroid hormone (PTH), allowing them to bind to the same type 1 PTH/PTHrP receptor [10, 29, 33, 34, 38]. Both PTHrP and PTH stimulate osteoclast-mediated bone resorption, renal reabsorption of calcium and 1,25(OH)$_2$D synthesis which further contributes to a hypercalcemic state. Moreover, recent studies have shown that PTHrP serves a normal function in the bone, cartilage, skeletal and heart muscle, pancreas, and breast [10, 29]. Although hypercalcemia due to PTHrP production has been frequently described in the context of non-endocrine carcinomas, it is infrequently reported in neuroendocrine tumors, with the first confirmed pancreatic *PTHrP-producing tumor* in 1989 by Drucker and colleagues [35, 39–41]. Cases of hypercalcemia caused by ectopic parathyroid hormone (*PTH*)-*producing neuroendocrine tumors* are more scarce, with only a single immunohistochemically confirmed pancreatic case in 2006 by VanHouten and colleagues [36, 42].

15.3 Epidemiology

Although pancreatic neuroendocrine tumors are rare, recent data from the National Cancer Institute's Surveillance, Epidemiology, and End Results (SEER) program show a twofold increase in the incidence since the 1980s, likely due to advancements made in diagnostic techniques and increased awareness among physicians [3, 6]. While accurate epidemiological data is lacking, reports from 2003 to 2006 suggest an annual incidence of 0.43 per 100 000 people [6, 7]. PanNETs are divided into nonfunctioning (90.8 %) and functioning tumors (9 %), which include gastrin (4.2 %)-, insulin (2.5 %)-, glucagon (1.6 %)-, and vasoactive intestinal polypeptide (0.9 %)-producing tumors [7]. Functioning GHRH-, GH-, ghrelin-, PTHrP-, and PTH-producing PanNETs are exceedingly rare and represent less than 1 % of cases.

Since its discovery in 1982, at least a hundred cases of *GHRH-producing neuroendocrine tumors* causing ectopic acromegaly have been reported in the literature (Table 15.2) [11, 19]. With the exception of a recent large French series of 21 cases, most of them were case reports [9, 11]. A review by Borson-Chazot et al. reported these 21 new cases, in addition to 53 cases that they identified in the literature [11]. In this cohort, functioning GHRH-producing tumors were found primarily in the pancreas (34 %) and lung (53 %); although in the recent French series alone, GHRH-producing tumors were reported more frequently in the pancreas than in the lung (57 % and 33 %, respectively) [9, 11]. Origin in the gastrointestinal tract, adrenal, thymus, pituitary, and mediastinum has also been described [11, 19, 43]. The median age at diagnosis was 39 years (range, 14–77 years), and there may be a predilection for these tumors to arise in women (60 %) [11]. An association between pancreatic GHRH-producing tumors and multiple endocrine neoplasia type 1 syndrome (MEN1) was first reported in 1987 by Asa and colleagues [44]. Since then, *MEN1* gene mutation has been described in 19 out of 25 (76 %) tested pancreatic cases, raising the question whether MEN1 status should be investigated in all patients presenting with a functioning pancreatic GHRH-producing tumor [9, 11]. In contrast, cases of extrapituitary growth hormone (*GH*)-*producing neuroendocrine tumors* causing acromegaly are seldom reported, with only two cases in the literature (one pancreas and one lung; Table 15.2) [15–19]. One case of ectopic acromegaly purportedly caused by a GH-producing non-Hodgkin's lymphoma has also been described [45].

Functioning *ghrelin-producing neuroendocrine tumors* ("ghrelinomas") have been recently described, on the basis of a putative ghrelin syndrome, consisting of extremely high levels of circulating ghrelin and vague clinical symptoms, including body mass index preservation despite widely disseminated disease [22, 25]. These neoplasms are exceptionally rare, with only two cases (one pancreatic and one gastric ghrelinoma) reported in the literature (Table 15.2) [22, 26–28].

With recent advances made in diagnostic techniques, *PTHrP-producing neuroendocrine tumors* causing hypercalcemia are increasingly detected, with at least 40 cases reported in the literature (~30 of which are described in the pancreas; Table 15.2) [10, 37, 46]. In particular, hypercalcemia caused by small-cell carcinoma of the gynecologic tract (cervix, ovary) producing PTHrP is increasingly recognized, although the exact incidence remains unclear [47, 48]. Of

note, ovarian small-cell carcinomas of the pulmonary type should be distinguished from those of the hypercalcemic type, as the latter lacks neuroendocrine differentiation [47–49]. Additionally, PTHrP expression has been widely reported in normal and neoplastic endocrine tissue of various origins, including pituitary, thyroid, parathyroid, adrenal, gastrointestinal tract, lung, testis, ovary, and cervix [40]. In the largest and most recent series of 895 patients with gastroenteropancreatic neuroendocrine tumors, ten patients (1.1 %) had proven hypercalcemia and PTHrP overproduction [10]. Nine of the ten functioning PTHrP-producing neuroendocrine tumors occurred in the pancreas (90 %) [10]. The median age at diagnosis was 50.4 years (range, 38.3–61.1 years) and a slight male predominance was noted [10]. In another series of four pancreatic PTHrP-producing tumors, the mean age at diagnosis was 52 years (range, 49–54 years), and three of the four patients were male [33]. In both series, pancreatic PTHrP-producing tumors were reported with metastatic disease at the time of diagnosis [10, 33]. These recent data appear to be somewhat in contrast with previous case reports and a series of five pancreatic PTHrP-producing tumors by Srirajaskanthan et al. in which the mean age of presentation was 38.6 years (range, 25–64 years), a female predominance was observed, and ~60 % of the patients had metastases on presentation [34]. Two cases of PTHrP-producing pancreatic tumors, with concomitant MEN1 syndrome and primary hyperparathyroidism, have been reported [34]. Hypercalcemia secondary to a functioning *PTH-producing extra-parathyroid neuroendocrine tumor* is exceptionally rare with less than ten cases reported in the literature, three of which are described in the pancreas (Table 15.2) [36, 42, 50]. However, their existence remains controversial because most cases were not confirmed biochemically with elevated PTH in the context of normal/decreased PTHrP serum levels, and only a single pancreatic case was confirmed by immunohistochemistry, in a patient presenting with concomitantly elevated PTH and PTHrP serum levels [36, 42, 50].

15.4 Diagnosis

Accurate diagnosis and subtyping of pancreatic neuroendocrine tumors producing GHRH, GH, ghrelin, PTHrP, or PTH require thorough integration of clinical, biochemical, imaging, pathologic, and molecular findings [1–6]. Given the subtle features of hormone excess that typically require months to years to become clinically florid, the diagnosis of these rare functioning tumors is usually delayed. In the past, most cases only became evident when the patient underwent investigations for local symptoms (abdominal pain, weight loss, jaundice, nausea, vomiting, and diarrhea) due to advanced tumor growth or metastatic disease [1–6, 8]. However, with recent advancement made in diagnostic techniques, including general neuroendocrine markers (e.g., chromogranins), tumor-specific serum biomarkers (e.g., hormones), and functional imaging modalities (e.g., octreotide scintigraphy), these neoplasms are increasingly detected incidentally for reasons unrelated to pancreatic disease, resulting in earlier diagnosis [1–6, 8, 51–53]. This section will focus on the preoperative (clinical, biochemical, radiologic) features of pancreatic tumors that produce GHRH, GH, ghrelin, PTHrP, or PTH.

15.4.1 Pancreatic Neuroendocrine Neoplasms Causing Ectopic Acromegaly

Functioning *GHRH- and GH-producing pancreatic neuroendocrine tumors* represent <1 % of cases of acromegaly, giving rise to a syndrome known as ectopic or extrapituitary acromegaly [8, 9, 11, 19]. From a clinical perspective, the overt acromegalic features associated with these tumors are indistinguishable from those of pituitary-dependent or classical acromegaly; patients exhibit acral overgrowth, soft tissue swelling, arthralgia, jaw prognathism, fasting hyperglycemia, hyperhidrosis, osteoarthritis, frontal bone bossing, diabetes mellitus, and hypertension [9, 11, 16, 19]. As is the case with

pituitary disease, the acromegalic features can be subtle and insidious, leading to a delay in diagnosis of 5–6 years from retrospective recognition of onset of symptoms [1–4, 8, 54]. Once acromegaly is suspected clinically, the diagnosis is confirmed biochemically on the basis of elevated insulin-like growth factor 1 (IGF-1), as well as the lack of suppression of GH during oral glucose tolerance testing (Table 15.3) [1, 9, 11, 15]. However, confirmation of an ectopic source requires clinical acumen, and unfortunately, many patients are only diagnosed after pituitary surgery fails to identify a pituitary adenoma, and instead, pituitary hyperplasia is diagnosed. The diagnosis can be made on MRI of the pituitary, which shows diffuse enlargement with no enhancing rim of normal adenohypophysis [55–57]. In some cases, the distinction between hyperplastic and adenomatous pituitary lesions can be challenging clinically and radiologically [9, 11, 19]. When the possibility of an ectopic source of GHRH is suspected, measurement of plasma GHRH using a threshold of 250–300 ng/L has been shown to have excellent specificity for the diagnosis of a GHRH-producing tumor and is also a biomarker for follow-up of patients after treatment [9, 11]. A recent review of 55 cases of functioning GHRH-producing tumors reported a median GHRH value of 860 ng/L (range 100–145,000 ng/L), with only three patients between 100 and 250 ng/L [11]. Lack of GH response to exogenous GHRH 1–44 has been proposed by some investigators as a mean to distinguish GHRH excess from a primary GH-producing pituitary tumor, as there is usually no response in ectopic acromegaly [11]. Moreover, an elevation of serum GH after thyrotropin releasing hormone (TRH) stimulation test has been described in ectopic acromegaly [19]. Elevated serum prolactin levels have also been frequently reported (up to 70 % in some studies), and in cases where pituitary pathology has been carefully investigated, this is attributed to mammosomatotroph hyperplasia, consistent with the findings in mice overexpressing GHRH [1, 9, 11, 58, 59]. Furthermore, GHRH-producing pancreatic tumors occasionally

Table 15.3 Clinical, biochemical, and radiologic features of functioning GHRH-, GH-, ghrelin-, PTHrP-, and PTH-producing PanNETs

PanNET type	GHRH	GH	Ghrelin	PTHrP	PTH
Clinical features	Acromegaly: acral and soft tissue overgrowth, skin thickening, macrognathia, swollen and enlarged hands/feet		Putative ghrelin syndrome: BMI preservation despite disseminated disease	Hypercalcemia of malignancy: anorexia, dehydration, nausea, vomiting, poor appetite, obstipation, polyuria, polydipsia, fatigue, muscle weakness, palpitations, cerebral symptoms, coma (late), renal failure (late)	
Biochemical features	Elevated IGF-1, elevated GH after OGTT, elevated prolactin levels, plasma GHRH >300 pg/mL	Elevated IGF-1, elevated GH after OGTT, elevated prolactin levels, plasma GHRH <100 pg/mL	Extremely elevated ghrelin levels, normal IGF-1 and normal GH levels	Hypercalcemia, hypophosphatemia, markedly elevated PTHrP, low PTH, low/normal 1,25(OH)2D levels	Hypercalcemia, hypophosphatemia, low/normal PTHrP, markedly elevated PTH and elevated 1,25(OH)2D levels
Radiologic features	Pituitary hyperplasia on MRI	Not defined[a]	Not defined[a]	PT imaging[b] and Pit MRI[b] usually within normal limits	
Tumor size	Median 5.5 (1–25) cm	~8 cm[a]	Not defined[a]	4–11 cm[a]	Not defined[a]
Metastases	Liver (~65 %)	Not defined[a]	Liver (100 %)	Liver (>90 %)[a]	Liver (100 %)[a]

Abbreviations: *GHRH* growth hormone-releasing hormone, *GH* growth hormone, *PTHrP* parathyroid hormone-related peptide, *PTH* parathyroid hormone, *PanNET* pancreatic neuroendocrine tumor, *IGF-1* insulin-like growth factor 1, *OGTT* oral glucose tolerance test, *MRI* magnetic resonance imaging, *PT* parathyroid, *Pit* pituitary
[a]Indicates scarce or controversial data
[b]In appropriate clinical context

secrete multiple hormones (gastrin, ACTH), leading to concomitant clinical syndromes (Zollinger-Ellison or Cushing's syndrome) [1, 2, 8, 11, 54]. Radiographically, GHRH-producing tumors are typically large and easy to localize on computed tomography (CT) or somatostatin receptor scintigraphy, with a reported median diameter of 5.5 cm (range, 1–25 cm), and over 65 % of cases presented with liver metastases in recent series [9, 11].

A single case of *GH-producing pancreatic neuroendocrine neoplasm* has been reported in a 63-year-old man, presenting with classic features of acromegaly and elevated serum GH and IGF-1 levels; CT scan of the pituitary was unremarkable, while that of the abdomen revealed a 8.1×6.6 cm mass in the head of the pancreas [17, 18]. Dynamic GH responses confirmed the functional autonomy of the GH-producing pancreatic tumor: serial GH sampling showed slight fluctuations with no discrete episodes of absent GH secretion, which is unlike pituitary acromegaly [18].

15.4.2 Pancreatic Neuroendocrine Tumors Causing Excess Ghrelin

Ghrelin-producing pancreatic neuroendocrine tumors are nearly impossible to detect on clinical grounds alone, due to the absence of distinct functional symptoms. Recently, a putative ghrelin syndrome has been proposed on the basis of vague clinical symptoms with body mass index (BMI) preservation despite widely disseminated disease, likely secondary to the orexigenic effect of extremely elevated serum ghrelin levels [5, 22–25]. A single case of ghrelin-producing pancreatic tumor was described in a 66-year-old woman, with a BMI of 29.9 kg/m [2], who was referred initially for an episode of intestinal subocclusion [27]. On further investigations, a pancreatic tumor with multiple hepatic metastases was detected on imaging; her circulating ghrelin levels were reported at 12 000 pM, with normal GH and IGF-1 serum levels (Table 15.3) [27]. A second case of gastric ghrelinoma was described in a 46-year-old Caucasian male, referred for occult gastrointestinal bleeding [26]. Similar to the first case, no evidence of acromegaly was found; the patient had a circulating ghrelin levels of 2,100 ug/L, with normal GH and IGF-1 serum levels [26]. Despite advanced disease with radiographic evidence of liver metastases, the patient maintained a stable BMI of 32 kg/m^2, and his appetite remained good even at his last follow-up appointment 1 year after diagnosis [26]. Recently, Walter and colleagues described three additional cases of metastatic neuroendocrine tumors (one pancreas, one rectum, one gallbladder) with elevated circulating ghrelin levels (respectively, 49 028, 63 711, and 101 996 pg/mL) [28]. However, no evidence of clinical or biological effects of ghrelin was reported in these cases [28].

15.4.3 Pancreatic Neuroendocrine Neoplasms Causing Hypercalcemia

Functioning *PTHrP- and PTH-producing pancreatic neuroendocrine tumors* give rise to hypercalcemia of malignancy, a paraneoplastic syndrome that encompasses a constellation of symptoms including anorexia, dehydration, nausea, vomiting, poor appetite, obstipation, polyuria, polydipsia, fatigue, muscle weakness, cerebral symptoms, and palpitations (Table 15.3) [10, 33, 34, 37]. In advanced stages, malignant hypercalcemia can lead to progressive mental impairment and renal failure [36]. The majority of cases (80 %) are attributed to PTHrP overproduction, causing a clinical syndrome known as humoral hypercalcemia of malignancy [36]. PTHrP-producing neuroendocrine tumors usually have an insidious onset, with hypercalcemia seen in late stages of the disease [4, 10, 33, 34, 38]. As a result, almost all cases of PTHrP-producing pancreatic tumors presenting with hypercalcemia have metastatic disease at the time of diagnosis [1, 4, 10, 33, 34, 38]. Given its non-specific clinical findings, hypercalcemia is typically detected on routine biochemical testing. The diagnosis of humoral hypercalcemia of malignancy is typically confirmed biochemically in conjunction with radiographic findings of malignancy, by demonstrating elevated serum calcium, ionized calcium, and PTHrP levels, as well as low PTH levels [10, 33, 37, 38]. In patients with elevated PTH serum levels, primary hyperparathyroidism as part of MEN1 syndrome should be considered [10, 34, 37]. Serum 25(OH) D and 1,25(OH)$_2$D levels, bone scan, skeletal survey, and parathyroid imaging may also be indicated to exclude alternative etiologies of hypercalcemia when appropriate [10, 36, 37].

Over the last 2 years, some of the largest series of clinically *functioning PTHrP-producing pancreatic neuroendocrine tumors* were described [10, 33]. In a recent study of ten PTHrP-producing neuroendocrine tumors (nine pancreatic and one unknown primary), all cases presented with metastases (liver 100 %, lymph nodes 40 %, bone 10 %); eight patients (80 %) had synchronous PTHrP secretion, while two patients (20 %) developed hypercalcemia later in their disease [10]. In another series of six PTHrP-producing tumors (four pancreatic), a single case presented with hypercalcemia, while others developed symptomatic hypercalcemia between 4 months and 6 years after diagnosis of the neuroendocrine tumor [33]. On imaging, PTHrP-producing tumors are usually large at the time of diagnosis, ranging from 4 to 11 cm in size, and all cases presented with liver metastases [33]. One case had concomitant somatostatin 160 pg/mL (normal, 10–22 pg/mL) and pancreatic polypeptide 3,870 pg/ml (<270 pg/ml) production, while another case had concomitant glucagon 363 ng/L (normal, 40–130 ng/L) production [33]. These recent findings appear to be in contrast with previous reports, where metastatic disease was only detected in three cases (50 %) at the time of diagnosis [34]. Plurihormonal production in PTHrP-producing pancreatic tumors was also reported in older series, with glucagon, somatostatin, and gastrin co-secreted in three different cases [34]. The clinical, biochemical, and radiological features of ectopic *PTH-producing neuroendocrine tumors* are quite similar to those reported in PTHrP-producing tumors, with the exception of elevated serum PTH and 1,25(OH)$_2$D levels and decreased serum PTHrP levels seen in cases of PTH-producing tumors (Table 15.3) [36, 42, 50].

15.5 Morphology

In conjunction with clinical, biochemical, and radiological investigations, pathologic evaluation is critical to grade, stage, prognosticate, and confirm the functional status of pancreatic neuroendocrine neoplasms [1–6]. Histopathologic examination should include immunohistochemistry with general neuroendocrine markers (chromogranin A, synaptophysin), cytokeratin (CAM5.2), common hormones (insulin, glucagon, somatostatin, gastrin, pancreatic polypeptide, peptide YY, glucagon-like peptide, serotonin, vasoactive intestinal peptide, and alpha-subunit), and specific hormone markers (GHRH, GH, ghrelin, PTHrP, and PTH) depending on the clinical syndrome [1–6]. In all cases, assessment of the mitotic activity and Ki-67 proliferation index is required to grade tumors according to the 2010 WHO classification system and guide treatment decision making [2–6].

Since most cases of clinically functioning pancreatic neoplasms producing GHRH, GH, ghrelin, PTHrP, or PTH are metastatic at the time of diagnosis and therefore not appropriate for surgery, the pathological assessment is often performed on biopsy specimens (instead of surgical resection specimens) either from liver metastases or from the primary tumor itself (endoscopic ultrasound-guided fine needle aspiration) [1–6, 10, 11, 26, 27, 36]. Consequently, the gross and microscopic findings of these rare tumors have not been extensively reported in the literature [1, 2]. This section will focus on the morphologic and ancillary features of pancreatic neuroendocrine neoplasms that produce GHRH, GH, ghrelin, PTHrP, or PTH.

15.5.1 Pancreatic Neuroendocrine Neoplasms Causing Ectopic Acromegaly

In ectopic acromegaly secondary to *GHRH-producing tumors*, the histological hallmark in the pituitary is somatotroph hyperplasia [11, 19, 54–57, 60–66]. Histologically, the hyperplastic cells are described as acidophilic densely granulated somatotrophs with prominent well-developed Golgi complex [54]. Secretory granules are often abundant and spherical, measuring 200–600 nm, although larger granules have been noted [54, 61]. The reticulin fiber network is irregularly expanded without any breakdown, and cases of pituitaries obtained from patients with ectopic GHRH production have been reported to show a morphological continuum from hyperplasia to areas of neoplastic transformation with evidence of reticulin framework disruption [54, 61–63]. Functioning GHRH-producing pancreatic neuroendocrine neoplasms are typically large in size, with a median diameter of 7 cm (range, 4–8 cm), and arise commonly in the tail of the pancreas [9, 11, 54, 61]. Previous reports have suggested that these tumors did not have a tendency to metastasize [54, 61]; however, in a recent French series of 12 pancreatic GHRH-producing tumors, which is the largest series up to date, 67 % of the cases presented with liver metastases at the time of diagnosis [9]. No relationship has been described between tumor size, duration of acromegaly, and plasma GHRH levels [54]. Histologically, tumors producing GHRH often have a trabecular, whorl-like meningotheliomatous, or "nested" growth patterns (Fig. 15.1) [2, 55]. GHRH-producing cells typically contain numerous small secretory cytoplasmic granules, ranging from 100 to 250 nm in diameter [54, 61]. Most series describe these neuroendocrine tumors as being "well differentiated," although grading with mitotic and Ki-67 proliferation index has not been consistently reported [9, 11, 54, 61]. Immunohistochemistry allows confirmation of the functional status of the pancreatic neoplasm, by demonstrating GHRH immunoreactivity in tumor cells (Fig. 15.1) [9, 11, 19, 54]. However, this should be correlated with clinical and biochemical findings, since GHRH expression has been reported in up to

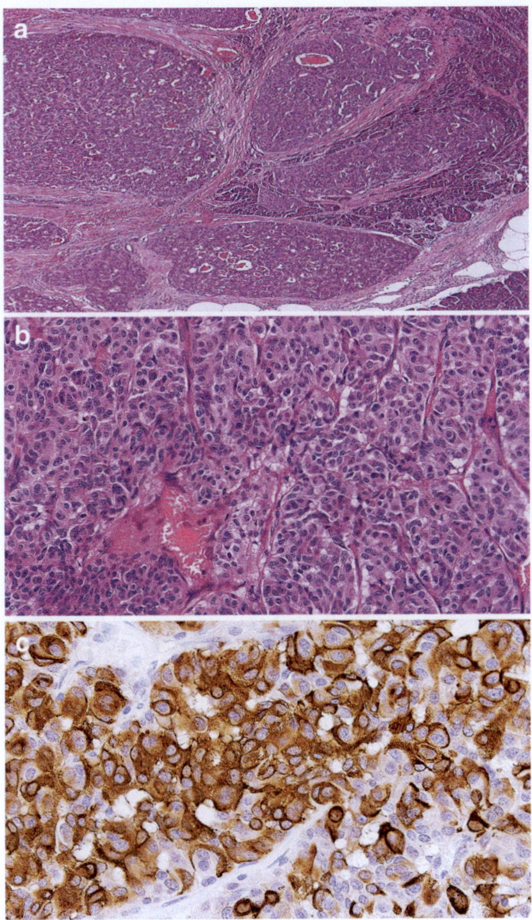

Fig. 15.1 Growth hormone-releasing hormone (*GHRH*)-producing well-differentiated pancreatic neuroendocrine tumor associated with multiple endocrine neoplasia-1 syndrome. In patients with MEN1 syndrome, multifocal neuroendocrine tumors are typically identified in the background of islet dysplasia and endocrine microadenomatosis (also known as well-differentiated pancreatic neuroendocrine microtumors) (**a**). Histologically, GHRH-producing neuroendocrine tumors often have a trabecular, whorl-like, or nested growth patterns (**b**). Immunohistochemistry allows confirmation of the functional status of the pancreatic neoplasm, by demonstrating GHRH immunoreactivity in tumor cells (**c**)

27 % of all pancreatic neuroendocrine tumors [11]. In the context of MEN1 syndrome, multifocal GHRH-producing neuroendocrine tumors have been described in the pancreas (Fig. 15.1) [54, 60, 61, 67]. Moreover, immunohistochemistry often demonstrates the expression of other peptides, including gastrin, gastrin-releasing peptide, calcitonin, pancreatic polypeptide, vasoactive intestinal polypeptide, glucagon, and insulin,

confirming the plurihormonal nature of GHRH-producing tumors [11, 54, 61].

A single case of *GH-producing pancreatic neuroendocrine* tumor causing acromegaly was reported, measuring 8.1 cm in size and located in the head of the pancreas [17, 18]. In vitro analysis of tumor tissue showed GH immunoreactivity, GH synthesis, and secretion, as well as expression of human GH mRNA [17, 18].

15.5.2 Pancreatic Neuroendocrine Tumors Causing Excess Ghrelin

Although pancreatic neuroendocrine tumors are commonly found to express ghrelin immunohistochemically (25–81 %) (Fig. 15.2), only a single case of a *metastatic pancreatic ghrelinoma* has been reported [22, 27]. In this unique case, pathologic evaluation was performed on samples obtained from the liver, lymph nodes, and peritoneal metastases [27]. Immunohistochemical staining for ghrelin, performed on metastatic peritoneal lesions, showed intense, focal cytoplasmic positivity in half of the neoplastic cells [27]. No additional information on the gross or microscopic findings of this tumor was provided in this isolated report [27]. In another report of gastric ghrelinoma, the tumor cells were described as small to intermediate size, arranged mainly in a nesting and irregular trabecular pattern with varying amount of stroma [26]. Nuclei were relatively uniform, and no mitosis was seen. On immunohistochemistry, half of the tumor cells showed chromogranin A and synaptic vesicle protein 2 immunoreactivity, while all the cells expressed synaptophysin and ghrelin [26]. Proliferation index with Ki-67 staining was approximately 12 % in this case [26].

15.5.3 Pancreatic Neuroendocrine Neoplasms Causing Hypercalcemia

The morphologic features of clinically functioning *PTHrP-producing pancreatic neuroendocrine tumors* are seldom reported. PTHrP production is

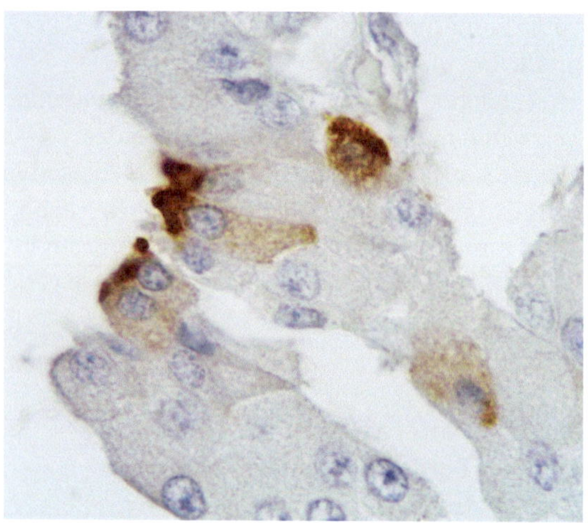

Fig. 15.2 Ghrelin-producing pancreatic neuroendocrine tumor. Immunohistochemically, pancreatic neuroendocrine tumors have been reported to express variably ghrelin in addition to other hormones. This photomicrograph provided by Dr. Stefano La Rosa illustrates focal ghrelin positivity in a vasoactive intestinal peptide (*VIP*)-producing pancreatic neuroendocrine tumor. While the identification of focal ghrelin immunoreactivity needs to be correlated with serum ghrelin levels, it is nearly impossible to detect a ghrelin-producing neuroendocrine tumor based on clinical grounds alone, due to the absence of distinct functional symptoms

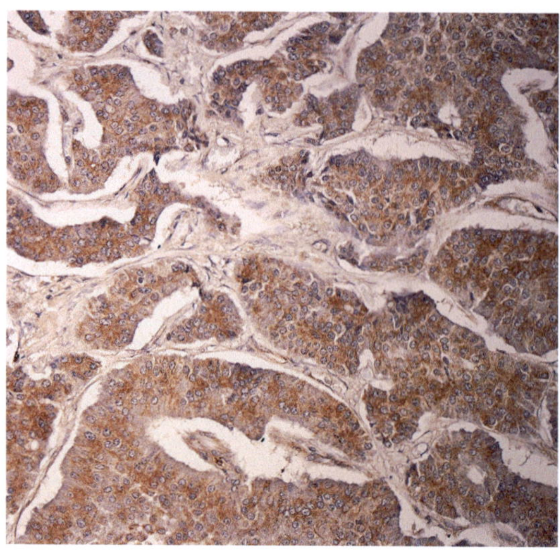

Fig. 15.3 Parathyroid hormone-related peptide (*PTHrP*)-producing pancreatic neuroendocrine tumor. PTHrP immunostain should always be interpreted in the context of biochemically proven elevated plasma PTHrP, ionized calcium, and suppressed PTH levels. A case of pancreatic neuroendocrine tumor presenting with hypercalcemia and PTHrP reactivity is illustrated

typically confirmed by showing PTHrP immunostain positivity in neuroendocrine tumor cells. Given the fact that PTHrP expression has been reported in over 80 % of nonfunctioning PanNETs, PTHrP immunostain should always be interpreted in the context of biochemically proven elevated plasma PTHrP, ionized calcium, and suppressed PTH levels (Fig. 15.3) [1, 5, 10, 33, 34, 38–40]. In a recent series of nine PTHrP-producing PanNETs, grading was reported in five cases: four were classified as well differentiated (grade 1, 80 %) and one was classified as poorly differentiated (grade 3, 20 %) [10]. All cases presented with metastases: liver (100 %), lymph nodes (44 %), and bone (11 %) [10]. An isolated report of metastatic PTHrP-producing PanNET causing metabolic bone disease, i.e., brown tumors, has also been described [38]. In another series of four metastatic pancreatic PTHrP-producing tumors, two cases were classified as grade 1, and two cases were classified as grade 2 [33]. In a third series of five PTHrP-producing pancreatic tumors, all of the tumors were classified as low-grade, well-differentiated pancreatic neuroendocrine carcinoma

with low mitotic rate (<2/10 high-power fields); Ki67 proliferation index was performed in four of five cases and varied between 1 and 10 % [34].

Only three cases of functioning *PTH-producing pancreatic neuroendocrine tumors* have been reported, presenting with metastatic disease at the time of diagnosis [36, 42, 50]. In all three cases, pathologic evaluation was performed on biopsy specimens of liver metastases, which revealed poorly differentiated neuroendocrine carcinomas of small-cell type in two cases and large-cell type in one case [36, 42, 50]. Only a single case was shown to have positive PTH immunostaining [42]. The distinction of PTH-producing neuroendocrine tumor from metastatic parathyroid carcinoma requires additional testing of the tumor for transcription factors that are commonly expressed in parathyroid neoplasms including GCM2 and GATA3 [68, 69].

15.6 Prognosis

The prognosis of pancreatic neuroendocrine neoplasms producing clinically detectable GHRH, GH, ghrelin, PTHrP, or PTH can be quite variable but tends to be quite poor when metastatic disease is present at the time of diagnosis, making them frequently ineligible for curative surgical intervention [1–6, 10, 11, 26, 27, 36]. Recently, several large series have reported treatment responses of these rare functioning pancreatic neuroendocrine tumors [9, 10, 32].

15.6.1 Pancreatic Neuroendocrine Neoplasms Causing Ectopic Acromegaly

Functioning *GHRH-producing neuroendocrine tumors* present with metastatic disease in more than 50 % of cases, but prognosis remains favorable in recent studies [11]. In the largest series, reported in 2012 by Garby et al., 66.6 % (8 of 12) of cases of pancreatic GHRH-producing tumors had metastasized at the time of diagnosis [9]. After a median follow-up of 5 years, 83 % of patients were alive [9]. Surgical management was feasible in 7 of 12 cases (58 %), and 5 cases were considered in remission after surgical intervention [9]. This is in keeping with the natural history of PanNETs, with cumulative survival, depending on grade and stage, of approximately 83 % at 5 years and 74 % at 10 years in the literature [9–11, 70]. In this series and in a subsequent review by Borson-Chazot et al., surgical resection of the primary tumor and, when feasible, of the metastases was shown to have the highest chance of inducing prolonged disease remission, with most patients achieving undetectable plasma GHRH levels postoperatively (<30 ng/L) [9, 11]. When complete surgical resection is not feasible because of extensive metastatic spread, somatostatin analog therapy (SSA) is recommended [9, 11]. Although somatostatin analog therapy had no significant effect on the tumor size, it led to IGF-1 level normalization in most cases, which is important in itself given the potential metabolic complications of acromegaly [9, 11]. Moreover, GHRH levels remained high (>250 ng/L) despite a median reduction of 61 % of IGF-1 levels after SSA therapy [9]. This observation, in concordance with the literature, illustrates a predominant action of somatostatin analogs on pituitary somatotrophs and on hepatic/ peripheral GH/IGF action [71, 72], with less potent direct influence on the GHRH-producing tumor [9, 11]. Progressive metastatic disease is treated with conventional chemotherapy, surgical debulking, or chemoembolization of liver metastases [11]. Plasma GHRH has been shown to accurately predict the likelihood of remission or recurrence after treatment and has been proposed as a monitoring tool [9, 11].

Ectopic acromegaly secondary to a *GH-producing pancreatic neuroendocrine tumor* was reported in one patient, who presented with localized disease at the time of diagnosis and achieved transient disease remission after surgical resection of the tumor [17, 18]. Unfortunately, the patient relapsed a year later with intraperitoneal metastases [18]. Treatment with combined dopaminergic and somatostatin analog was initiated but did not sustain GH suppression [18]. Consecutive courses of chemotherapy with streptozocin and 5-fluorouracil, doxorubicin, and dacarbazine were attempted unsuccessfully. The patient subsequently died 3 years after the initial diagnosis [18].

15.6.2 Pancreatic Neuroendocrine Tumors Causing Excess Ghrelin

A single case of *ghrelin-producing pancreatic neuroendocrine tumor* was reported as a ghrelinoma, with liver metastases at the time of presentation [27]. The patient underwent chemotherapy (epirubicin, 5-fluorouracil, dacarbazine), leading to decreased levels of ghrelin from 12 000 to 6 600 pM, without change in chromogranin A and pancreatic polypeptide serum levels [27]. The patient died 28 months after diagnosis of the tumor [27].

15.6.3 Pancreatic Neuroendocrine Neoplasms Causing Hypercalcemia

Pancreatic neuroendocrine neoplasms causing hypercalcemia present almost exclusively with metastatic disease at the time of diagnosis [1, 5,

10, 33, 36, 38]. Acute management is focused on lowering calcium levels, while long-term control can only be achieved by targeting the primary tumor and inhibiting PTHrP release [10, 33–37]. Data on the treatment response of *PTHrP-producing pancreatic neuroendocrine tumors* remains limited, given the rarity of this tumor. Recently, Kamp and colleagues published the largest single-center case series of functioning PTHrP-producing pancreatic tumors with a median follow-up of 57.2 months [10]. The median survival after the diagnosis of PTHrP overproduction was 52.2 months [10]. The estimated 5- and 10-year survival of patients with PTHrP-producing pancreatic tumors were 70 % and <40 %, respectively, which is worse than the cumulative survival of approximately 83 % at 5 years and 74 % at 10 years for PanNETs reported in the literature [10, 70]. Although rarely feasible, resection of the primary tumor and its metastases should be undertaken and has been shown to result in prolonged disease remission, varying from 2 to 3 years in isolated cases [10, 34]. Other surgical interventions, such as hepatic artery embolization and ethanol injection of liver metastases, showed limited effectiveness [10]. In the largest series of PTHrP-producing pancreatic tumors, the most successful treatment modalities are somatostatin analog (SSA) and peptide receptor radiotherapy (PRRT) using radiolabeled somatostatin analogs [10, 33, 34]. In seven of ten patients (70 %), somatostatin analog (SSA) treatment resulted in a temporary normalization of serum calcium levels, with long-term response observed in two patients (up to 35.2 months) [10]. Peptide receptor radiotherapy (PRRT) with radiolabeled SSAs induced long-term responses ranging from 9.0 to 49.0 months in four of six patients [10]. Chemotherapy has been shown to have response rates varying from 35 % to 65 % in pancreatic neuroendocrine tumors [34]. Other treatment modalities, such as debulking surgery to treat hypercalcemia and liver transplantation for patients with metastases confined to the liver, have been reported with variable response rates, although data on this topic remains scarce [34].

The prognosis of *PTH-producing pancreatic neuroendocrine neoplasms* remains unclear. In all three cases reported up to date, the patients presented with metastatic disease at the time of diagnosis [36, 42, 50]. Chemotherapy (cisplatinum and etoposide) was initiated in one patient with good response [36]. However, the treatment was stopped at the patient's request after six cycles, and the disease recurred 8 months later. Despite resuming chemotherapy, the patient died 15 months after diagnosis [36]. In a second case, the patient died from multiorgan failure several days after admission for hypercalcemic crisis, despite vigorous treatment with bisphosphonates, calcitonin, and forced saline diuresis [42]. A third case was treated with chemotherapy (cyclophosphamide, adriamycin, and etoposide) with good response, although long-term follow-up data was not provided [50].

References

1. Jensen R (2009) Endocrine neoplasms of the pancreas. In: Yamada T, Alpers DH, Kalloo AN et al (eds) Textbook of gastroenterology, 5th edn. Wiley-Blackwell, Oxford, pp 1875–1920
2. La Rosa S, Furlan D, Sessa F, Capella C (2010) The endocrine pancreas. In: Lloyd R (ed) Endocrine pathology: differential diagnosis and molecular advances. Springer, New York, pp 367–413
3. Tsolakis A, Kanakis G (2014) Pancreatic neuroendocrine tumors. In: Islam S (ed) Islets of langerhans, 2nd ed. Springer Netherlands, pp 1–29
4. O'Toole D, Salazar R, Falconi M et al (2006) Rare functioning pancreatic endocrine tumors. Neuroendocrinology 84(3):189–195
5. Ito T, Igarashi H, Jensen RT (2012) Pancreatic neuroendocrine tumors: clinical features, diagnosis and medical treatment: advances. Best Pract Res Clin Gastroenterol 26(6):737–753
6. Sadaria MR, Hruban RH, Edil BH (2013) Advancements in pancreatic neuroendocrine tumors. Expert Rev Gastroenterol Hepatol 7(5):477–490
7. Halfdanarson TR, Rabe KG, Rubin J, Petersen GM (2008) Pancreatic neuroendocrine tumors (PNETs): incidence, prognosis and recent trend toward improved survival. Ann Oncol 19(10):1727–1733
8. Kaltsas G, Androulakis II, De Herder WW, Grossman AB (2010) Paraneoplastic syndromes secondary to neuroendocrine tumours. Endocr Relat Cancer 17(3):R173–R193
9. Garby L, Caron P, Claustrat F et al (2012) Clinical characteristics and outcome of acromegaly induced by ectopic secretion of growth hormone-releasing hormone (GHRH): a French nationwide series of 21 cases. J Clin Endocrinol Metab 97(6):2093–2104

10. Kamp K, Feelders RA, Van Adrichem RC et al (2014) Parathyroid hormone-related peptide (PTHrP) secretion by gastroenteropancreatic neuroendocrine tumors (GEP-NETs): clinical features, diagnosis, management, and follow-up. J Clin Endocrinol Metab 99(9):3060–3069

11. Borson-Chazot F, Garby L, Raverot G et al (2012) Acromegaly induced by ectopic secretion of GHRH: a review 30 years after GHRH discovery. Ann Endocrinol (Paris) 73(6):497–502

12. Guillemin R, Brazeau P, Böhlen P, Esch F, Ling N, Wehrenberg WB (1982) Growth hormone-releasing factor from a human pancreatic tumor that caused acromegaly. Science 218(4572):585–587

13. Rivier J, Spiess J, Thorner M, Vale W (1982) Characterization of a growth hormone-releasing factor from a human pancreatic islet tumour. Nature 300(5889):276–278

14. Kovacs K, Ryan N, Horvath E et al (1984) Somatoliberinoma: morphologic characteristics. Arch Pathol Lab Med 108(5):355–356

15. Katznelson L, Laws ER, Melmed S et al (2014) Acromegaly: an endocrine society clinical practice guideline. J Clin Endocrinol Metab 99(11):3933–3951

16. Melmed S (2006) Medical progress: acromegaly. N Engl J Med 355(24):2558–2573

17. Melmed S, Ezrin C, Kovacs K, Goodman RS, Frohman LA (1985) Acromegaly due to secretion of growth hormone by an ectopic pancreatic islet-cell tumor. N Engl J Med 312(1):9–17

18. Ezzat S, Ezrin C, Yamashita S, Melmed S (1993) Recurrent acromegaly resulting from ectopic growth hormone gene expression by a metastatic pancreatic tumor. Cancer 71(1):66–70

19. Ghazi AA, Amirbaigloo A, Dezfooli AA et al (2013) Ectopic acromegaly due to growth hormone releasing hormone. Endocrine 43(2):293–302

20. Kojima M, Hosoda H, Date Y, Nakazato M, Matsuo H, Kangawa K (1999) Ghrelin is a growth-hormone-releasing acylated peptide from stomach. Nature 402(6762):656–660

21. Sato T, Nakamura Y, Shiimura Y, Ohgusu H, Kangawa K, Kojima M (2012) Structure, regulation and function of ghrelin. J Biochem 151(2):119–128

22. Papotti M, Duregon E, Volante M (2013) Ghrelin and tumors. Endocr Dev 25:122–134

23. Vu JP, Wang HS, Germano PM, Pisegna JR (2011) Ghrelin in neuroendocrine tumors. Peptides 32(11):2340–2347

24. Molfino A, Formiconi A, Rossi fanelli F, Muscaritoli M (2014) Ghrelin: from discovery to cancer cachexia therapy. Curr Opin Clin Nutr Metab Care 17(5):471–476

25. Wang HS, Oh DS, Ohning GV, Pisegna JR (2007) Elevated serum ghrelin exerts an orexigenic effect that may maintain body mass index in patients with metastatic neuroendocrine tumors. J Mol Neurosci 33(3):225–231

26. Tsolakis AV, Portela-Gomes GM, Stridsberg M et al (2004) Malignant gastric ghrelinoma with hyperghrelinemia. J Clin Endocrinol Metab 89(8):3739–3744

27. Corbetta S, Peracchi M, Cappiello V et al (2003) Circulating ghrelin levels in patients with pancreatic and gastrointestinal neuroendocrine tumors: identification of one pancreatic ghrelinoma. J Clin Endocrinol Metab 88(7):3117–3120

28. Walter T, Chardon L, Hervieu V et al (2009) Major hyperghrelinemia in advanced well-differentiated neuroendocrine carcinomas: report of three cases. Eur J Endocrinol 161(4):639–645

29. Wysolmerski JJ (2012) Parathyroid hormone-related protein: an update. J Clin Endocrinol Metab 97(9):2947–2956

30. Suva LJ, Winslow GA, Wettenhall RE et al (1987) A parathyroid hormone-related protein implicated in malignant hypercalcemia: cloning and expression. Science 237(4817):893–896

31. Strewler GJ, Stern PH, Jacobs JW et al (1987) Parathyroid hormonelike protein from human renal carcinoma cells. Structural and functional homology with parathyroid hormone. J Clin Invest 80(6):1803–1807

32. Burtis WJ, Wu T, Bunch C et al (1987) Identification of a novel 17,000-dalton parathyroid hormone-like adenylate cyclase-stimulating protein from a tumor associated with humoral hypercalcemia of malignancy. J Biol Chem 262(15):7151–7156

33. Milanesi A, Yu R, Wolin EM (2013) Humoral hypercalcemia of malignancy caused by parathyroid hormone-related peptide-secreting neuroendocrine tumors. Report of six cases. Pancreatology 13(3):324–326

34. Srirajaskanthan R, Mcstay M, Toumpanakis C, Meyer T, Caplin ME (2009) Parathyroid hormone-related peptide-secreting pancreatic neuroendocrine tumours: case series and literature review. Neuroendocrinology 89(1):48–55

35. Matsen SL, Yeo CJ, Hruban RH, Choti MA (2005) Hypercalcemia and pancreatic endocrine neoplasia with elevated PTH-rP: report of two new cases and subject review. J Gastrointest Surg 9(2):270–279

36. Doyle MA, Malcolm JC (2013) An unusual case of malignancy-related hypercalcemia. Int J Gen Med 7:21–27

37. Stewart AF (2005) Clinical practice. Hypercalcemia associated with cancer. N Engl J Med 352(4):373–379

38. Kanakis G, Kaltsas G, Granberg D et al (2012) Unusual complication of a pancreatic neuroendocrine tumor presenting with malignant hypercalcemia. J Clin Endocrinol Metab 97(4):E627–E631

39. Drucker DJ, Asa SL, Henderson J, Goltzman D (1989) The parathyroid hormone-like peptide gene is expressed in the normal and neoplastic human endocrine pancreas. Mol Endocrinol 3(10):1589–1595

40. Asa SL, Henderson J, Goltzman D, Drucker DJ (1990) Parathyroid hormone-like peptide in normal

and neoplastic human endocrine tissues. J Clin Endocrinol Metab 71(5):1112–1118

41. Wynick D, Ratcliffe WA, Heath DA, Ball S, Barnard M, Bloom SR (1990) Treatment of a malignant pancreatic endocrine tumour secreting parathyroid hormone related protein. BMJ 300(6735):1314–1315

42. VanHouten JN, Yu N, Rimm D et al (2006) Hypercalcemia of malignancy due to ectopic transactivation of the parathyroid hormone gene. J Clin Endocrinol Metab 91(2):580–583

43. Asa SL, Kovacs K, Thorner MO, Leong DA, Rivier J, Vale W (1985) Immunohistological localization of growth hormone-releasing hormone in human tumors. J Clin Endocrinol Metab 60(3):423–427

44. Asa SL, Singer W, Kovacs K et al (1987) Pancreatic endocrine tumour producing growth hormone-releasing hormone associated with multiple endocrine neoplasia type I syndrome. Acta Endocrinol 115(3):331–337

45. Beuschlein F, Strasburger CJ, Siegerstetter V et al (2000) Acromegaly caused by secretion of growth hormone by a non-Hodgkin's lymphoma. N Engl J Med 342(25):1871–1876

46. Brzozowska MM, Wolmarans L, Conaglen JV (2009) Hypercalcaemia caused by a carcinoid tumour. Intern Med J 39(6):415–418

47. Gamwell LF, Gambaro K, Merziotis M et al (2013) Small cell ovarian carcinoma: genomic stability and responsiveness to therapeutics. Orphanet J Rare Dis 8:33

48. Gardner GJ, Reidy-lagunes D, Gehrig PA (2011) Neuroendocrine tumors of the gynecologic tract: a Society of Gynecologic Oncology (SGO) clinical document. Gynecol Oncol 122(1):190–198

49. Cohen JG, Chan JK, Kapp DS (2012) The management of small-cell carcinomas of the gynecologic tract. Curr Opin Oncol 24(5):572–579

50. Vacher-Coponat H, Opris A, Denizot A, Dussol B, Berland Y (2005) Hypercalcaemia induced by excessive parathyroid hormone secretion in a patient with a neuroendocrine tumour. Nephrol Dial Transplant 20(12):2832–2835

51. Kanakis G, Kaltsas G (2012) Biochemical markers for gastroenteropancreatic neuroendocrine tumours (GEP-NETs). Best Pract Res Clin Gastroenterol 26(6):791–802

52. Van Essen M, Sundin A, Krenning EP, Kwekkeboom DJ (2014) Neuroendocrine tumours: the role of imaging for diagnosis and therapy. Nat Rev Endocrinol 10(2):102–114

53. De Herder WW (2014) GEP-NETS update: functional localisation and scintigraphy in neuroendocrine tumours of the gastrointestinal tract and pancreas (GEP-NETs). Eur J Endocrinol 170(5):R173–R183

54. Losa M, Von Werder K (1997) Pathophysiology and clinical aspects of the ectopic GH-releasing hormone syndrome. Clin Endocrinol (Oxf) 47(2):123–135

55. Kovacs K, Horvath E (1986) Tumors of the pituitary gland, Atlas of Tumor Pathology, Second Series, Fascicle 21. Armed Forces Institute of Pathology, Washington, DC

56. Asa SL (1998) Tumors of the pituitary gland, Atlas of Tumor Pathology, Third Series, Fascicle 22. Armed Forces Institute of Pathology, Washington, DC

57. Asa SL (2011) Tumors of the pituitary gland, AFIP Atlas of Tumor Pathology. Series 4, Fascicle 15. ARP Press, Silver Spring

58. Stefaneanu L, Kovacs K, Horvath E et al (1989) Adenohypophysial changes in mice transgenic for human growth hormone-releasing factor: a histological, immunocytochemical, and electron microscopic investigation. Endocrinology 125(5): 2710–2718

59. Asa SL, Kovacs K, Stefaneanu L et al (1990) Pituitary mammosomatotroph adenomas develop in old mice transgenic for growth hormone-releasing hormone. Proc Soc Exp Biol Med 193(3):232–235

60. Solcia E, Klöppel G, Capella C (1997) Tumors of the endocrine pancreas. In: Rosai J, Sobin LH (eds) Tumors of the pancreas. Atlas of tumor pathology, 3rd edn. Armed Forces Institute of Pathology, Washington, pp 145–209

61. Sano T, Asa SL, Kovacs K (1988) Growth hormone-releasing hormone-producing tumors: clinical, biochemical, and morphological manifestations. Endocr Rev 9(3):357–373

62. Ramsay JA, Kovacs K, Asa SL, Pike MJ, Thorner MO (1988) Reversible sellar enlargement due to growth hormone-releasing hormone production by pancreatic endocrine tumors in a acromegalic patient with multiple endocrine neoplasia type I syndrome. Cancer 62(2):445–450

63. Ezzat S, Asa SL, Stefaneanu L et al (1994) Somatotroph hyperplasia without pituitary adenoma associated with a long standing growth hormone-releasing hormone-producing bronchial carcinoid. J Clin Endocrinol Metab 78(3):555–560

64. Othman NH, Ezzat S, Kovacs K et al (2001) Growth hormone-releasing hormone (GHRH) and GHRH receptor (GHRH-R) isoform expression in ectopic acromegaly. Clin Endocrinol (Oxf) 55(1):135–140

65. Nasr C, Mason A, Mayberg M, Staugaitis SM, Asa SL (2006) Acromegaly and somatotroph hyperplasia with adenomatous transformation due to pituitary metastasis of a growth hormone-releasing hormone-secreting pulmonary endocrine carcinoma. J Clin Endocrinol Metab 91(12):4776–4780

66. Colak Ozbey N, Kapran Y, Bozbora A, Erbil Y, Tascioglu C, Asa SL (2009) Ectopic growth hormone-releasing hormone secretion by a neuroendocrine tumor causing acromegaly: long-term follow-up results. Endocr Pathol 20(2):127–132

67. Sala E, Ferrante E, Verrua E et al (2013) Growth hormone-releasing hormone-producing pancreatic

neuroendocrine tumor in a multiple endocrine neoplasia type 1 family with an uncommon phenotype. Eur J Gastroenterol Hepatol 25(7):858–862

68. Nonaka D (2011) Study of parathyroid transcription factor GCM2 expression in parathyroid lesions. Am J Surg Pathol 35(1):145–151

69. Ordóñez NG (2014) Value of GATA3 immunostaining in the diagnosis of parathyroid tumors. Appl Immunohistochem Mol Morphol 22(10):756–761

70. Rindi G, Falconi M, Klersy C et al (2012) TNM staging of neoplasms of the endocrine pancreas: results from a large international cohort study. J Natl Cancer Inst 104(10):764–777

71. Ezzat S, Ren SG, Braunstein GD, Melmed S (1992) Octreotide stimulates insulin-like growth factor-binding protein-1: a potential pituitary-independent mechanism for drug action. J Clin Endocrinol Metab 75(6):1459–1463

72. Ezzat S, Pahl-Wostl C, Rudin M, Harris AG (1994) [13C]NMR studies of the effect of the somatostatin analogue octreotide on hepatic glycogenesis and glycogenolysis. Peptides 15(7):1223–1227

Nonfunctioning Pancreatic Neuroendocrine Neoplasms (Including PP-Producing and Calcitonin-Producing Tumors)

Alessandro Vanoli and Enrico Solcia

16.1 Historical Background and Epidemiology

Nonfunctioning pancreatic neuroendocrine neoplasms are pancreatic neoplasms with endocrine differentiation in the absence of a clinical syndrome of hormone hyperfunction. Neoplasms with increased hormone levels in blood but without evidence of a hyperfunctional syndrome, which in principle should be called "functioning nonsyndromic neoplasms," are also currently reported as nonfunctioning neoplasms. Among nonfunctioning neuroendocrine neoplasms, those presenting with symptoms of an expanding mass in the upper abdomen should be separated from clinically silent neoplasms.

Clinically silent neuroendocrine neoplasms have been reported in 0.3–1.6 % of unselected *autopsies* in which only a few sections of the pancreas were examined and in up to 10 % of autopsies in which the whole pancreas was systematically investigated. Most such tumors were, in elderly subjects (mean age, 70 years), small (less than 1 cm, mostly a few millimeters) mainly composed of well-granulated islet A and PP cells, forming thin trabeculae, usually diagnosed as islet cell microadenomas [1, 2].

The majority of nonfunctioning neoplasms from *surgical series* are large, e.g., more than 5 cm in 72 % of cases from the Mayo Clinic series [3] and present with symptoms of an expanding mass or metastatic growth. Older series suggested an overall incidence of about 30–35 %, a figure second only to that of insulinomas (about 40 %) and higher than that of remaining types of pancreatic neuroendocrine neoplasms [4]. Incidentally discovered nonfunctioning neoplasms have been increasingly detected in recent years due to high-resolution imaging techniques [5]. In a recent study they accounted for 35 % of 355 nonfunctioning cases, with lower tumor stage at diagnosis and better progression-free survival for each tumor stage, when compared with symptomatic nonfunctioning tumors [6].

Clinically symptomatic nonfunctioning neuroendocrine neoplasms arise more frequently (65 % of 82 cases) in the head of the pancreas, a pattern comparable to that of gastrinomas (71 % of 56 cases) and at variance with that of insulinomas (35 % of 1,519 cases), glucagonomas (25 % of 65 cases), and VIPomas (23 % of 66 cases) [7]. The more prominent local symptoms produced by tumors in the head of the gland (due for instance to main pancreatic duct and/or biliary three obstruction), rather than in the body or tail, may account in part for the head concentration of nonfunctioning neoplasms; however, this would

A. Vanoli (✉) • E. Solcia
Department of Molecular Medicine,
University of Pavia, and Fondazione IRCCS
Policlinico San Matteo di Pavia,
Via Forlanini, 16, Pavia, Italy
e-mail: ale.vanol@virgilio.it; solciae@smatteo.pv.it

S. La Rosa, F. Sessa (eds.), *Pancreatic Neuroendocrine Neoplasms: Practical Approach to Diagnosis, Classification, and Therapy*, DOI 10.1007/978-3-319-17235-4_16,
© Springer International Publishing Switzerland 2015

not explain the body-tail concentration of glucagonomas or VIPomas, usually about as large as locally symptomatic nonfunctioning neoplasms and even less of insulinomas, generally much smaller in size. The preponderance of normal islet tissue and some cell types (with special reference to glucagon-producing A cells) in the body-tail of the pancreas may contribute to such differences.

The most frequent presenting signs of nonfunctioning neuroendocrine neoplasms are abdominal pain, jaundice, a palpable abdominal mass, ascites, steatorrhea, and intestinal bleeding. More than half of the cases have their malignancy proven by metastases or local invasion [3, 7, 8]. Incidentally found neoplasms, compared with symptomatic ones, show significantly lower size (65 % vs. 35 % being ≤35 mm in diameter) and TNM stage (68 % vs. 30 % in stage I to IIb) at diagnosis [6].

16.2 Morphology

No significant difference in *histologic pattern* has been found in nonfunctioning as compared to functioning neoplasms, with trabecular, micronodular, and solid structures formed by monomorphic small- to medium-sized cells being more frequently represented.

Several rare morphologic variants have been described which could cause difficulties in distinction with non-neuroendocrine neoplasms, especially in nonfunctioning tumors. The *clear cell (or lipid-rich) variant* of pancreatic neuroendocrine tumors is characterized by the presence of abundant cytoplasm with a foamy appearance, due to lipid-containing cytoplasmic vesicles (Fig. 16.1a). Clear cell pancreatic neuroendocrine tumors should be distinguished from renal cell carcinoma metastatic to the pancreas and seem more common in patients with von Hippel-Lindau or MEN1 syndromes [9, 10]. In the *oncocytic variant*, the tumor cells contain abundant granular eosinophilic cytoplasm, because of the accumulation of mitochondria (Fig. 16.1b). Oncocytic pancreatic neuroendocrine tumors should not be confused with the oncocytic and hepatoid variants of ductal adenocarcinoma [11]. In the *pleomorphic variant*, the tumor cells exhibit marked nuclear atypia, which may obscure the neuroendocrine nature of the neoplasm; however, they are not usually associated with an increased proliferative activity or a more aggressive biological behavior than pancreatic neuroendocrine tumors with conventional histology [12]. Spindle cell, hepatoid, and rhabdoid morphology are also found occasionally, often as focal pattern, in nonfunctioning pancreatic neuroendocrine tumors. In addition, it should be

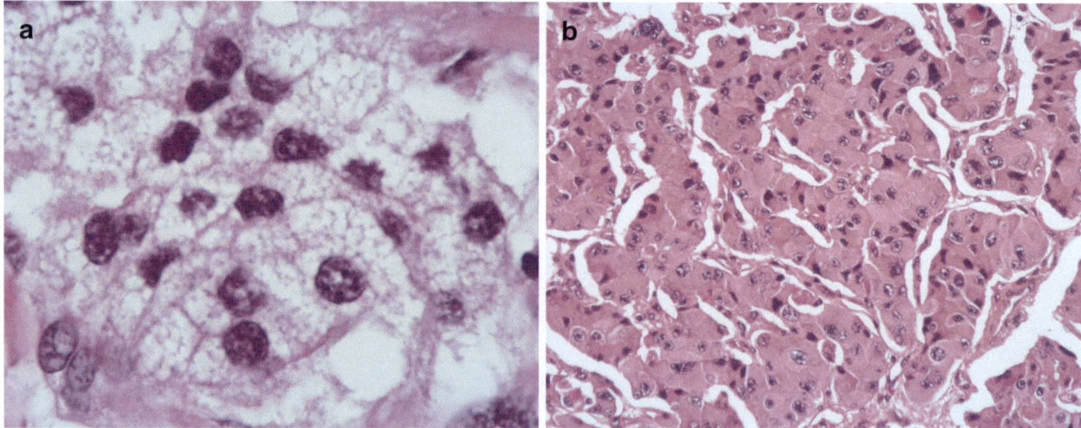

Fig. 16.1 Clear cell (lipid-rich) variant of pancreatic neuroendocrine tumor in (**a**). Oncocytic variant of pancreatic nonfunctioning neuroendocrine tumor in (**b**)

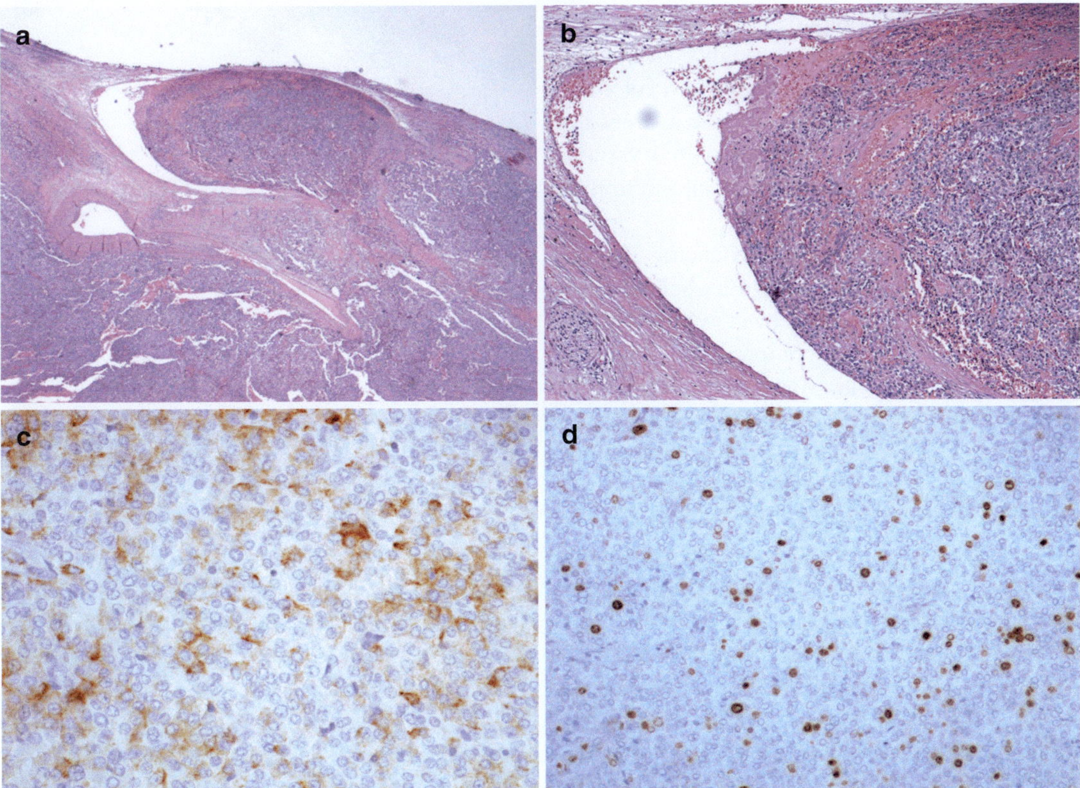

Fig. 16.2 Nonfunctioning pancreatic neuroendocrine tumor, grade 2 (WHO 2010), showing angioinvasion (**a**, high magnification in **b**). This tumor is immunoreactive for chromogranin A (**c**) and exhibits a Ki67 proliferative index of 20 % (**d**). The mitotic index is 10 mitoses/10 HPFs. The differential diagnosis with a neuroendocrine carcinoma (NEC) is challenging

mentioned that a minority of nonfunctioning pancreatic neuroendocrine tumors may present as grossly cystic lesions, thus making radiological diagnosis challenging. Worth noting, cystic tumors usually present at a lower pathologic stage as compared with solid pancreatic neuroendocrine tumors [13, 14].

Among prognostically relevant histologic findings, there are vascular invasion (Fig. 16.2), perineural invasion, focal necrosis, mitotic index, and the percentage of cells reactive for proliferative markers like *Ki67 protein* [8, 15–17]. In general no difference has been found in nonfunctioning compared to functioning neoplasms, with the Ki67 index proving more sensitive and effective than the mitotic index to grade neuroendocrine neoplasms as grade 1 or 2.

Of special interest is the histologic evaluation of incidentally found neoplasms, most of which proved to be grade 1, in the absence of microvascular or perineural invasion and of macroscopic signs of invasion or metastasis [6]. Indeed, incidental grade 1 cases (with 0–2 % of Ki67 index and a mitotic index less than 2/10 HPFs, high-power fields) less than 2 cm in size seem to be appropriate candidates for studies concerning conservative managements of pancreatic neuroendocrine neoplasms, especially in patients at increased surgical risk due to coexisting morbidities.

Immunohistochemical tests showed a variety of hormones in nonfunctioning neoplasms, including pancreatic polypeptide (PP), glucagon, somatostatin, insulin, serotonin, calcitonin, gastrin, vasoactive intestinal peptide (VIP), ghrelin, neurotensin, and ACTH in a roughly decreasing order of frequency [8, 18]. They often coexisted in the same "multihormonal" tumor as minor or major cell populations, together with a variable (often large and overwhelming) proportion of hormone-unreactive cells.

It appears that neoplasms producing PP, glucagon, and somatostatin have a higher tendency to remain nonfunctioning, even when showing high hormone contents, compared to neoplasms producing powerful hormones like insulin, gastrin, or VIP, affecting clinically more relevant functions. Consequently, in multihormone-producing neoplasms, the predominant hormone produced or tumor cell type expressed is not necessarily the one accounting for the associated hyperfunctional syndrome. This has been repeatedly observed for predominantly PP cell neoplasms, whose associated watery diarrhea, hypokalemia, and achlorhydria (WDHA) or Zollinger-Ellison (ZE) syndromes were often found to be accounted for the minority populations of VIP-producing cells or gastrin-producing cells, respectively [19–23]. Similar findings have been obtained for neurotensin-producing tumors in respect to WDHA or ZE syndromes [24–26].

Given their large proportion of hormonally unreactive cells and/or the limited clinical impact of the hormones they actually produce, the diagnosis of nonfunctioning neoplasms should be based chiefly on their reactivity toward general neuroendocrine markers like chromogranin A, synaptophysin, neuron-specific enolase, or PGP 9.5 (i.e., ubiquitin hydrolase L1), more than on the individual hormones produced.

Besides being observed in neoplastic cells, *pancreatic polypeptide* has been frequently found to be increased in serum of patients bearing neuroendocrine neoplasms, though in the absence of any sign of pertinent hyperfunction [23, 24]. Based on these findings, serum PP level measurements have been proposed as a useful test to detect occult pancreatic neuroendocrine neoplasms. Although it has been suggested that the majority of neoplasms purely or predominantly

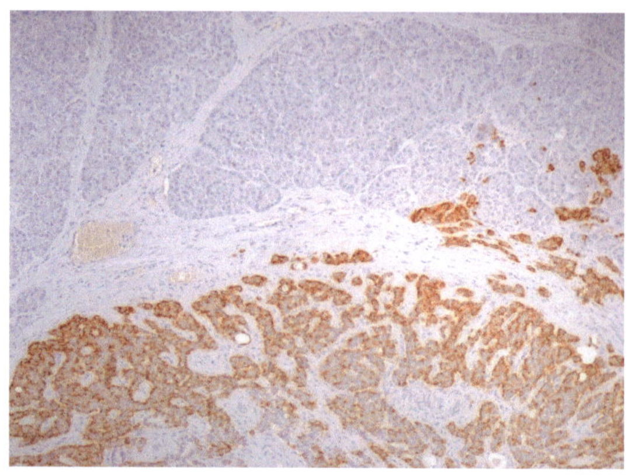

Fig. 16.3 PP-producing pancreatic neuroendocrine tumor (microadenoma) in a MEN1 patient: PP immunostain shows a diffuse and strong positivity

composed of PP cells (Fig. 16.3) have a benign behavior, it should be outlined that several malignant cases causing patient death have been also reported [18, 20–23].

Calcitonin-producing pancreatic neoplasms are quite rare. A search in 2011 identified 37 cases, many of which, in addition to calcitonin, also produced multiple other hormones, among which somatostatin, VIP, PP, insulin, gastrin, and glucagon, like most other nonfunctioning neoplasms [27]. However, a frequent (19/37 cases) association with watery diarrhea (WDHA) syndrome was noted, in several cases coupled with, and likely due to, increased blood levels of VIP produced by tumor tissue. In other cases, no VIP increase in serum was detected and a possible role of calcitonin itself was proposed, also considering the frequent association of the watery diarrhea syndrome with calcitonin-producing thyroid medullary carcinoma, with or without associated VIP production. The rare pancreatic metastases from thyroid medullary carcinoma should be considered in the differential diagnosis [28]. Most (60 %) calcitonin-secreting pancreatic neoplasms proved metastatic [27], a finding confirming previous suggestions on histochemical grounds that calcitonin expression by tumor cells may represent an unfavorable prognostic sign [8].

16.3 Diagnosis

The distinction between functioning and nonfunctioning pancreatic neuroendocrine tumors is made solely on the basis of the clinical picture, as nonfunctioning pancreatic neuroendocrine tumors are not associated with a distinct clinical syndrome. However, they may produce hormones that can be detected as abnormally increased serum levels or by immunohistochemical stainings on tumor tissue. Incidentally discovered nonfunctioning tumors have been increasingly detected in recent years due to high-resolution imaging techniques [5] and should be separated from those presenting with symptoms of an expanding mass in the upper abdomen or of tumor infiltration of neighboring organs.

16.4 Prognosis

In nonfunctioning pancreatic neuroendocrine neoplasm, the most important factors predictive of aggressive behavior include grade and stage. As a rule, production of specific peptides has no major impact on survival. Recent data from 1,072 patients who underwent surgery for neuroendocrine neoplasms of the pancreas suggest that the European Neuroendocrine Tumor Society (ENETS) TNM staging system is superior to the International Union for Cancer Control/American Joint Cancer Committee/World Health Organization (UICC/AJCC/WHO 2010) TNM staging system and, for nonfunctioning tumors, reported a death rate per 100 person-years of 4.5 [17].

References

1. Grimelius L, Hultquist GT, Stenkvist B (1975) Cytological differentiation of asymptomatic pancreatic islet cell tumours in autopsy material. Virchows Arch A Pathol Anat Histol 365:275–288
2. Kimura W, Kuroda A, Morioka Y (1991) Clinical pathology of endocrine tumors of the pancreas. Analysis of autopsy cases. Dig Dis Sci 36:933–942
3. Kent RB 3rd, van Heerden JA, Weiland LH (1981) Nonfunctioning islet cell tumors. Ann Surg 193:185–190
4. Klöppel G, Heitz PU (1988) Pancreatic endocrine tumors. Pathol Res Pract 183:155–168
5. Yao JC, Hassan M, Phan A et al (2008) One hundred years after "carcinoid": epidemiology of and prognostic factors for neuroendocrine tumors in 35,825 cases in the United States. J Clin Oncol 26:3063–3072
6. Crippa S, Partelli S, Zamboni G et al (2014) Incidental diagnosis as prognostic factor in different tumor stages of nonfunctioning pancreatic endocrine tumors. Surgery 155:145–153
7. Solcia E, Capella C, Klöppel G (1997) Atlas of tumor pathology. Tumors of the pancreas. Armed Forces Institute of Pathology, Washington, DC
8. La Rosa S, Sessa F, Capella C et al (1996) Prognostic criteria in nonfunctioning pancreatic endocrine tumours. Virchows Arch 429:323–333
9. Singh R, Basturk O, Klimstra DS et al (2006) Lipid-rich variant of pancreatic endocrine neoplasms. Am J Surg Pathol 30:194–200
10. Fryer E, Serra S, Chetty R (2012) Lipid-rich ("clear cell") neuroendocrine tumors of the pancreas in MEN I patients. Endocr Pathol 23:243–246
11. Volante M, La Rosa S, Castellano I et al (2006) Clinico-pathological features of a series of 11 oncocytic endocrine tumours of the pancreas. Virchows Arch 448:545–551
12. Zee SY, Hochwald SN, Conlon KC et al (2005) Pleomorphic pancreatic endocrine neoplasms: a variant commonly confused with adenocarcinoma. Am J Surg Pathol 29:1194–1200
13. Boninsegna L, Partelli S, D'Innocenzio MM et al (2010) Pancreatic cystic endocrine tumors: a different morphological entity associated with a less aggressive behavior. Neuroendocrinology 92:246–251
14. Singhi AD, Chu LC, Tatsas AD et al (2012) Cystic pancreatic neuroendocrine tumors: a clinicopathologic study. Am J Surg Pathol 36:1666–1673
15. La Rosa S, Klersy C, Uccella S et al (2009) Improved histologic and clinicopathologic criteria for prognostic evaluation of pancreatic endocrine tumors. Hum Pathol 40:30–40
16. Rindi G, Klöppel G, Alhman H et al (2006) TNM staging of foregut (neuro)endocrine tumors: a consensus proposal including a grading system. Virchows Arch 449:395–401
17. Rindi G, Falconi M, Klersy C et al (2012) TNM staging of neoplasms of the endocrine pancreas: results from a large international cohort study. J Natl Cancer Inst 104:764–777
18. Heitz PU, Kasper M, Polak JM et al (1982) Pancreatic endocrine tumors. Hum Pathol 13:263–271
19. Larsson LI, Schwartz T, Lundqvist G et al (1976) Occurrence of human pancreatic polypeptide in pancreatic endocrine tumors. Possible implication in the watery diarrhea syndrome. Am J Pathol 85:675–684
20. Tomita T, Friesen SR, Kimmel JR et al (1983) Pancreatic polypeptide-secreting islet-cell tumors. A study of three cases. Am J Pathol 113:134–142

21. Nobin A, Berg M, Ericsson M et al (1984) Pancreatic polypeptide-producing tumors. Report on two cases. Cancer 53:2688–2691
22. Strodel WE, Vinik AI, Lloyd RV et al (1984) Pancreatic polypeptide-producing tumors. Silent lesions of the pancreas? Arch Surg 119:508–514
23. Bordi C, Azzoni C, D'Adda T et al (2002) Pancreatic polypeptide-related tumors. Peptides 23:339–348
24. Gutniak M, Rosenqvist U, Grimelius L et al (1980) Report on a patient with watery diarrhoea syndrome caused by a pancreatic tumour containing neurotensin, enkephalin and calcitonin. Acta Med Scand 208:95–100
25. Feurle GE, Helmstaedter V, Tischbirek K et al (1981) A multihormonal tumor of the pancreas producing neurotensin. Dig Dis Sci 26:1125–1133
26. Theodorsson-Norheim E, Oberg K, Rosell S et al (1983) Neurotensinlike immunoreactivity in plasma and tumor tissue from patients with endocrine tumors of the pancreas and gut. Gastroenterology 85:881–889
27. Schneider R, Waldmann J, Swaid Z et al (2011) Calcitonin-secreting pancreatic endocrine tumors: systematic analysis of a rare tumor entity. Pancreas 40:213–221
28. Hyodo M, Nagai H, Sata N et al (2003) Long-term survivor without recurrence after resection of simultaneous solitary pancreatic metastasis from thyroid medullary carcinoma. Hepatogastroenterology 50:1687–1688

Poorly Differentiated Neuroendocrine Carcinoma of the Pancreas

17

Olca Basturk and David S. Klimstra

17.1 Definition

In the current (2010) World Health Organization (WHO) classification system, pancreatic poorly differentiated neuroendocrine carcinomas (PD-NECs) are included in the grade 3 category along with well-differentiated neuroendocrine tumors (NETs) that have more than 20 mitoses per 10 HPFs or a Ki-67 index greater than 20 % [1]. This system suggests that PD-NECs are part of a continuum with well-differentiated NETs, and therefore the two entities are closely related, and that grade should be based entirely on proliferation rate. However, evolving evidence strongly suggests that morphologic differentiation is also relevant and that PD-NECs should be regarded as a separate entity [2–5], and as such they will be discussed separately.

PD-NECs of the pancreas are clinically highly aggressive, poorly differentiated carcinomas with neuroendocrine differentiation. They are characterized and defined by high mitotic activity (by definition more than 20 mitoses per 10 HPFs, and usually 40–50 per 10 HPFs) and usually exhibit necrosis, in addition to their distinctive morphology and high-grade cytology. Morphologically, some PD-NECs are almost identical to pulmonary small cell carcinomas, but others more resemble large cell neuroendocrine carcinomas. Immunoexpression of chromogranin and synaptophysin is typical and required for the diagnosis of large cell neuroendocrine carcinoma [6–8].

17.2 Clinical Features

Primary pancreatic PD-NECs are extremely rare, accounting less than 1 % of all pancreatic carcinomas [9] and at most 2–3 % of all pancreatic neuroendocrine neoplasms [6].

Most patients are in their late 50s and there is a slight male predilection. In contrast to pancreatic well-differentiated NETs, the PD-NECs are not associated with hereditary syndromes and are usually clinically nonfunctioning [3], although individual cases with paraneoplastic syndromes such as carcinoid syndrome [10], Cushing syndrome [11], hypercalcemia [12], or hyperinsulinism [3] have been reported. The patients present with symptoms similar to those of exocrine pancreatic neoplasms such as back pain, weight lost, and jaundice, due to obstruction of the common bile duct.

O. Basturk, MD (✉)
Department of Pathology,
Memorial Sloan Kettering Cancer Center,
1275 York Avenue, New York, NY 10065, USA
e-mail: basturko@mskcc.org

D.S. Klimstra, MD
Department of Pathology, Memorial Sloan Kettering
Cancer Center, New York, NY, USA

S. La Rosa, F. Sessa (eds.), *Pancreatic Neuroendocrine Neoplasms: Practical Approach to Diagnosis, Classification, and Therapy*, DOI 10.1007/978-3-319-17235-4_17,
© Springer International Publishing Switzerland 2015

17.3 Pathologic Features

PD-NECs are more common in the head of the pancreas and present as a large (median tumor size of 4 cm), relatively circumscribed, tan-yellow, fleshy mass. Hemorrhage and necrosis are common [3].

Morphologically, these poorly differentiated carcinomas are subdivided into small and large cell variants, based on cell size. The small cell variant (small cell carcinoma) is characterized by small to intermediate cells with finely granular chromatin, high nucleus-to-cytoplasm ratio, inconspicuous nucleoli, prominent nuclear molding, and crush artifact (Fig. 17.1). These carcinomas display predominantly a diffuse, sheetlike growth pattern with confluent areas of necrosis and entrapment of pancreatic parenchyma [3, 13, 14]. Scattered tumor giant cells with hyperchromatic, bizarre nuclei or rosettes may be seen in some tumors. In a recent series of 44 histologically confirmed primary pancreatic PD-NECs, the average mitotic count and Ki-67 labeling index of small cell carcinomas were found to be 51 per 10 high power fields and 75 % (Fig. 17.2), respectively [3].

The large cell variant (large cell neuroendocrine carcinoma) is more common and characterized by large cells with prominent nucleoli and variable amounts of cytoplasm. Diffuse, nested, trabecular, gland-forming, and peripheral palisading growth patterns, often intermingled in varying proportions, are seen in most large cell neuroendocrine carcinomas (Fig. 17.3). Some tumors display pseudopapillae, composed of viable tumor cells surrounding fibrovascular cores, usually at the periphery of necrotic areas. Apoptotic cells and mitotic figures are abundant, but mitotic figures in the large cell neuroendocrine carcinomas are usually not as numerous as in the small cell carcinomas. In the aforementioned study, the average mitotic count and Ki-67 labeling index of large cell neuroendocrine carcinomas were found to be 37 per 10 high power fields and 66 %, respectively [3].

In cases with the typical cytologic features of small cell carcinoma, it is not necessary to document neuroendocrine differentiation by immu-

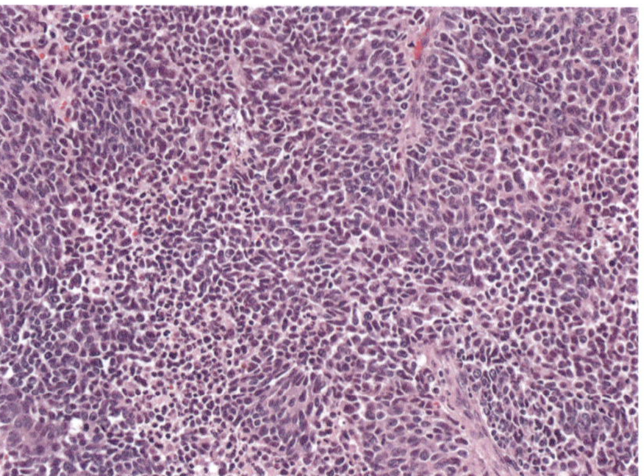

Fig. 17.1 Small cell carcinomas are characterized by loosely arranged sheets of small cells with a high N:C ratio, hyperchromatic and finely granular chromatin, inconspicuous nucleoli, and nuclear molding. High mitotic activity and necrosis are also present

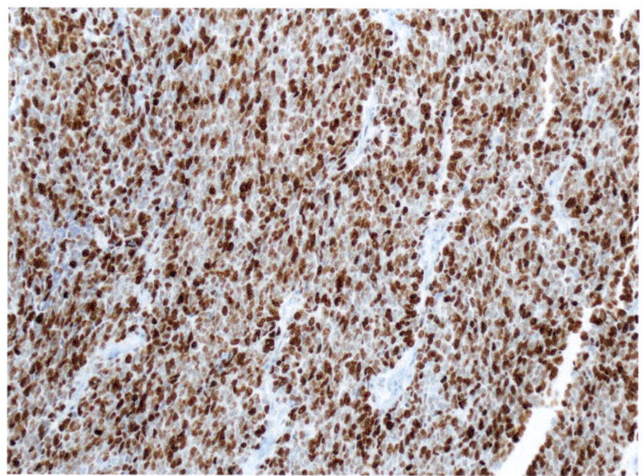

Fig. 17.2 Ki-67 labeling index of poorly differentiated neuroendocrine carcinomas is much higher than the WHO-recommended threshold (>20 %) for the grade 3 category. A small cell carcinoma with >95 % Ki-67 labeling index is depicted here

nohistochemistry, provided alternative diagnoses (primitive neuroectodermal tumor, desmoplastic small round cell tumor, etc.) can be excluded. However, for large cell neuroendocrine carcinomas, positive immunohistochemical staining for chromogranin or synaptophysin should be obtained to confirm the diagnosis [1, 6, 15], although the extent and intensity of staining are usually less than in well-differentiated NETs of the pancreas.

Some PD-NECs may be associated with exocrine pancreatic neoplasm component, in the form

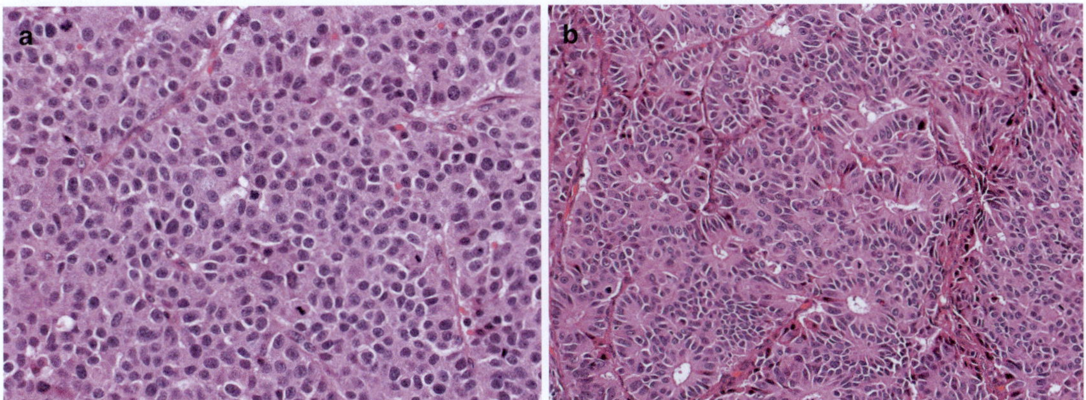

Fig. 17.3 Large cell neuroendocrine carcinoma may reveal various growth patterns (**a**, trabecular; **b**, gland-forming pattern). Compared to small cell carcinoma, their cells are larger and round to polygonal with round nuclei that have vesicular chromatin or prominent nucleoli

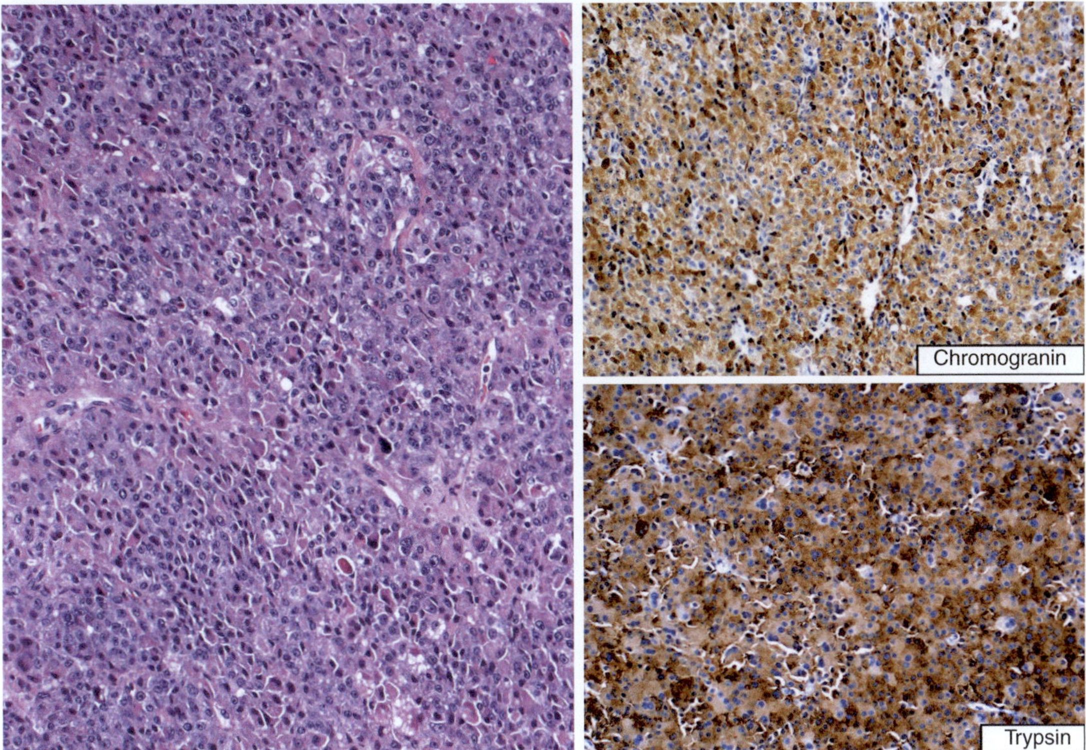

Fig. 17.4 Mixed acinar-neuroendocrine carcinomas are usually composed of morphologically homogenous population of cells, and the divergent differentiation cannot be detected without immunohistochemical labeling for both neuroendocrine and acinar differentiation markers (chromogranin and trypsin immunohistochemical stains are depicted here)

of acinar cell carcinoma (Fig. 17.4) or in the form of ductal adenocarcinoma (Fig. 17.5), intraductal papillary mucinous neoplasm, or even squamous cell carcinoma [1, 3, 6, 16–19]. The 2010 WHO classification system recommends that at least 30 % of either component be present in order to qualify a tumor as "mixed carcinoma" [1], although the figure of 25 % has also been

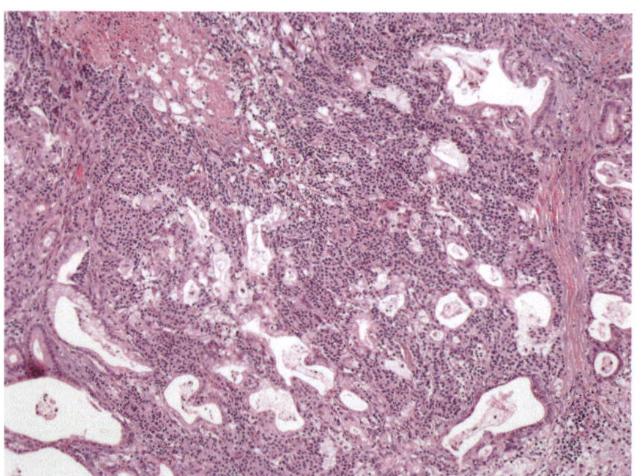

Fig. 17.5 In contrast to mixed acinar-neuroendocrine carcinomas, different components are morphologically recognizable in mixed ductal-neuroendocrine carcinomas, even if they are intimately admixed as illustrated here, as gland formations and presence of abundant intracellular mucin are striking

advocated in the AFIP fascicle on tumors of the pancreas [6].

In mixed ductal- or squamous-neuroendocrine carcinomas, different components, sharply segregated or intimately admixed, are usually morphologically recognizable (Fig. 17.4). Of note, PD-NECs, especially large cell neuroendocrine carcinomas, with gland formations should not be mistaken for mixed ductal-neuroendocrine carcinomas. Absence of detectable mucin and careful attention to the cytologic appearance aid in proper diagnosis in the former (see Chap. 18 for detailed discussion). In contrast, mixed acinar-neuroendocrine carcinomas display less segregation of the two cell types (Fig. 17.4). In fact, in most cases, it is not possible to recognize with certainty that two lines of differentiation are present without immunohistochemical staining for both neuroendocrine and acinar differentiation markers [3, 6, 19]. If only neuroendocrine staining is performed, these cases can be misinterpreted as neuroendocrine carcinomas. Therefore, it is not surprising that many cases that are diagnosed as PD-NECs prove to be mixed acinar-neuroendocrine carcinoma once studied more carefully [3, 19].

On cytology, small cell carcinoma is characterized by often crushed, small- to intermediate-sized tumor cells with irregular nuclear borders, high nucleus-to-cytoplasm ratio, and nuclear molding. In addition to brisk mitotic activity, there is extensive single-cell and background necrosis. For large cell neuroendocrine carcinoma, tumor cells are usually larger with variable cytoplasm as well as prominent central nucleoli. However, these tumors may resemble a poorly differentiated adenocarcinoma and may not show the classical coarsely clumped chromatin of well-differentiated NETs or the nuclear molding of their small cell counterpart. If a neuroendocrine carcinoma is not suspected at the time of evaluation, the diagnosis may be easily missed [20].

17.4 Differential Diagnosis

Primary pancreatic PD-NECs are extremely rare and must be distinguished from metastatic PD-NECs from another organ or direct invasion from a contiguous site, particularly the ampulla of Vater [21] or stomach. When there is a single mass in the pancreas and, after critical evaluation, no convincing clinical, radiographic, or pathologic evidence of a lung primary (or another site), then pancreatic origin is reasonable. It should be kept in mind that TTF1 immunohistochemical staining is not helpful, as small cell carcinomas from both pulmonary and a variety of extrapulmonary sites are TTF1 positive. Clinical information and a history of a previous carcinoma are especially important in the accurate diagnosis of such cases.

Pancreatic well-differentiated NETs can show significant nuclear pleomorphism or small cell change (high nuclear/cytoplasmic ratio resembling small cell carcinoma) [22], and features such as a markedly infiltrative growth pattern and necrosis can also be identified [6]. On casual examination, these findings falsely suggest a PD-NEC. If thorough mitotic counting as well as immunolabeling for Ki-67 are not performed, misclassification can occur, which can have therapeutic consequences [2, 23]. A recent landmark study has shown that not all patients with a grade 3 NEC defined based on WHO 2010 criteria benefit from the platinum-based chemotherapy typically used for PD-NECs. In this study, grade 3 tumors with a Ki-67 index <55 % were less responsive than grade 3 NECs with a Ki-67 index ≥55 %, although the latter group experienced early recurrence of shorter ultimate survival than the group with a Ki-67 in the 20–55 % range [2], supporting the concept that the 2010 WHO grade 3 category is heterogeneous, and the tumors at the lower end of the grade 3 range are in fact well-differentiated NETs with an elevated proliferation rate. These well-differentiated NETs typically have a Ki-67 index around 40 %, whereas PD-NECs' Ki-67 index is about 70 % [3, 4]. Also, a recent study has shown that most pancreatic PD-NECs abnormally immunolabel for p53 (nuclear expression) and Rb (loss of expression) in 95 % and 74 % of cases, respectively. In that study, the abnormal expression of these proteins correlated with intragenic mutations in the *TP53* and *retinoblastoma* genes coding for these proteins. By contrast, immunohistochemical studies only detect rare p53 abnormalities and Rb immunolabeling is intact in pancreatic well-differentiated NETs [5, 24]. In addition, approximately 45 % of sporadic pancreatic well-differentiated NETs show mutually exclusive loss of expression of DAXX (death-domain-associated protein) or ATRX (α-thalassemia/mental retardation syndrome X-linked) immunohistochemical stains, which correlates with mutations in the *DAXX* and *ATRX* genes [5, 25] (see Molecular Pathology section for more details).

As discussed above, the distinction of acinar cell carcinoma and mixed acinar-neuroendocrine carcinomas from PD-NECs is also problematic [3]. Both entities usually have a high proliferation rate; acinar cell carcinomas can have a diffuse growth pattern and, along with large cell neuroendocrine carcinomas, can have prominent nucleoli. The correct diagnosis may not be established without immunohistochemical evaluation using acinar and neuroendocrine differentiation markers. Given the rarity of primary pancreatic PD-NECs, relative to acinar neoplasms, it is thus recommended that a diagnosis of PD-NEC should not be rendered unless acinar differentiation has been excluded immunohistochemically.

The crushed and molded tumor cells of small cell carcinoma may resemble a high-grade lymphoma. Morphologic distinction is often impossible and immunohistochemistry is required for diagnosis. Other small, round, blue cell tumors, such as primitive neuroectodermal tumor (PNET) and desmoplastic small round cell tumor, may also involve the pancreas primarily or secondarily and need to be distinguished from small cell carcinoma, especially in younger patients [14]. PNETs generally have small, round, monotonous nuclei with inconspicuous nucleoli and scant cytoplasm, although pancreatic examples can be more epithelioid and can express keratin strongly [14]. The proliferation rate is variable but can overlap with that of PD-NEC. Immunolabeling for CD99 can be helpful, since most PNETs show strong, diffuse membranous staining. CD99 does label a subset of well-differentiated NETs of the pancreas, however. In questionable cases, molecular studies can be performed to search for the diagnostic [t(11;22)] translocation of PNETs [14, 26].

17.5 Molecular Pathology

Recently, pancreatic small cell carcinomas and large cell neuroendocrine carcinomas were shown to be genetically related but distinct from pancreatic well-differentiated NETs. The genetic changes frequently seen in these poorly differentiated carcinomas, such as inactivation of the TP53 and the retinoblastoma/p16 pathways [5], are rarely observed in well-differentiated NETs, with only 4 % of well-differentiated NETs revealing a mutation in the *TP53* gene and none in the *retinoblastoma* gene [25]. In addition, immunohistochemical studies only detect rare p53 abnormalities in well-differentiated NETs [5, 24]. Of note, dysregulation of the TP53 pathway – through aberrant activation of its negative regulators (MDM2, MDM4, and WIP1) – may still be involved in pancreatic well-differentiated NETs as gene amplification and protein overexpression of these negative regulators are detected in some pancreatic well-differentiated NETs [24]. Conversely, approximately 45 % of sporadic pancreatic well-differentiated NETs harbor mutually exclusive mutations in either *DAXX* (death-domain-associated protein) or

ATRX (α-thalassemia/mental retardation syndrome X-linked) genes [25]. *DAXX* and *ATRX* encode nuclear proteins, which form a chromatin remolding complex and are involved in chromatin remolding at telomeric and pericentromeric regions. Mutations of these genes are associated with loss of DAXX/ATRX protein expression.

Of note, BCL2 protein, which is overexpressed in small cell carcinoma of the lung, is also overexpressed in PD-NECs (100 % of small cell carcinoma and 50 % of large cell neuroendocrine carcinomas) but is variably expressed in well-differentiated NETs [5].

17.6 Prognosis

The clinical course of pancreatic PD-NECs is worse than that of morphologically well-differentiated NETs that would be classified as 2010 WHO grade 3 on the basis of proliferation rate [4]. Most cases are rapidly fatal with widespread metastases involving regional and distant lymph node as well as intra- and extra-abdominal organs such as the liver and lung [2, 3]. Cisplatin- and etoposide-based regimens have shown some promise in controlling their growth; however, their overall prognosis remains grim [2, 27–30] with a median survival of 11 months [3]. Of note, there is no difference in survival among the morphologic subtypes of PD-NEC (small cell carcinoma vs. large cell neuroendocrine carcinoma) [2, 3]. The recent demonstration of BCL2 overexpression by PD-NECs [5] suggests that BCL2 antagonists may prove useful in their treatment in a manner similar to their current use in small cell carcinoma of the lung, which also expresses BCL2.

References

1. Bosman FT, Carneiro F, Hruban RH, Theise ND (2010) Neuroendocrine tumors of the GI tract. WHO Press, Lyon
2. Sorbye H, Welin S, Langer SW et al (2013) Predictive and prognostic factors for treatment and survival in 305 patients with advanced gastrointestinal neuroendocrine carcinoma (WHO G3): the NORDIC NEC study. Ann Oncol 24:152–160
3. Basturk O, Tang L, Hruban RH et al (2014) Poorly differentiated neuroendocrine carcinomas of the pancreas: a clinicopathologic analysis of 44 cases. Am J Surg Pathol 38(4):437–447
4. Basturk O, Yang Z, Tang LH et al (2015) The high-grade (WHO G3) pancreatic neuroendocrine tumor category is morphologically and biologically heterogenous and includes both well differentiated and poorly differentiated neoplasms. Am J Surg Pathol [Epub ahead of print]
5. Yachida S, Vakiani E, White CM et al (2012) Small cell and large cell neuroendocrine carcinomas of the pancreas are genetically similar and distinct from well-differentiated pancreatic neuroendocrine tumors. Am J Surg Pathol 36:173–184
6. Hruban R, Pitman MB, Klimstra DS (2007) Tumors of the pancreas. American Registry of Pathology, Washington, DC
7. Klimstra DS, Adsay V (2014) Tumors of the pancreas. In: Odze RD, Goldblum JR (eds) Surgical pathology of the GI tract, liver, biliary tract and pancreas. Saunders, Philadelphia
8. Thompson LDR, Basturk O, Adsay NV (2015) Pancreas. In: Mills SE, Carter D, Greenson JK et al (eds) Sternberg's diagnostic surgical pathology. Wolters Kluwer Health, Philadelphia
9. Morohoshi T, Held G, Klöppel G (1983) Exocrine pancreatic tumours and their histological classification. A study based on 167 autopsy and 97 surgical cases. Histopathology 7:645–661
10. Gordon DL, Lo MC, Schwartz MA (1971) Carcinoid of the pancreas. Am J Med 51:412–415
11. Corrin B, Gilby ED, Jones NF, Patrick J (1973) Oat cell carcinoma of the pancreas with ectopic ACTH secretion. Cancer 31:1523–1527
12. Hobbs RD, Stewart AF, Ravin ND, Carter D (1984) Hypercalcemia in small cell carcinoma of the pancreas. Cancer 53:1552–1554
13. Ordóñez NG, Silva EG (1997) Islet cell tumour with vacuolated lipid-rich cytoplasm: a new histological variant of islet cell tumour. Histopathology 31: 157–160
14. Movahedi-Lankarani S, Hruban RH, Westra WH, Klimstra DS (2002) Primitive neuroectodermal tumors of the pancreas. A report of seven cases of a rare neoplasm. Am J Surg Pathol 26:1040–1047
15. Shi C, Klimstra DS (2014) Pancreatic neuroendocrine tumors: pathologic and molecular characteristics. Semin Diagn Pathol 31:498–511
16. Klimstra DS, Rosai J, Heffess CS (1994) Mixed acinar-endocrine carcinomas of the pancreas. Am J Surg Pathol 18:765–778
17. Ohike N, Kosmahl M, Kloppel G (2004) Mixed acinar-endocrine carcinoma of the pancreas. A clinicopathological study and comparison with acinar-cell carcinoma. Virchows Arch 445:231–235
18. Ohike N, Basturk O, Klöppel G, Morohoshi T (2010) Mixed acinar-endocrine carcinoma of the pancreas. Pathol Case Rev 15:205–209

19. Basturk O, Adsay V, Hruban RH et al (2014) Pancreatic acinar cell carcinomas with prominent neuroendocrine differentiation: clinicopathologic analysis of a distinct and diagnostically challenging neoplasm (Abstract). Mod Pathol 27:447A

20. Reid MD, Balci S, Saka B, Adsay NV (2014) Neuroendocrine tumors of the pancreas: current concepts and controversies. Endocr Pathol 25:65–79

21. Nassar H, Albores-Saavedra J, Klimstra DS (2005) High-grade neuroendocrine carcinoma of the ampulla of vater: a clinicopathologic and immunohistochemical analysis of 14 cases. Am J Surg Pathol 29:588–594

22. Zee SY, Hochwald SN, Conlon KC et al (2005) Pleomorphic pancreatic endocrine neoplasms: a variant commonly confused with adenocarcinoma. Am J Surg Pathol 29:1194–1200

23. Strosberg JR, Coppola D, Klimstra DS et al (2010) The NANETS consensus guidelines for the diagnosis and management of poorly differentiated (high-grade) extrapulmonary neuroendocrine carcinomas. Pancreas 39:799–800

24. Hu W, Feng Z, Modica I et al (2010) Gene amplifications in well-differentiated pancreatic neuroendocrine tumors inactivate the p53 pathway. Genes Cancer 1:360–368

25. Jiao Y, Shi C, Edil BH et al (2011) DAXX/ATRX, MEN1, and mTOR pathway genes are frequently altered in pancreatic neuroendocrine tumors. Science 331:1199–1203

26. Bulchmann G, Schuster T, Haas JR, Joppich I (2000) Primitive neuroectodermal tumor of the pancreas: an extremely rare tumor. Case report and review of the literature. Klin Padiatr 2:185–188

27. Sellner F, Sobhian B, De Santis M et al (2008) Well or poorly differentiated nonfunctioning neuroendocrine carcinoma of the pancreas: a single institution experience with 17 cases. Eur J Surg Oncol 34:191–195

28. Kulke MH, Anthony LB, Bushnell DL et al (2010) NANETS treatment guidelines: well-differentiated neuroendocrine tumors of the stomach and pancreas. Pancreas 39:735–752

29. Gupta A, Duque M, Saif MW (2013) Treatment of poorly differentiated neuroendocrine carcinoma of the pancreas. JOP 14:381–383

30. Smith J, Reidy-Lagunes D (2013) The management of extrapulmonary poorly differentiated (high-grade) neuroendocrine carcinomas. Semin Oncol 40:100–108

Mixed Adenoneuroendocrine Carcinoma of the Pancreas

Michelle D. Reid, Gizem Akkas, Olca Basturk, and Volkan Adsay

18.1 Introduction: Definition

Pancreatic tumors typically differentiate into one of the three cell types that constitute this organ, ductal, acinar, or neuroendocrine (previously also called "endocrine"), and their classification is also based on the tumor's primary cell lineage. However, as in any other organ, a combination of different cell populations can be encountered in tumors involving the pancreas. This occurs through different mechanisms: (1) entrapment of native host cells within the neoplasm (e.g., peri-islet invasion by ductal adenocarcinomas, or the so-called ductulo-insular neuroendocrine tumors), (2) collision of two independent tumor types (serous cystadenomas and pancreatic neuroendocrine neoplasms seen in patients with von Hippel Lindau (VHL) disease), and (3) differentiation of the neoplastic cells along multiple lineages, such as in pancreatoblastomas and in mixed adenoneuroendocrine carcinomas, which will be discussed in detail in the ensuing text.

Neuroendocrine (NE) cells are particularly prone to occur as a second cell population in a variety of neoplasms, virtually in any organ. This may be due in part to the "stem-cell-ness" of neoplastic cells and the immature nature of the NE cells [1, 2]. In the pancreas, scattered NE cells are seen not uncommonly in non-neuroendocrine tumors, including adenocarcinomas, intraductal neoplasms, and acinar cell carcinomas. NE cells are especially notorious for occurring in the latter tumor (see Chap. 17), presumably related to their developmental kinship. In acinar cell carcinoma NE cells can manifest in a variety of patterns, ranging from scattered cells, to distinct clusters, to large zones, and, in some cases, even to dual differentiation within a given cell, as evidenced immunohistochemically by coexpression of the respective markers or the coexistence of neurosecretory and zymogen granules within the same cells.

Among the "mixed" carcinomas of the pancreas, *mixed adenoneuroendocrine carcinomas* are the least common and in fact are extremely rare epithelial neoplasms. They are characterized by an intimate mixture of dual ductal (glandular) component and a NE component, both of which show variable degrees of differentiation (well–poorly differentiated) and have distinct respective immunoprofiles. The World Health Organization (WHO) book for classification of

M.D. Reid • G. Akkas • V. Adsay, MD (✉)
Department of Pathology and Laboratory Medicine, Emory University School of Medicine, 1364 Clifton Rd NE, Atlanta, GA 30322, USA
e-mail: michelle.reid@emory.edu; Gizem.akkas@emory.edu; nadsay@emory.edu

O. Basturk
Department of Pathology, Memorial Sloan-Kettering Cancer Center, 1275 York Avenue, New York, NY 10065, USA
e-mail: basturko@mskcc.org

S. La Rosa, F. Sessa (eds.), *Pancreatic Neuroendocrine Neoplasms: Practical Approach to Diagnosis, Classification, and Therapy*, DOI 10.1007/978-3-319-17235-4_18,
© Springer International Publishing Switzerland 2015

gastrointestinal neoplasms recommends that at least 30 % of either component be present in order for a tumor to qualify as *mixed adenoneuroendocrine carcinoma* (MANEC) [3], although the figure of 25 % has also been advocated in some other texts.

Interestingly, NE carcinomas elsewhere in the gastrointestinal tract are commonly associated with a glandular precursor lesion or an adenocarcinoma component [4], but the pancreas seems to be different in the sense that poorly differentiated NE carcinomas (PDNECs) of the pancreas often do not have a glandular component [5]. Thus, it may not be surprising that MANECs as described in organs including the nasal cavity [6], stomach [4], small bowel [7], colon [4, 8, 9], gallbladder [10], and ampulla [11] are actually exceedingly uncommon in the pancreas [5, 12–15].

MANECs are known by a variety of synonyms including mixed adenoneuroendocrine carcinoma, mixed carcinoid-adenocarcinoma, mucinous carcinoid tumor, and mixed exocrine-endocrine tumor. The multiplicity of terms used to describe them in the literature has led to considerable confusion among pathologists, clinicians, and surgeons and has limited the accuracy of information regarding their true frequency, behavior, and prognosis. We believe it is advisable to refrain from using any of these names other than MANEC and the terms carcinoid-adenocarcinoma and mucinous carcinoid tumor ought to be avoided, especially in the pancreas.

18.2 Epidemiology

Pancreatic MANECs are said to account for less than 2 % of all gastroenteropancreatic neuroendocrine tumors [7]; however, in reality they may be even more uncommon, because it appears that a variety of cases described in the literature would not qualify using the current definition of 30 %. Many of the cases that appeared to have been recorded under the heading of "MANEC" ranged from predominant neuroendocrine neoplasms with focal exocrine cells to predominant

exocrine carcinomas with only isolated neuroendocrine cells, at the other extreme.

In pancreatic MANECs, both epithelial components are considered malignant, hence the term "mixed *carcinoma*." In the vast majority of cases, the NE component of the tumor is also high grade (Fig. 18.1), i.e., an overt carcinoma but with NE differentiation. However, occasionally a well-differentiated NE tumor (WDNET), qualifying as grade 1 or 2 of the 2010 WHO/European Neuroendocrine Tumor Society (ENETS), may be encountered in combination with an adenocar-

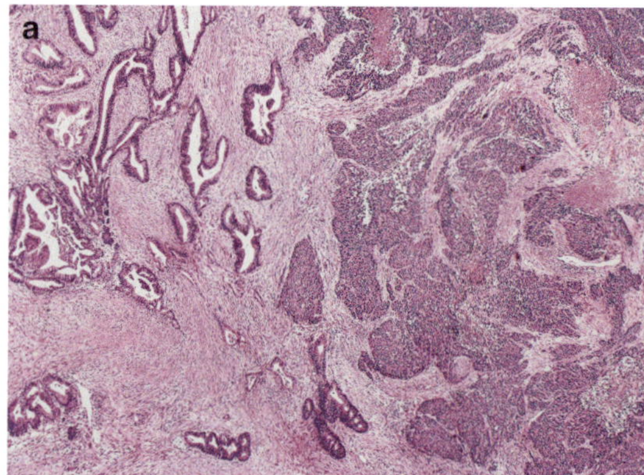

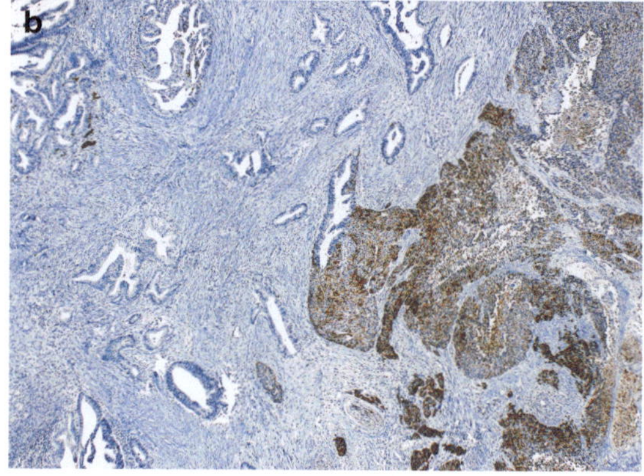

Fig. 18.1 Mixed adenoneuroendocrine carcinoma (MANEC) of the pancreas. (**a**) In the *left half* of the image, the pancreatic ductal adenocarcinoma component is composed of well-differentiated glandular structures within desmoplastic stroma (hematoxylin and eosin stain, magnification ×40). In the *right half* of the image, neuroendocrine carcinoma tumor cells have a high nuclear-to-cytoplasmic ratio with focal comedo necrosis. (**b**) The neuroendocrine cells are positive for chromogranin while the adenocarcinoma component is negative (magnification ×40)

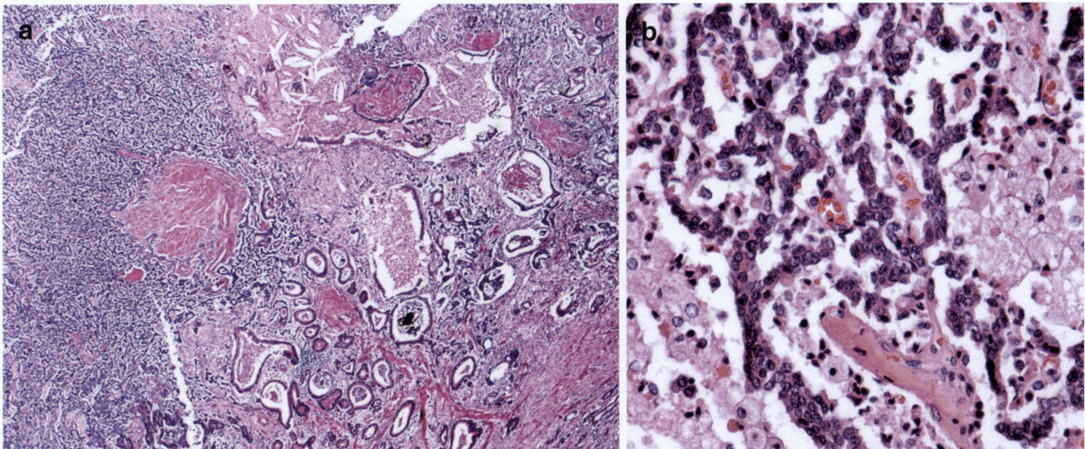

Fig. 18.2 (**a**) Mixed adenoneuroendocrine tumor (MANET) of the pancreas. In the right half of the image, the adenocarcinoma component is composed of well-differentiated glands within desmoplastic stroma (hematoxylin and eosin stain, magnification ×20). In the *left half* of the image, a second population of neuroendocrine tumor cells is seen which has high nuclear-to-cytoplasmic ratio and anastomosing ribbon-like network. (**b**) Image shows that these neuroendocrine cells are bland with only mild atypia (hematoxylin and eosin stain, magnification ×200)

cinoma. These may be alternatively termed "*mixed adenoneuroendocrine tumors* (MANETs)" [16], in a manner similar to their pure pancreatic and gastrointestinal counterparts (Fig. 18.2), as proposed by the 2010 WHO nomenclature used for (the neuroendocrine component of) these tumors [17]. These are even less common than PDNEC-predominant MANECs [13, 18].

18.3 Clinicopathologic Features

Patients with pancreatic MANEC range in age from 21 (unpublished data) to 84 years (mean of 68 years) and males and females are equally affected [5, 12–14, 18–25]. Tumors may arise anywhere in the pancreas, but are most common in the head, followed by the tail and body. They are often fairly cellular circumscribed tumors and range in size from 2 to 12 cm (mean 5.6 cm) [5, 13, 19].

18.3.1 Diagnosis and Morphology

The distribution of the two constituent tumor types is highly variable in MANECs. The two components may occur as separate and distinct

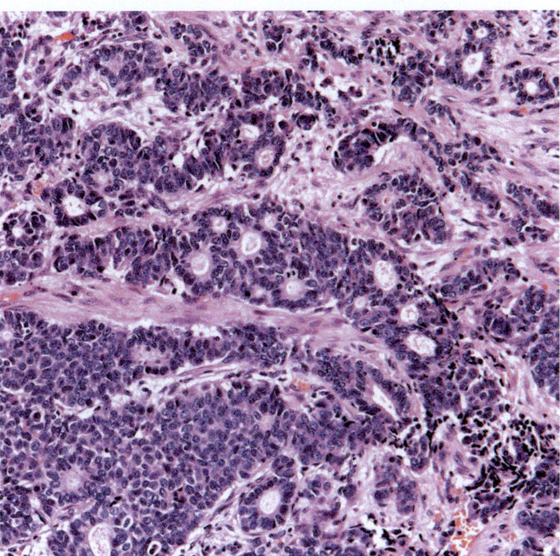

Fig. 18.3 Mixed adenoneuroendocrine carcinoma (MANEC) of the pancreas. Malignant glands are intimately admixed with large neuroendocrine cells showing high nuclear-to-cytoplasmic ratio and coarse salt-and-pepper chromatin (hematoxylin and eosin stain, magnification ×200)

(Fig. 18.1) or composite foci [4, 13, 19] or may be more intricately mixed (Fig. 18.3). The former group (the presence of distinct components) has also been termed "collision" tumors in the literature, but we prefer to reserve this term for neoplasms in which the two components are believed to be independent of each other (such as a serous adenoma and a NE tumor), presumably arising from different cell types. In contrast, in MANECs, the two components seem to be the product of the same neoplasm, even though they may appear as, and form distinct foci.

In some MANECs, the two cell types may not be clearly recognizable as distinct on cursory histologic examination and may require immunostains to more clearly identify a dual or divergent immunoprofile, while in other cases, the dual differentiation may be identified within the very same cells (true "amphicrine" carcinomas).

The ductal adenocarcinoma (PDAC) component of pancreatic MANECs typically shows variable differentiation ranging from well-differentiated tumors with well-formed glands (Fig. 18.1) to poorly differentiated carcinomas with ill-defined glandular units (Fig. 18.3), as well as clusters and sheets of highly malignant epithelial cells with marked nuclear pleomorphism and prominent nucleoli. These are typically embedded in abundant desmoplastic stroma. High-grade pancreatic intraepithelial neoplasia (PanIN-3) may be identified in the background pancreatic parenchyma [5].

The NE component is more frequently a poorly differentiated neuroendocrine carcinoma (PDNEC) of small or large cell type, as defined in the lungs. The small cell type is characterized by sheets or islands of small cells with high nuclear-to-cytoplasmic ratio, hyperchromatic nuclei with coarse chromatin, inconspicuous nucleoli, and irregular nuclear contours, with nuclear molding, single-cell and confluent necrosis, and brisk mitotic activity (>20/10 high power fields). The NE nature of the large cell type is often more readily evident in many examples by the more nested pattern and cytologic uniformity characteristic of NE carcinomas and is also often more successfully highlighted by immunohistochemical evaluation. Typically large cell types have more abundant cytoplasm and large nuclei with open chromatin and prominent nucleoli.

Among the six pancreatic MANECs described by Basturk et al. [5], five had a large cell PDNEC component and one had a small cell PDNEC com-

ponent. Four of the tumors showed lymphovascular and perineural invasion, as well as positive resection margins. All tumors had lymph node metastasis and by Union for International Cancer Control (UICC) guidelines were stage pT3N1 with two showing liver metastasis at diagnosis.

18.3.2 Immunohistochemistry

The PDAC component expresses a range of keratins including pancytokeratin, cytokeratin 7, and Cam5.2 as well as the glycoproteins of carcinoembryonic antigen (CEA), CA19-9, MUC1, and B72.3 [23]. Poorly differentiated forms show nuclear positivity for p53 [13, 26] (indicative of *p53* gene mutation), loss of DPC4 (indicative of *DPC4* gene mutations), and brisk mitotic activity corresponding to high Ki-67 indices [5]. The epithelial cells of glandular origin typically do not express NE markers.

In contrast, the NE cells in the NE component of the tumor, whether well or poorly differentiated, often express NE markers (synaptophysin, chromogranin A, and CD56), typically in more than 10 % of the tumor cells (Fig. 18.1), in addition to epithelial markers such as pancytokeratin. NE marker expression may be sparser in higher-grade examples. Synaptophysin is more sensitive than chromogranin A, but the latter is more specific [4]. CD56 antibody targets neural cell adhesion molecules (NCAMs), and although it is the least specific neuroendocrine marker, it may be useful in the differential diagnosis of these tumors. TTF1 is also often expressed in the PDNEC component, especially in those with a small cell pattern. p53 is positive in the NE cells and Rb is lost in up to 90 % [27]. In fact, some advocate the use of Rb loss as evidence of NE lineage in this setting. The pancreatic duodenal homeobox protein 1 (PDX-1) immunostain may also be positive in up to 40 % of PDNECs. BCL2 protein is also positive in PDNECs (100 % in small cell types and 50 % in large cell types), but is negative or focally positive in WDNETs [27]. By definition, the Ki-67 labeling index is typically high (greater than 50 %) in PDNECs and in fact is typically even greater than 80 % [5] but is between 0 and 20 % in WDNETs [17].

18.3.3 Cytopathology

The cytologic features of MANEC have only rarely been described [11, 22]. Tumors have both glandular and neuroendocrine features, the amount of which is highly variable depending on the component sampled during fine needle aspiration. This has significant implications for the accurate cytologic diagnosis of these tumors and may partly explain their underrepresentation in the cytology literature.

The ductal component has a variety of features depending on the degree of differentiation. For well-differentiated PDAC, tumor cells are usually present in flat or folded sheets composed of focally crowded and overlapping bland-appearing cells with only slight nuclear membrane irregularity and hyper- or hypochromasia. For poorly differentiated PDAC, cells form three-dimensional groups with nuclear pleomorphism, anisonucleosis, high nuclear-to-cytoplasmic ratio, marked nuclear contour irregularity, hypo- or hyperchromasia, and prominent (sometimes macro-) nucleoli. Single intact malignant cells, single-cell necrosis, abnormal mitotic figures, and background necrosis are typically seen in poorly differentiated tumors [11].

The neuroendocrine component also shows variable cytology depending on the degree of differentiation of the tumor. For tumors with a WDNET component, tumor cells are typically singly dispersed and bland, with plasmacytoid features. Focal rosettes may be seen both on cell blocks and on smears [11]. Nuclei are round to oval and bland and on Papanicolaou stain have characteristic salt-and-pepper chromatin. Nucleoli, if present, are usually small in well-differentiated neuroendocrine tumors. In small cell-type PDNEC, tumor cells resemble their counterparts in the lung. They are small to intermediate with high nuclear-to-cytoplasmic ratio, inconspicuous nucleoli, nuclear contour irregularity, salt-and-pepper chromatin, nuclear molding, single-cell and confluent necrosis, as well as crush artifact. Large cell-type PDNEC is characterized by large cells with abundant cytoplasm and nuclei with open, vesicular chromatin, and prominent nucleoli. The latter may be especially difficult to distinguish from the poorly differentiated PDAC component of the tumor without the help of immunohistochemical stains.

18.4 Differential Diagnosis

18.4.1 Ordinary Pancreatic Ductal Adenocarcinoma with Isolated Neuroendocrine Cells

PDACs can have rare isolated nonneoplastic neuroendocrine cells (best identified by immunohistochemical staining). In most instances, they are represented as rare scattered cells and, by definition, account for far less than 30 % of the tumor volume [4, 23]. These should not be categorized as MANECs nor should NE neoplasms that have focal non-neuroendocrine ductal cells.

It should be noted here that in many PDACs, adenocarcinoma cells invade into, and partially replace, the native islets of Langerhans and are intimately admixed with the islet cells (peri-isletic invasion; Fig. 18.4). When the adenocarcinoma is well differentiated and subtle, these foci can be dismissed as benign ductulo-insular complexes. Conversely, when carcinoma is prominent and

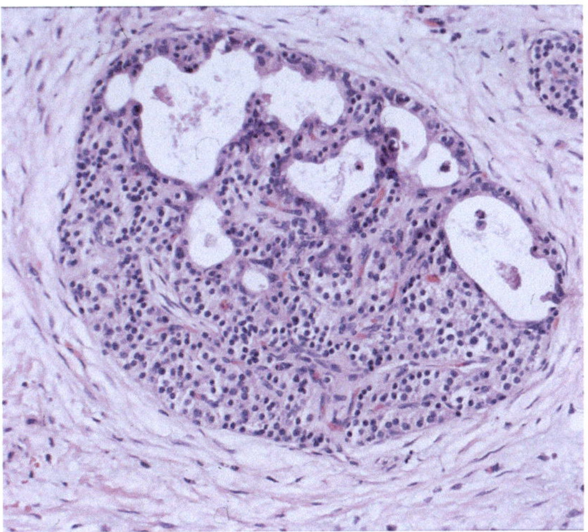

Fig. 18.4 Pancreatic ductal adenocarcinoma with malignant glands invading and partially replacing a native islet of Langerhans, the so-called peri-isletic invasion (hematoxylin and eosin stain, magnification ×100)

massively replaces the islet, the remaining islet cells can be mistaken as evidence of "mixed" differentiation.

18.4.2 Pancreatic "Ductulo-Insular"-Type Neuroendocrine Tumors

Some otherwise classical pancreatic neuroendocrine neoplasms show a striking admixture of benign ductular units. This phenomenon is known by a variety of names including pancreatic neuroendocrine tumors with ductulo-insular differentiation, duct-islet cell tumor, mucin-producing islet cell adenoma, and ductulo-insular tumors. These NE tumors are typically well differentiated with classical morphology, and the ducts are generally believed to be benign native ducts (Fig. 18.5) that are proliferative (hyperplastic), presumably under the induction of local tumor factors [23, 28–30]. Although some authors had speculated in the past on the neoplastic nature of the ducts [29], more recent studies showed that the ductal cells were morphologically, immunohistochemically (p53-negative), and genetically nonneoplastic (negative for *KRAS*, *DPC4*, and *ERBB2* mutations, all early genetic events in the development of PDAC) and likely represent preexisting entrapped ductules

[30]. This is in contrast to MANECs in which both the glandular and neuroendocrine components are not only neoplastic but also malignant. Additionally, when ductulo-insular tumors metastasize, it is only the neuroendocrine component that metastasizes, unlike MANECs in which either or both components may metastasize [14, 22]. Therefore, the interchangeable use of the terminology mixed ductular-insular tumor and MANECs is incorrect and misleading since the latter are morphologically malignant tumors with uniformly poor prognosis. In MANECs, the coexistence of ductular and neuroendocrine cells has been postulated to be due to transdifferentiation of neuroendocrine cells or divergent differentiation of pancreatic stem cells along ductal and endocrine lines.

This phenomenon of ductulo-insular NETs (in which there are benign ductules within a WDNET) is reported in variable amounts in 16 % of all neuroendocrine tumors in the pancreas; however, the examples with more abundant ductal units as illustrated in Fig. 18.5 are far less common in our experience. They are typically smaller than classical pancreatic neuroendocrine tumors (<2 cm), have prominent intratumoral sclerosis, and are insulin-positive (by immunohistochemistry), and the benign ductules can be distributed centrally, peripherally, or diffusely

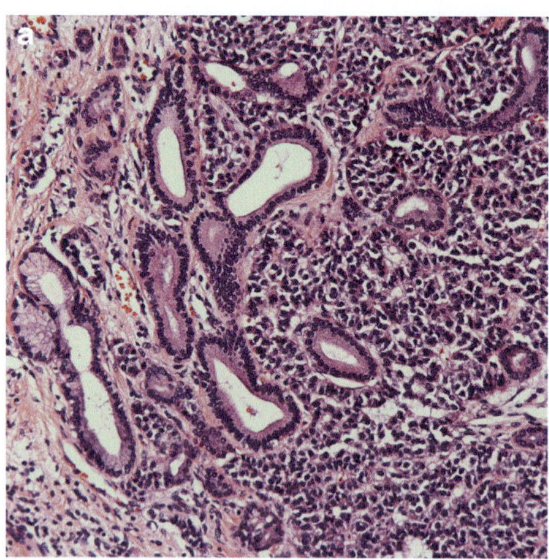
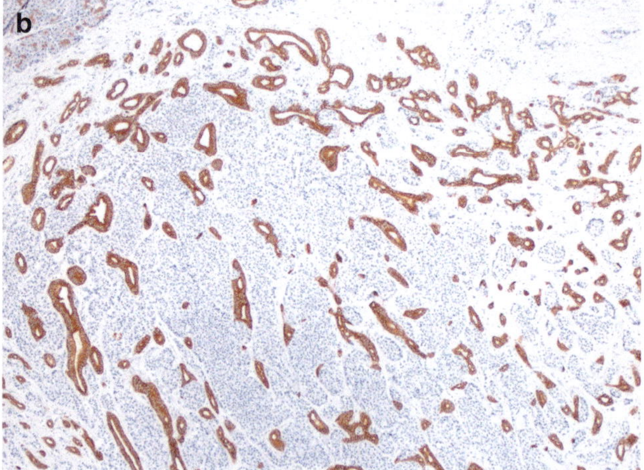

Fig. 18.5 Ductulo-insular tumor of the pancreas. (**a**) Neuroendocrine tumor cells are dispersed as aggregates of plasmacytoid cells with high nuclear-to-cytoplasmic ratio. Benign pancreatic ductules surround them peripherally (hematoxylin and eosin stain, magnification ×200). (**b**) The benign ductules are positive for cytokeratin 19, while the well-differentiated neuroendocrine component is negative (magnification ×40)

within the tumor. Ductules stain positively with cytokeratin 7 and 19 and are negative for neuroendocrine markers [28, 29].

18.4.3 Pancreatoblastoma

Pancreatoblastoma which is an extremely rare primary pancreatic neoplasm that shows trilineage differentiation can show predominant ductal and NE differentiation, thus simulating a MANEC on histology. Although pancreatoblastomas are generally regarded as tumors of childhood, they certainly also occur in adults, with a second peak in the mid-30s. In addition to glandular and neuroendocrine components, tumors typically have a significant acinar component, which would stain for pancreatic enzymes trypsin and chymotrypsin, as well as BCL10. More importantly squamoid morules, which are meningothelial-like or squamoid cell clusters, often but not always with optically clear biotin rich nuclei [31], are pathognomonic of pancreatoblastoma.

18.5 Molecular Pathology

Unfortunately few definitive molecular studies have been done on MANECs. The genetic alterations in these tumors thus would have to be extrapolated from the work that has previously been done on ordinary PDACs and neuroendocrine neoplasms.

A variety of somatic mutations involving four *key driver genes* have been implicated in PDAC including *KRAS*, *P16/CDKN2A*, *TP53*, and *SMAD4/DPC4* [32]. The frequency of these genetic mutations is somewhat variable, with *KRAS* and *p16/CDKN2A* mutations being most frequent (over 90 % of PDACs), while *TP53* (75 %) and *SMAD4/DPC4* (55 %) mutations are more variable.

Small and large cell-type PDNECs often show abnormal immunolabeling with p53 and Rb proteins (95 % and 74 % of cases, respectively) [27]. This correlates with intragenic mutant *TP53* and retinoblastoma *RB-1* genes. As a result p53

immunostain is frequently positive in the PDNEC component. Rb protein is lost in 60–90 % of PDNECs and tumors that retain Rb usually show concomitant loss of p16 staining [27], unlike WDNETs, in which Rb and p16 are retained. PDNECs retain DAXX and ATRX protein on immunohistochemical staining, indicative of the absence of inactivating *DAXX* (death-domain associated protein) and *ATRX* (alpha thalassemia/mental retardation syndrome X-linked) gene mutations. This is in contrast to WDNETs in which these mutations are frequently present and result in loss of DAXX and ATRX staining [33].

Gastrointestinal MANECs have been shown to harbor *TP53* mutations (92 %), with less frequent mutations in *ATM*, *CTNNB1*, *ERBB4*, *JAK3*, *KDR*, *KRAS*, and *RB1* genes [34]. The glandular and neuroendocrine components of some gastrointestinal MANECs have been shown to have overlapping mutations, suggesting a monoclonal origin of both tumor components. One reported colonic MANEC (with a PDNEC component) showed identical *KRAS*, *BCL9*, and *FOXP1* gene mutations in both components, further supporting the clonal relationship between the two [9]. These have not been tested in pancreatic MANECs.

18.6 Cell of Origin

Numerous authors have proposed that MANECs arise from pluripotent endodermal precursor stem cells within the pancreatic ducts and islets and give rise to both the ductal and neuroendocrine components [13, 15, 26]. As yet unknown stimuli are thought to then lead to the differentiation of these stem cells into exocrine and neuroendocrine primitive cells which later differentiate into ductal and neuroendocrine tumor cells.

This is a compelling proposal and is somewhat supported by the fact that the neuroendocrine component of MANECs expresses several transcription factors, including TTF-1 and PDX1. Positivity for these markers alludes to the "stem cell-like" nature of these tumor cells and the precursors from which they arise. PDX1 transcription factor plays a critical role in embryologic development of primal pancreatic ductal, neuro-endocrine, and acinar cells. Interestingly it is also expressed by pancreatic PDNECs, which further supports the possible development of these tumors from primal stem cells.

Additionally, the hematopoietic stem cell markers CD117 (75 %), CD34 (8 %), and PAX5 (17 %) have been identified in colorectal MANECs, suggesting a relationship with pro-genitor cells [8]. To our knowledge, these have not been tested systematically in pancreatic MANECs.

18.7 Management

The optimal management of MANECs remains unknown as too few cases have been studied in the literature. However, most MANECs are clearly high-grade malignancies, and the treatment of these tumors should be guided by the more aggressive tumor component. For the rare WDNETs with associated PDAC, the treatment should be focused on the ductal adenocarcinoma, while for MANECs in which the NE component is high grade, consideration may have to be given to the use of cis-platinum-based NE protocols [16].

18.8 Prognosis

Because few have examined pancreatic MANECs in detail, the assessment of their overall survival and behavior compared to their "pure" counter-parts is difficult. In the largest series of pancreatic MANECs published to date (six cases), it was shown that compared to pure pancreatic PDNECs, pancreatic MANECs had a slightly longer median survival of 20 months (versus 12 months for pure PDNECs) [5]. However the 2- and 5-year survival rates of these MANECs were 25 % and 0 %, respectively, which was not significantly different from those of pure pancreatic PDNECs (22 % and 9 %, respectively) [5]. Others have also shown similar results in colorectal MANECs, with better survival rates in the MANEC tumors versus pure PDNECs [8]. Thus, it is being specu-

lated that the ability of the neoplasm to form dif-ferent cell lineages may be a sign of differentiation (better grade). This, however, remains to be veri-fied in larger cohorts.

Pancreatic and colorectal MANECs both tend to present at advanced stage (stage III-IV by UICC/ENETS) [5, 8], and tumors with large neu-roendocrine cells seem to have better survival than small cell or mixed small and large cell types. CD117 (immunohistochemical) expression and vascular invasion have been shown to negatively affect survival in colorectal tumors [8].

18.9 Other Neoplasms with "Mixed" Glandular-Neuroendocrine Lineages

18.9.1 "Mixed" Intraductal Papillary Mucinous Neoplasm and Neuroendocrine Neoplasms

There is an interesting and rather unique associa-tion between pancreatic neuroendocrine neo-plasms and, another pancreatic exocrine neoplasm, intraductal papillary mucinous neo-plasm (IPMN) [5, 35–42]. While coexistence between these tumors is not considered MANEC, the frequent association (incidence rates range from 2.8 % to 4.8 %) [35, 38] provides compel-ling evidence that their coexistence is more than coincidental.

Tumors typically occur in the sixth decade and are more common in females (F:M, 2:1) [37]. The NE component ranges from well [36, 37, 40] to poorly differentiated [39] and is either separate from or intimately admixed with the IPMN com-ponent. The NE component ranges from minute (<10 mm) to approximately 3 cm, with the larg-est tumors occurring in PDNECs.

Those IPMNs with a WDNET are generally regarded as two separate neoplasms that arose independently (as is the case for those with serous adenomas; see below), presumably due to the patient's propensity to develop various tumor types, which end up "colliding" in the same area. However, those with PDNECs may represent true

MANECs [35, 43] (recognized as such if the NE carcinoma component is >30 % of invasion), as is the case for similar tumors in the tubular gastrointestinal tract [4].

18.9.2 "Mixed" Serous Cystic Neoplasms and Neuroendocrine Neoplasms

Pancreatic serous cystic neoplasms are rare benign non-mucinous tumors that may occasionally be seen in association with neuroendocrine neoplasms. In our experience, this occurs in 7 % of SCNs [44]. The NE component is usually well differentiated (WDNET) and is either intimately admixed with the serous component of the tumor or arises as a separate neoplasm. These so-called coexistent neoplasms are most commonly seen in patients with an underlying genetic disposition (most specifically VHL disease). In VHL disease, a rare autosomal dominant genetic disease, individuals have germline mutations in the von Hippel Lindau (*VHL*) tumor suppressor gene located on chromosome 3p(3p25–3p26) [45]. *VHL* gene mutations lead to the development of multiple extra-pancreatic (cerebellar hemangioblastoma, clear cell renal cell carcinoma, retinal angiomas) and pancreatic neoplasms including serous cystadenomas (11 % of patients) and neuroendocrine neoplasms (15 % of patients) [46], a higher frequency than that of sporadic cases. Unlike the loose association between IPMNs and neuroendocrine pancreatic neoplasms, the germline *VHL* mutations (and secondary somatic *VHL* mutations) are clearly linked to the development of the pancreatic serous neoplasms seen in these patients [47, 48].

References

1. Palapattu GS, Wu C, Silvers CR et al (2009) Selective expression of CD44, a putative prostate cancer stem cell marker, in neuroendocrine tumor cells of human prostate cancer. Prostate 69:787–798
2. Zhang Z, Zhou Y, Qian H et al (2013) Stemness and inducing differentiation of small cell lung cancer NCI-H446 cells. Cell Death Dis 4:e633
3. Rindi G, Arnold R, Bosman F et al (2010) Nomenclature and classification of neuroendocrine neoplasms of the digestive system. In: Bosman F, Carneiro F, Hruban R et al (eds) WHO classification of tumours of the digestive system, 4th edn. IARC Press, Lyon, pp 13–14
4. Shia J, Tang LH, Weiser MR et al (2008) Is nonsmall cell type high-grade neuroendocrine carcinoma of the tubular gastrointestinal tract a distinct disease entity? Am J Surg Pathol 32:719–731
5. Basturk O, Tang L, Hruban RH et al (2014) Poorly differentiated neuroendocrine carcinomas of the pancreas: a clinicopathologic analysis of 44 cases. Am J Surg Pathol 38:437–447
6. La Rosa S, Furlan D, Franzi F et al (2013) Mixed exocrine-neuroendocrine carcinoma of the nasal cavity: clinico-pathologic and molecular study of a case and review of the literature. Head Neck Pathol 7:76–84
7. Mandys V, Jirasek T (2014) Spectrum of gastroenteropancreatic NENs in routine histological examinations of bioptic and surgical specimen: a study of 161 cases collected from 17 departments of pathology in the Czech Republic. Gastroenterol Res Pract 2014:373828
8. La Rosa S, Marando A, Furlan D et al (2012) Colorectal poorly differentiated neuroendocrine carcinomas and mixed adenoneuroendocrine carcinomas: insights into the diagnostic immunophenotype, assessment of methylation profile, and search for prognostic markers. Am J Surg Pathol 36: 601–611
9. Vanacker L, Smeets D, Hoorens A et al (2014) Mixed adenoneuroendocrine carcinoma of the colon: molecular pathogenesis and treatment. Anticancer Res 34:5517–5521
10. Paniz Mondolfi AE, Slova D, Fan W et al (2011) Mixed adenoneuroendocrine carcinoma (MANEC) of the gallbladder: a possible stem cell tumor? Pathol Int 61:608–614
11. Zhang L, Demay RM (2014) Cytological features of mixed adenoneuroendocrine carcinoma of the ampulla: two case reports with review of literature. Diagn Cytopathol 42:1075–1084
12. Ahmad Z, Mumtaz S, Fatima S et al (2011) Mixed ductal-endocrine carcinoma of pancreas. BMJ Case Rep
13. Chang SM, Yan ST, Wei CK et al (2010) Solitary concomitant endocrine tumor and ductal adenocarcinoma of pancreas. World J Gastroenterol 16:2692–2697
14. Kloppel G (2000) Mixed exocrine-endocrine tumors of the pancreas. Semin Diagn Pathol 17:104–108
15. Leteurtre E, Brami F, Kerr-Conte J et al (2000) Mixed ductal-endocrine carcinoma of the pancreas: a possible pathogenic mechanism for arrhythmogenic right ventricular cardiomyopathy. Arch Pathol Lab Med 124:284–286
16. La Rosa S, Marando A, Sessa F et al (2012) Mixed Adenoneuroendocrine Carcinomas (MANECs) of the gastrointestinal tract: an update. Cancer Basel 4:11–30

17. Klimstra D, Arnold R, Capella C (2010) Neuroendocrine neoplasms of the pancreas. In: Bosman F, Carneiro F, Hruban R et al (eds) WHO classification of tumours of the digestive system, 3rd edn. IARC Press, Lyon, pp 322–326

18. Hirano H, Terada N, Yamada N et al (2011) A case of mixed ductal-endocrine carcinoma of the pancreas. Med Mol Morphol 44:58–62

19. Ballas KD, Rafailidis SF, Demertzidis C et al (2005) Mixed exocrine-endocrine tumor of the pancreas. JOP 6:449–454

20. Carter RR, Woodall CE 3rd, McNally ME et al (2008) Mixed ductal-endocrine carcinoma of the pancreas with synchronous papillary carcinoma-in-situ of the common bile duct: a case report and literature review – synchronous pancreatic and bile duct tumors. Am Surg 74:338–340

21. Eusebi V, Capella C, Bondi A et al (1981) Endocrine-paracrine cells in pancreatic exocrine carcinomas. Histopathology 5:599–613

22. Lennerz JK, Fernandez-Del Castillo C, Pitman MB (2011) Mixed ductal-endocrine carcinoma of the pancreas metastatic to the liver. Pancreas 40:319–321

23. Ohike N, Jurgensen A, Pipeleers-Marichal M et al (2003) Mixed ductal-endocrine carcinomas of the pancreas and ductal adenocarcinomas with scattered endocrine cells: characterization of the endocrine cells. Virchows Arch 442:258–265

24. Schron DS, Mendelsohn G (1984) Pancreatic carcinoma with duct, endocrine, and acinar differentiation. A histologic, immunocytochemical, and ultrastructural study. Cancer 54:1766–1770

25. Sessa F, Bonato M, Frigerio B et al (1990) Ductal cancers of the pancreas frequently express markers of gastrointestinal epithelial cells. Gastroenterology 98:1655–1665

26. Chatelain D, Parc Y, Christin-Maitre S et al (2002) Mixed ductal-pancreatic polypeptide-cell carcinoma of the pancreas. Histopathology 41:122–126

27. Yachida S, Vakiani E, White CM et al (2012) Small cell and large cell neuroendocrine carcinomas of the pancreas are genetically similar and distinct from well-differentiated pancreatic neuroendocrine tumors. Am J Surg Pathol 36:173–184

28. Chetty R, Serra S, Asa SL et al (2006) Pancreatic endocrine tumour with ductules: further observations of an unusual histological subtype. Pathology 38:5–9

29. Deshpande V, Selig MK, Nielsen GP et al (2003) Ductulo-insular pancreatic endocrine neoplasms: clinicopathologic analysis of a unique subtype of pancreatic endocrine neoplasms. Am J Surg Pathol 27:461–468

30. van Eeden S, de Leng WW, Offerhaus GJ et al (2004) Ductuloinsular tumors of the pancreas: endocrine tumors with entrapped nonneoplastic ductules. Am J Surg Pathol 28:813–820

31. Tanaka Y, Ijiri R, Yamanaka S et al (1998) Pancreatoblastoma: optically clear nuclei in squamoid corpuscles are rich in biotin. Mod Pathol 11:945–949

32. Jones S, Zhang X, Parsons DW et al (2008) Core signaling pathways in human pancreatic cancers revealed by global genomic analyses. Science 321:1801–1806

33. Heaphy CM, de Wilde RF, Jiao Y et al (2011) Altered telomeres in tumors with ATRX and DAXX mutations. Science 333:425

34. Scardoni M, Vittoria E, Volante M et al (2014) Mixed Adenoneuroendocrine Carcinomas (MANECs) of the gastrointestinal tract: targeted next generation sequencing suggests a monoclonal origin of the two components. Neuroendocrinology 100:310–316

35. Goh BK, Ooi LL, Kumarasinghe MP et al (2006) Clinicopathological features of patients with concomitant intraductal papillary mucinous neoplasm of the pancreas and pancreatic endocrine neoplasm. Pancreatology 6:520–526

36. Hashimoto Y, Murakami Y, Uemura K et al (2008) Mixed ductal-endocrine carcinoma derived from intraductal papillary mucinous neoplasm (IPMN) of the pancreas identified by human telomerase reverse transcriptase (hTERT) expression. J Surg Oncol 97:469–475

37. Kadota Y, Shinoda M, Tanabe M et al (2013) Concomitant pancreatic endocrine neoplasm and intraductal papillary mucinous neoplasm: a case report and literature review. World J Surg Oncol 11:75

38. Marrache F, Cazals-Hatem D, Kianmanesh R et al (2005) Endocrine tumor and intraductal papillary mucinous neoplasm of the pancreas: a fortuitous association? Pancreas 31:79–83

39. Stukavec J, Jirasek T, Mandys V et al (2007) Poorly differentiated endocrine carcinoma and intraductal papillary-mucinous neoplasm of the pancreas: description of an unusual case. Pathol Res Pract 203:879–884

40. Gill KR, Scimeca D, Stauffer J et al (2009) Pancreatic neuroendocrine tumors among patients with intraductal papillary mucinous neoplasms: real association or just a coincidence? JOP 10:515–517

41. Larghi A, Stobinski M, Galasso D et al (2009) Concomitant intraductal papillary mucinous neoplasm and pancreatic endocrine tumour: report of two cases and review of the literature. Dig Liver Dis 41:759–761

42. Mortele KJ, Peters HE, Odze RD et al (2009) An unusual mixed tumor of the pancreas: sonographic and MDCT features. JOP 10:204–208

43. Terada T, Ohta T, Kitamura Y et al (1997) Endocrine cells in intraductal papillary-mucinous neoplasms of the pancreas. A histochemical and immunohistochemical study. Virchows Arch 431:31–36

44. Hyejeong C, Memis B, Akkas G et al (2015) Serous neoplasms of pancreas (SNs): analysis of 231 cases with emphasis on variants and reappraisal of "serous cystadenocarcinoma". Mod Pathol 28:443A

45. Latif F, Tory K, Gnarra J et al (1993) Identification of the von Hippel-Lindau disease tumor suppressor gene. Science 260:1317–1320

46. Charlesworth M, Verbeke CS, Falk GA et al (2012) Pancreatic lesions in von Hippel-Lindau disease? A systematic review and meta-synthesis of the literature. J Gastrointest Surg 16:1422–1428
47. Mohr VH, Vortmeyer AO, Zhuang Z et al (2000) Histopathology and molecular genetics of multiple cysts and microcystic (serous) adenomas of the pancreas in von Hippel-Lindau patients. Am J Pathol 157:1615–1621
48. Vortmeyer AO, Lubensky IA, Fogt F et al (1997) Allelic deletion and mutation of the von Hippel-Lindau (VHL) tumor suppressor gene in pancreatic microcystic adenomas. Am J Pathol 151:951–956

Hyperplastic and Microadenomatous Pancreatic Neuroendocrine Lesions

19

Günter Klöppel, Martin Anlauf, Aurel Perren, and Bence Sipos

19.1 Introduction

Hyperplastic lesions of the neuroendocrine pancreas are based in their definition on a numerical increase in islets or certain islet cell types compared to the situation in the "normal pancreas." The diagnosis of islet hyperplasia therefore requires a quantitative approach. However, in almost all the pancreatic conditions that have been associated with hyperplastic islet lesions, the quantitations of the islets or the islet types have not been based on morphometric assessments but rather on subjective estimates or semiquantitative calculations. The reason for this lack of objective quantitative assessments is the difficulty to determine the normality of islet distribution, islet density, islet size, and islet cell type quantitation. These parameters not only differ very much with the age of the subjects whose pancreas is used as "control" tissue (e.g., infants versus adults or adults younger than 40 years versus older individuals), but also because of changes of the exocrine pancreas that increasingly occur with age and alter the affected islets. In theory, islet cell hyperplasia can be defined as an increase of the islet cell mass of more than 2 % (in adults) or 10 % (in infants) of that what is usually observed, but in practice, particularly if only portions of pancreatic tissue are available, all morphometric measurements are so variable that they only represent a rough approach to reality. Because of these inherent difficulties in determining the endocrine cell number, and even more, the cell mass, most diagnoses and descriptions of islet cell hyperplasia in the pancreas are based on estimates or rough semiquantitative calculations. It is therefore probably right to say that undisputed islet hyperplasia or hyperplasia of certain islet cell types are rare conditions but so distinct that they are recognized without the application of any sophisticated morphometry.

Microadenomatous lesions are, in the era of immunohistochemistry, much easier to define than islet hyperplasia. They are characterized as round islet cell clusters with a solid or trabecular pattern and a monohormonal (or almost monohormonal) cell composition. Their diameter is usually (but not strictly) greater than 300 μm

G. Klöppel (✉)
Department of Pathology, Consultation Center
for Pancreatic and Endocrine Tumors,
Technical University Munich,
Ismaningerstr. 22, 81675 Munich, Germany
e-mail: guenter.kloeppel@alumni.uni-kiel.de

M. Anlauf
Überregionale Gemeinschaftspraxis,
Institut für Pathologie und Zytologie,
St. Vincenz Krankenhaus, Limburg, Germany

A. Perren
Institute of Pathology, University Hospital Bern,
Bern, Switzerland

B. Sipos
Department of Pathology and Neuropathology,
University Hospital Tübingen, Tübingen, Germany

S. La Rosa, F. Sessa (eds.), *Pancreatic Neuroendocrine Neoplasms: Practical Approach to Diagnosis,
Classification, and Therapy*, DOI 10.1007/978-3-319-17235-4_19,
© Springer International Publishing Switzerland 2015

and less than 5 mm. In the "normal" pancreas, such microadenomas are encountered in up to 10 % of the cases [1] and are usually composed of glucagon cells. Some of them are found in fibrotic areas of the pancreas, where they are, because of the absence of the acinar cells, often in close contact with small ducts – a finding frequently regarded as an indication of islet cell neogenesis from ductal cells, although this has never been clearly proven.

In this chapter, we discuss hyperplastic lesions of the islets in conditions in which they are associated with subsequent neoplastic changes, i.e., microadenomas, whose forerunner they probably are (hyperplasia–neoplasia sequence) [2]. Beta-cell hyperplasia in newborns of diabetic mothers, or the beta-cell changes observed in "congenital hypoglycemic hyperinsulinism" [3, 4] and "non-insulinoma pancreatogenous hypoglycemia," also called "adult nesidioblastosis" are not discussed [5]. The insulin cell alterations of the latter diseases are usually included among the hyperplastic changes of the endocrine pancreas [6, 7], where they however do not belong, since they are characterized by hypertrophy of single beta cells rather than by diffuse insulin cell hyperplasia [3, 8]. Considered are reports on PP-cell hyperplasia which in retrospect most likely describe pseudohyperplasia of pancreatic polypeptide-rich islets in the pancreatic head [9].

19.2 MEN 1

The pancreas of patients with MEN1 (multiple endocrine neoplasia type 1) typically contains multiple small (<5 mm) NETs (neuroendocrine tumors), a finding referred to as microadenomatosis [10]. Islet hyperplasia and ductuloinsular proliferations, once described as key findings in addition to tumors in the MEN1 pancreas, have not been confirmed in more recent publications and seem not to be a feature of the MEN1 pancreas [10]. The pancreatic microadenomas that characterize MEN1 are often accompanied by one or more macrotumors (diameter >5 mm). Multihormonality is a common finding in these tumors, with one hormone usually prevailing (Fig. 19.1). Most frequent are tumors that are mainly glucagon positive, followed by PP, and then insulin or somatostatin-expressing tumors [10].

In MEN1 patients, all somatic cells harbor a heterozygous germline mutation of the *MEN1* tumor suppressor gene. By combining fluorescence in situ hybridization of the *MEN1* locus at 11q13 and the centromeric region of chromosome 11q with hormone immunostaining, it was demonstrated that microadenomas, defined as compact neuroendocrine cell aggregates lacking the typical islet architecture and expressing usually only one hormone, show loss of heterozygosity (LOH) at 11q13 and thus lack one *MEN1* allele which characterizes the neoplastic stage in MEN1 [11]. Normal islet cells were found to retain both MEN1 alleles. Interestingly, a few islets were identified that exhibited glucagon cell hyperplasia compared to the number of insulin cells in the same islets. As these glucagon cells also hold a central position in the islets, these intraislet glucagon cell clusters were regarded as precursors to microadenomas. The glucagon cells in these lesions either still retained both MEN1 alleles or already showed LOH at 11q [11] (Fig. 19.2). This suggested that the hyperplastic glucagon cells, that carry, like all cells of the body, the MEN1 germline mutation on one allele, were in a transient stage. While some had not yet assumed the neoplastic genotype, others had already performed the transition from the non-neoplastic to the neoplastic stage characterized by the allelic loss of 11q13. We do not know what mechanisms and factors force some islet cells, in particular glucagon cells, into proliferation and produce hyperplastic changes, but this process could be related to an increased responsiveness of the glucagon cell in the setting of MEN1 to certain growth factors or some other growth-enhancing mechanisms. The glucagon cells obviously share this ability with gastrin cells in the duodenal mucosa where focal gastrin cell hyperplasias were identified as precursors to gastrin microadenomas [12].

These results implicate first that the allelic loss at 11q13 in an islet cell sets the stage for NET development; second, it seems that the glucagon cell is the islet cell type that is most respon-

Fig. 19.1 Multihormonal microadenoma in the MEN1 pancreas immunostained for (**a**) glucagon and (**b**) pancreatic polypeptide

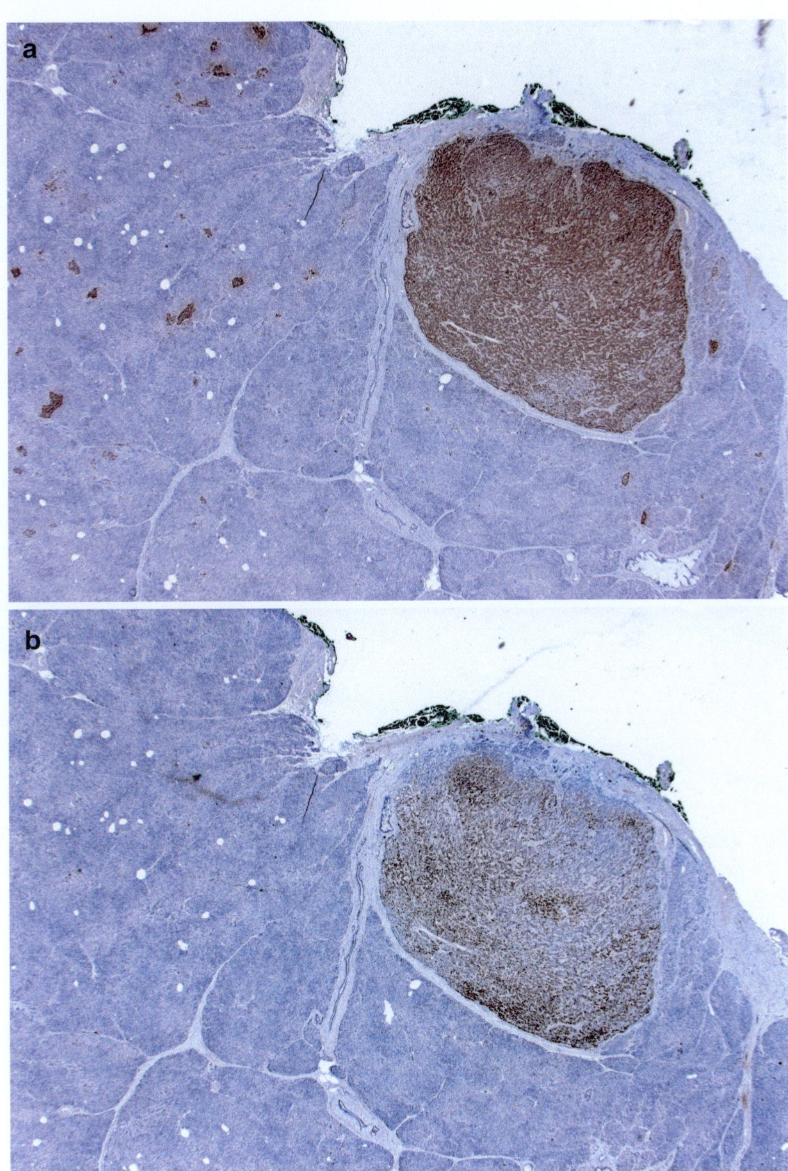

sive to hyperplastic and finally neoplastic stimuli. The reason why glucagon cells are particularly prone to these changes is yet not known.

Of the many microadenomas that are developing in the MEN1 pancreas, apparently only a small fraction proceeds to macrotumors (>0.5 cm and larger). This selective tumor evolution seems to be related to additional genetic alteration. When MEN1 microadenomas and macrotumors were analyzed for *ATRX/DAXX* mutations that correlate with alternate lengthening of telomeres and chromosomal instability [13], and are commonly found in advanced sporadic PanNETs [13, 14], microadenomas lacked the *ATRX/DAXX* mutations, while advanced macrotumors carried them [15]. This suggests that *ATRX* and *DAXX* mutations are late events in the tumorigenesis of pancreatic neuroendocrine neoplasms, and only those microadenomas may progress to macrotumors that acquire these genetic alterations.

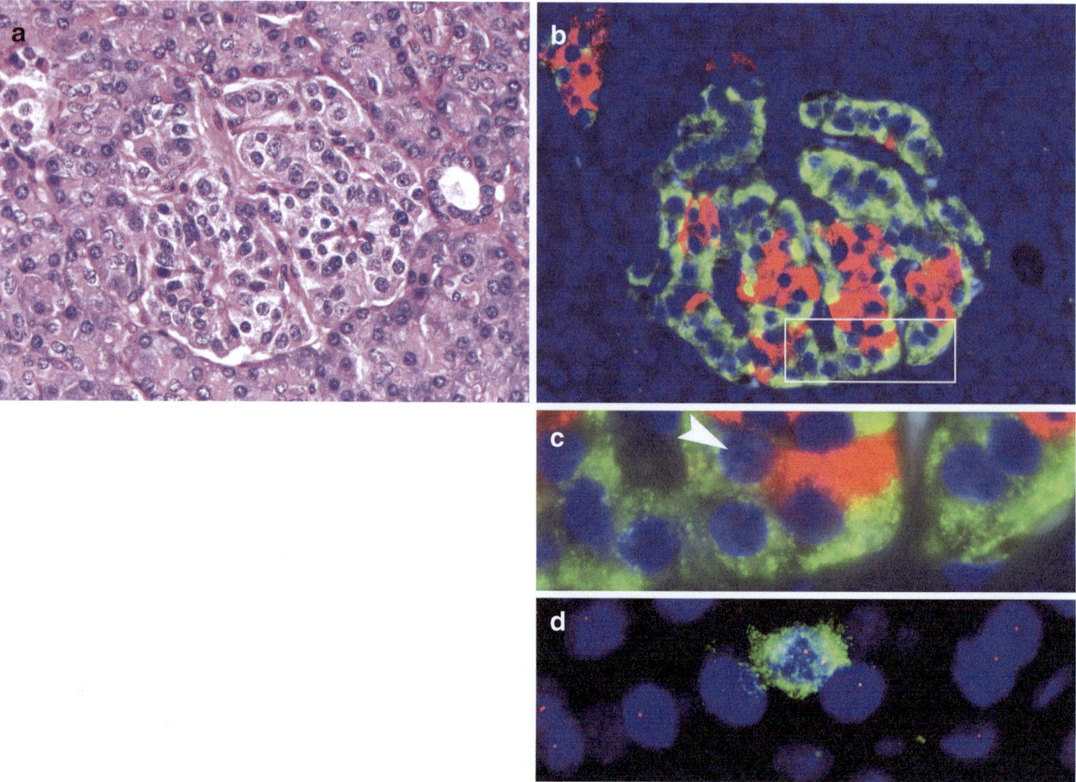

Fig. 19.2 Islet with glucagon cell hyperplasia turning into monoclonal cell proliferation. (**a**) H&E-stained islet with almost normal structure. (**b**) Serial section showing glucagon cell hyperplasia (immunofluorescence: glucagon in *green*, insulin in *red*). (**c**) *Enlarged box*-labeled area in **b**. Arrow head indicates the insulin cell marked in green in panel **d**. (**d**) Retention of heterozygosity of 11q13 in a single insulin cell (*green*) and LOH on 11q13 in unstained glucagon cells (From Perren et al. [11] with permission of publisher)

19.3 Glucagon Cell Adenomatosis (GCA)

Recently, GCA has been described as a distinct multicentric neoplastic disease of the pancreas that is preceded by glucagon cell hyperplasia of the islets [16, 17] (Fig. 19.3). There may be earlier reports on GCA (see [7]), but the descriptions of the changes are often difficult to classify. GCA is a disease that involves the entire pancreas, except for the so-called PP lobe in the head of the pancreas, where glucagon cells are infrequent [17a]. In the remaining pancreas, the islets are looking normal, when they are small. The bigger islets, however, display glucagon cell hyperplasia that correlates in its extent with the islet diam-

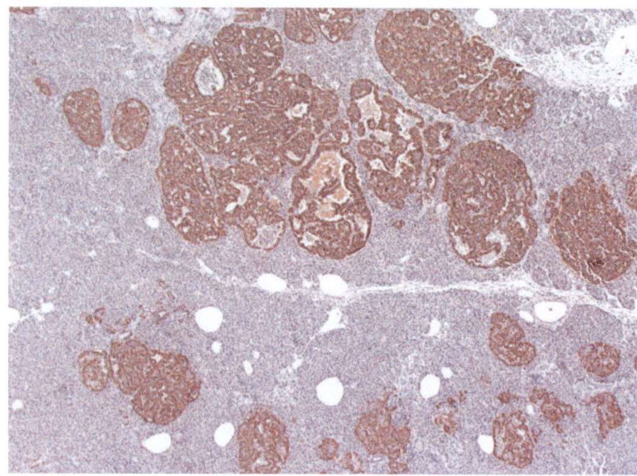

Fig. 19.3 Glucagon cell adenomatosis: islets with glucagon cell hyperplasia (lower part) next to multiple small glucagon-positive microadenomas (upper part of the illustration)

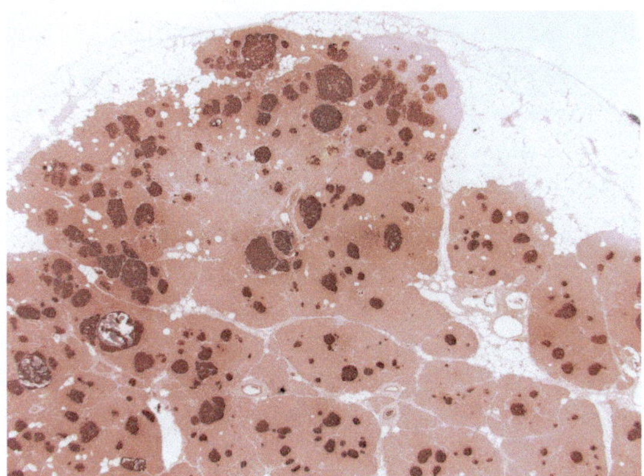

Fig. 19.4 Glucagon cell adenomatosis: immunostaining for glucagon shows islets with glucagon cell hyperplasia that imperceptibly transforms into microadenomas

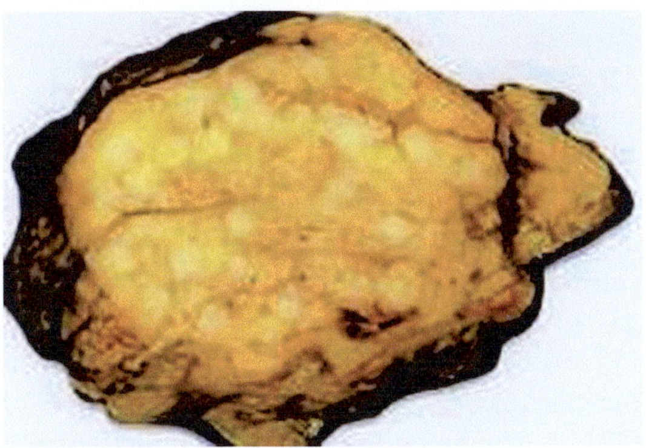

Fig. 19.5 Glucagon cell adenomatosis: cut surface of a pancreatic resection specimen shows multiple whitish small tumors

eter (Fig. 19.3). The largest islets then imperceptibly transform into glucagon cell microadenomas (Fig. 19.4). Rarely, the tumors may also contain a considerable number of PP cells. In the most advanced cases, there are single macrotumors (5–20 mm in size) (Fig. 19.5), some of them with cystic changes, as it is typical for glucagon-producing tumors [18]. All tumors were well differentiated, with a Ki67 index below 2 %. However, despite these benign features, lymph node micrometastases were detected in one patient. Clinically, the patients who were tested were found to have elevated glucagon serum levels, but usually presented without signs of a glucagonoma syndrome [7, 16].

Genetically, the disease was found to be unrelated to MEN1 and VHL. In half of the six patients of our GCA series, however, it was associated with inactivating homozygous and double-heterozygous germline mutations of the glucagon receptor (GCGR) gene, that were probably inherited in an autosomal, recessive mode as demonstrated in the parents of one of our patients [17a]. This suggests that a single heterozygous mutation of the *GCGR* gene probably does not cause the disease.

Analysis of the *GCGR* gene alterations suggests that the mutations cause a loss of receptor function, an assumption which is also supported by murine models [19], in which the deletion of the *GCGR* gene results in glucagon cell hyperplasia and finally also neoplasia [20]. While a dysfunctioning GCGR nicely explains the absence of a glucagonoma syndrome in the presence of elevated glucagon levels in the serum, the mechanisms that lead to the proliferative glucagon cell changes are unclear. It can be, however, postulated that there is a factor that stimulates the growth of glucagon cells. Since gluconeogenesis in the liver particularly depends on the effect of glucagon and thus on a functioning GCGR, it might be that the liver is the source of the postulated factor which is secreted in order to increase glucagon production by increasing glucagon cell number.

The mechanisms that lead to GCA in the patients of our series, in whom no *GCGR* mutations were detected, are also not known. However, the fact that GCA seems to occur without *GCGR* mutation, as has also been described in a recent case report on GCA [21], implies that probably alternate mechanisms exist that indirectly affect the GCGR signaling. GCA seems therefore to be a heterogeneous disease. If the patients with and without *GCGR* mutations are compared with each other, it appears that the mutation-positive patients have a more severe disease in terms of tumor size and number than the mutation-negative patients [17a].

If disturbed GCGR signaling, either directly or via an alternate pathway, plays an important role in the initiation of the disease, the question that has to be addressed next is what stimulates the development of the subsequent neoplastic changes. Most likely, additional genetic changes are required for this development, but so far, no findings are available explaining this second step in the tumorigenesis of GCA. Since in rare cases GCA may cause lymph node metastases, its name has perhaps to be changed in the future to glucagon cell hyperplasia and neoplasia.

19.4 Insulinomatosis

Insulinomatosis has been described as a distinct neoplastic disease of the pancreas, in which, syn- and metachronously, multiple small and single large insulin-producing tumors develop [22] (Fig. 19.6). The affected patients present with hyperinsulinemic hypoglycemia which, after removal of the large visible insulinoma(s), has a great risk of recurrence because of the development of new large tumors in the remaining pancreas. The patients therefore often have a history of repeated pancreatic surgery that finally results in total removal of the pancreas. It seems that the tumors are not preceded by an insulin cell hyperplasia in the islets, but rather originate from compact insulin cell clusters, often with a trabecular pattern, devoid of any other islet cell type. In all but one patient of our series, the disease followed a benign course. The patient with malignant disease developed lymph node and liver metastases. So far, no genetic defect has been discovered, but familiarity may occur.

19.5 Microadenomatosis in Von Hippel-Lindau Disease (VHL)

In patients with *VHL* gene mutations, the pancreas may show multiple neuroendocrine tumors, sometimes in addition to multicentric serous cystic neoplasms. These tumors that are commonly positive for somatostatin and may show clear cell features also appear to arise on a background of microadenomatosis [23] (Fig. 19.7). Not known so far is whether the microadenomas evolve from a hyperplasia of islet cells.

19.6 Pseudohyperplasia of PP-Rich Islets

The dorsal portion of the head of the pancreas is densely populated by pancreatic polypeptide cell-rich islets (PPRIs). This physiologic finding has often given rise to the false diagnosis of PP-cell hyperplasia, although the "PP lobe" in the pancreas has already been described in 1979 [24]. It was found that PP cells are not equally distributed in the human pancreas. They are abundant in the posterior part of the pancreatic head, where they account for 70–80 % of the islet

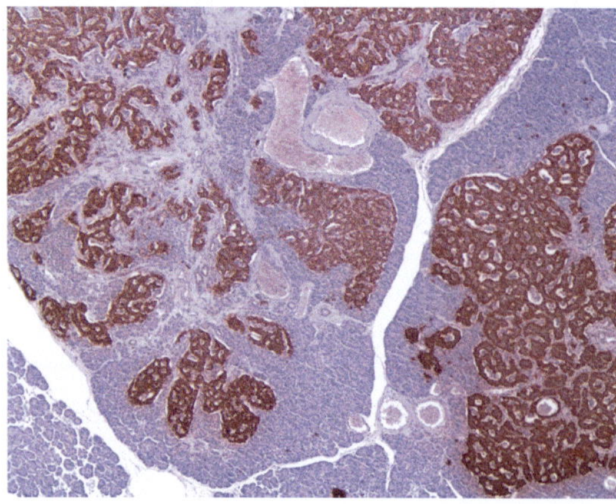

Fig. 19.6 Insulinomatosis: immunostaining for insulin reveals multiple trabecular microadenomas

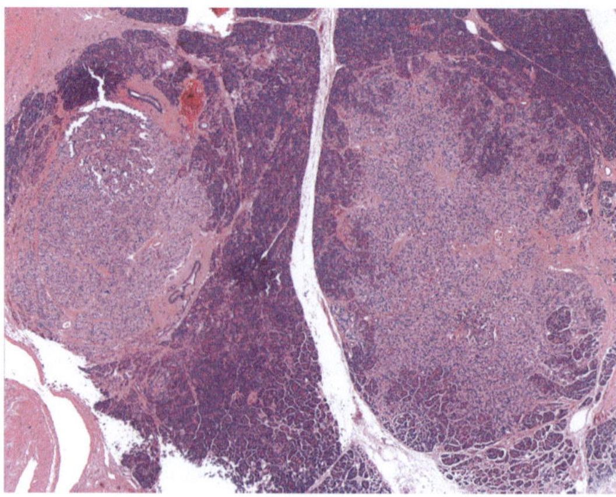

Fig. 19.7 Pancreatic microadenomas in von Hippel-Lindau disease

cells ("PP-rich islets," PPRIs), but scarce in the remaining gland. This distinct distribution of the PP cells in the pancreas is explained by the gland's complex ontogeny. The posterior portion of the pancreatic head that harbors the PPRI stems from the ventral pancreatic anlage, which accounts for approximately 10 % of the total pancreas parenchyma [25], while the remainder of the gland that contains the insulin-rich islets derives from the dorsal anlage. In subjects older than 50 years, the PPRI appears to be larger and more numerous because of a reduction of the surrounding acinar cells. The reason for this change is unclear, but it leads to pseudohyperplasia of the PPRI that may be misinterpreted as true hyperplasia or even neoplasia. Thus, the hyperplasia-like changes of the PP lobe represent a normal condition in elderly people. In the literature, eight cases of "PP-cell hyperplasia" have been reported (for review, see [7]). In retrospect, it seems that all these reports describe pseudohyperplastic PPRI aggregates in the pancreatic head. Why some of the cases were associated with a Zollinger-Ellison syndrome (ZES) or the syndrome of watery diarrhea is not known. However, what is clear from the reports is that the pseudohyperplastic islet aggregates in the pancreatic head neither produced gastrin nor VIP and could therefore not have caused the syndrome, which in case of a ZES was most likely be due to a small gastrinoma in the duodenum [26].

Regarding the question why in elderly people PPRI clusters in pseudohyperplastic aggregates, it is of interest that insulin exerts a trophic effect on acinar cells (Fig. 19.8). This is known from the pancreas of type 1 diabetics with long-lasting disease, which shows atrophic acinar cells surrounding the islets without insulin cells [27]. The islets of the PP lobe still contain their insulin cells in elderly people, but as the insulin cells account only for 30 % of the islet cell population, this insulin cell number might not provide a sufficient lifelong trophic effect on all the surrounding acinar cells. The result might be a cellular and numeric atrophy of the acinar cells in the PP lobe resulting in a clustering of PPRI in elderly subjects. Since PP cells and all other islet cells in the PPRI clusters strongly express somatostatin receptors, a signal may be recognized in somatostatin receptor scintigraphy

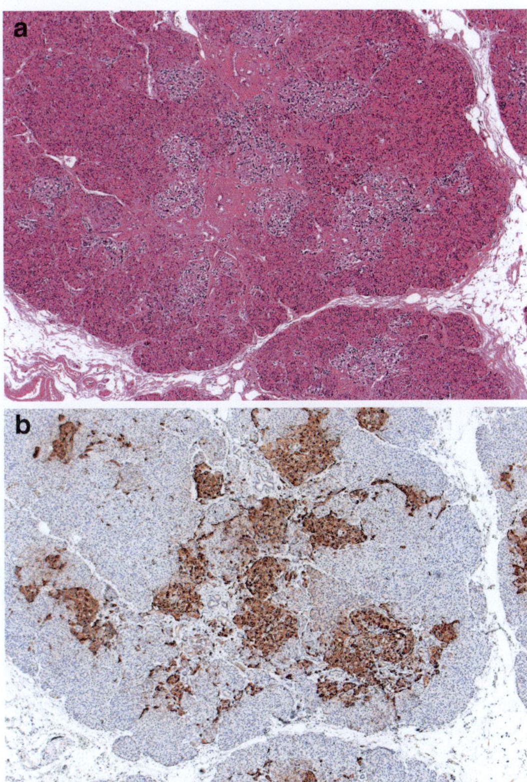

Fig. 19.8 Pseudohyperplasia of pancreatic polypeptide (PP)-rich islets in the posterior portion of the head of the pancreas of a 75-year-old patient. (**a**) H&E-stained section. (**b**) Consecutive section stained for PP

that mimics the uptake associated with a tumor and may therefore lead to the false diagnosis of a pancreatic NET [9].

Conclusions

The two distinct neuroendocrine diseases of the pancreas that show a hyperplasia–neoplasia sequence are MEN1 and the recently discovered glucagon cell adenomatosis that is associated with a germline mutation in the glucagon receptor gene. Diseases characterized by microadenomatosis, in which however a hyperplasia–neoplasia sequence has not (yet) been established, are insulinomatosis and VHL-associated microadenomatosis.

The clustering of islets rich in PP cells in the dorsal portion of the pancreatic head is a physiological age-dependent change that shows no evolution into a hyperplasia–neoplasia sequence.

References

1. Kimura W, Kuroda A, Morioka Y (1991) Clinical pathology of endocrine tumors of the pancreas. Analysis of autopsy cases. Dig Dis Sci 36:933–942

2. Kloppel G, Anlauf M, Perren A, Sipos B (2014) Hyperplasia to neoplasia sequence of duodenal and pancreatic neuroendocrine diseases and pseudohyperplasia of the PP-cells in the pancreas. Endocr Pathol 25:181–185

3. Kloppel G, Reinecke-Luthge A, Koschoreck F (1999) Focal and diffuse beta cell changes in persistent hyperinsulinemic hypoglycemia of infancy. Endocr Pathol 10:299–304

4. Sempoux C, Guiot Y, Jaubert F, Rahier J (2004) Focal and diffuse forms of congenital hyperinsulinism: the keys for differential diagnosis. Endocr Pathol 15:241–246; Rahier J, Guiot Y, Sempoux C (2011) Morphologic analysis of focal and diffuse forms of congenital hyperinsulinism. Semin Pediatr Surg 20:3–12

5. Anlauf M, Wieben D, Perren A et al (2005) Persistent hyperinsulinemic hypoglycemia in 15 adults with diffuse nesidioblastosis: diagnostic criteria, incidence and characterization of á-cell changes. Am J Surg Pathol 29:524–533

6. Starke A, Saddig C, Kirch B, Tschahargane C, Goretzki P (2006) Islet hyperplasia in adults: challenge to preoperatively diagnose non-insulinoma pancreatogenic hypoglycemia syndrome. World J Surg 30:670–679

7. Ouyang D, Dhall D, Yu R (2011) Pathologic pancreatic endocrine cell hyperplasia. World J Gastroenterol: WJG 17:137–143

8. Kloppel G, Anlauf M, Raffel A, Perren A, Knoefel WT (2008) Adult diffuse nesidioblastosis: genetically or environmentally induced? Hum Pathol 39:3–8

9. Albers MB, Maurer E, Kloppel G, Bartsch DK (2014) Pancreatic polypeptide-rich islets in the posterior portion of the pancreatic head–a tumor mimic in somatostatin receptor scintigraphy. Pancreas 43:648–650

10. Anlauf M, Schlenger R, Perren A et al (2006) Microadenomatosis of the endocrine pancreas in patients with and without the multiple endocrine neoplasia type 1 syndrome. Am J Surg Pathol 30:560–574

11. Perren A, Anlauf M, Henopp T et al (2007) Multiple endocrine neoplasia type 1: loss of one MEN1 allele in tumors and monohormonal endocrine cell clusters, but not in islet hyperplasia of the pancreas. A combined FISH and immunofluorescence study. J Clin Endocrinol Metab 92:1118–1128

12. Anlauf M, Perren A, Henopp T et al (2007) Allelic deletion of the MEN1 gene in duodenal gastrin and somatostatin cell neoplasms and their precursor lesions. Gut 56:637–644

13. Marinoni I, Kurrer AS, Vassella E et al (2014) Loss of DAXX and ATRX are associated with chromosome instability and reduced survival of patients with pancreatic neuroendocrine tumors. Gastroenterology 146:453–460.e455

14. Jiao Y, Shi C, Edil BH et al (2011) DAXX/ATRX, MEN1, and mTOR pathway genes are frequently altered in pancreatic neuroendocrine tumors. Science 331:1199–1203

15. de Wilde RF, Heaphy CM, Maitra A et al (2012) Loss of ATRX or DAXX expression and concomitant acquisition of the alternative lengthening of telomeres phenotype are late events in a small subset of MEN-1 syndrome pancreatic neuroendocrine tumors. Mod Pathol: Off J U S Can Acad Pathol Inc 25:1033–1039

16. Henopp T, Anlauf M, Schmitt A et al (2009) Glucagon cell adenomatosis: a newly recognized disease of the endocrine pancreas. J Clin Endocrinol Metab 94:213–217

17. Zhou C, Dhall D, Nissen NN, Chen CR, Yu R (2009) Homozygous P86S mutation of the human glucagon receptor is associated with hyperglucagonemia, alpha cell hyperplasia, and islet cell tumor. Pancreas 38:941–946

17a. Sipos B, Sperveslage J, Anlauf M, Hoffmeister M, Henopp T, Buch S, Hampe J, Weber A, Hammel P, Couvelard A, Höbling W, Lieb W, Böhm BO, Klöppel G. (2015) Glucagon cell hyperplasia and neoplasia with and without glucagon receptor mutations. J Clin Endocrinol Metab. jc20144405. [Epub ahead of print]

18. Konukiewitz B, Enosawa T, Kloppel G (2011) Glucagon expression in cystic pancreatic neuroendocrine neoplasms: an immunohistochemical analysis. Virchows Archiv: Int J Pathol 458:47–53

19. Yu R (2014) Pancreatic alpha-cell hyperplasia: facts and myths. J Clin Endocrinol Metab 99:748–756

20. Yu R, Dhall D, Nissen NN, Zhou C, Ren SG (2011) Pancreatic neuroendocrine tumors in glucagon receptor-deficient mice. PLoS ONE 6:e23397

21. Al-Sarireh B, Haidermota M, Verbeke C, Rees DA, Yu R, Griffiths AP (2013) Glucagon cell adenomatosis without glucagon receptor mutation. Pancreas 42:360–362

22. Anlauf M, Bauersfeld J, Raffel A et al (2009) Insulinomatosis. A multicentric insulinoma disease that frequently causes early recurrent hyperinsulinemic hypoglycemia. Am J Surg Pathol 33:339–346

23. Perigny M, Hammel P, Corcos O et al (2009) Pancreatic endocrine microadenomatosis in patients with von Hippel-Lindau disease: characterization by VHL/HIF pathway proteins expression. Am J Surg Pathol 33:739–748

24. Malaisse-Lagae F, Stefan Y, Cox J, Perrelet A, Orci L (1979) Identification of a lobe in the adult human pancreas rich in pancreatic polypeptide. Diabetologia 17:361–365

25. Bommer G, Friedel U, Heitz PU (1980) Kl''ppel G Pancreatic PP cell distribution and hyperplasia: immunocytochemical morphology in normal pancreas, chronic pancreatitis and pancreatic carcinoma. Virchows Archiv [A] Pathol Anat 387:319–331

26. Anlauf M, Garbrecht N, Henopp T et al (2006) Sporadic versus hereditary gastrinomas of the duodenum and pancreas: distinct clinico-pathological and epidemiological features. World J Gastroenterol 12:5440–5446

27. Löhr M, Klöppel G (1987) Residual insulin positivity and pancreatic atrophy in relation to duration of chronic type 1 (insulin-dependent) diabetes mellitus and microangiopathy. Diabetologia 30:757–762

Daniela Furlan

20.1 Hereditary Pancreatic Neuroendocrine Tumors

Approximately 5–10 % of PanNETs have a hereditary background, and they may occur as part of four hereditary syndromes: multiple endocrine neoplasia type1 (MEN1; OMIM 131100), von Hippel-Lindau disease (VHL; OMIM 193300), and, less frequently, neurofibromatosis type 1 (NF1; OMIM 162200) or tuberous sclerosis (TS; OMIM 191100) (Table 20.1).

MEN1 is a rare autosomal dominant disorder characterized by a greatly elevated risk of a variety of endocrine tumors involving the pituitary, parathyroid, endocrine pancreas, and duodenum. Hereditary PanNETs occur in 20–70 % of MEN1-affected patients [1], and they are frequently small, nonfunctioning, multiple, and benign. Moreover, they have an earlier age of onset and a much higher rate of postoperative recurrences compared with their sporadic counterparts. MEN1 patients typically harbor multiple small pancreatic neuroendocrine microadenomas, thought to be precursor lesions to malignant PanNETs. A genetic locus associated with MEN1

syndrome was localized to the long arm of chromosome 11 (11q13), and the gene responsible (*MEN1*) was identified by positional cloning techniques [2, 3]. *MEN1* spans 9.8 kb with ten exons and encodes a 610-amino-acid protein named menin [4] which is a ubiquitously expressed nuclear protein. Heterozygous germline mutations scattered throughout the *MEN1* coding region have been identified in over 80 % of probands/families with patients sharing at least three major lesions of the syndrome and first-degree relatives affected by one (or more) MEN1-related lesions. More than 1,300 mutations in *MEN1* have been identified to date, with the majority of mutations resulting in the loss of function of the protein [5].

Menin is critical to normal pancreatic β cell homeostasis and glucose sensing. High glucose levels activate PI3K/Akt, through phosphorylation of the transcription factor FoxO1 [6, 7]. FoxO1 has decreased binding affinity to the *MEN1* promoter, resulting in inhibition of menin expression and

D. Furlan
Department of Surgical and Morphological Sciences,
Section of Anatomic Pathology,
University of Insubria, O. Rossi 9, Varese,
Varese 21100, Italy
e-mail: daniela.furlan@uninsubria.it

Table 20.1 Genetic syndromes associated with PanNETs

Syndrome	Affected gene	Prevalence in PanNETs (%)
Multiple endocrine neoplasia type 1	*MEN1*	20–70
Von Hippel-Lindau	*VHL*	<20
Neurofibromatosis type 1	*NF1*	<10
Tuberous sclerosis complex	*TSC2*	Rare (~1)

S. La Rosa, F. Sessa (eds.), *Pancreatic Neuroendocrine Neoplasms: Practical Approach to Diagnosis, Classification, and Therapy*, DOI 10.1007/978-3-319-17235-4_20,
© Springer International Publishing Switzerland 2015

enhanced proliferation. Homozygous deletion of the *MEN1* gene is embryonic lethal [8]. Mice with heterozygous deletion of the *MEN1* gene develop multiple endocrine tumors, reminiscent of the human syndrome [9–11]. Moreover, menin promotes the expression of cell-cycle inhibitors being an essential component of the mixed lineage leukemia (MLL) histone methyl transferase complex that regulates chromatin remodeling [12, 13]. In normal pancreatic islet cells, the tumor suppressor activity of menin is due to the inhibition of proliferation, through H3K4 methylation at promoters of *CDKN2C* and *CDKN1B* [14, 15]. In addition, menin may also be involved in the response to DNA damage. Genome-wide chromatin studies have found menin to be associated with promoter and coding regions of hundreds of genes [16, 17]. In particular it associates with the 5′ regions of genes whose protein products are involved in DNA repair, implicating menin in the DNA damage response and therefore genomic stability [18, 19]. Taken together, these data suggest that loss of menin causes deregulation of normal cell growth control in conjunction with increased genomic instability.

Von Hippel-Lindau syndrome is the second autosomal dominant predisposition syndrome featuring an elevated rate of NETs [20]. VHL-related pancreatic tumors are mostly exocrine microcystic adenomas, but 5–17 % of patients with VHL could be affected by PanNETs [21–23]. These tumors have typical morphological characteristics, consisting of solid, trabecular, or glandular structures composed in about 60 % of cases of clear cells with vacuolated lipid-rich cytoplasm [24, 25]. Most VHL PanNETs are multiple and nonfunctioning, and 30–40 % of them demonstrate focal positivity for pancreatic polypeptide, somatostatin, glucagon, and/or insulin [24]. Like VHL-associated renal tumors and retinal and/or cerebellar neoplasms, pancreatic islet-cell tumors are markedly vascular. Most of these tumors are slow-growing and asymptomatic, but some cases can grow rapidly or metastasize. Despite the variety of tumor types observed clinically in this disorder, progression to malignancy in VHL disease is associated primarily with the development of renal carcinomas and PanNETs [24, 25]. VHL syndrome results from germline mutations in the *VHL* gene, a tumor suppressor gene located at 3p25 with three coding exons [23]. That has been shown to be involved in multiple functions including ubiquitination and the regulation of angiogenesis, as well as a gatekeeper function in the G0/G1 checkpoint. A crucial function of VHL protein is the oxygen-regulated degradation of hypoxia-inducible factor (HIF) alpha, a transcription factor that regulates gene expression in response to low-oxygen conditions [26, 27]. Lack of degradation of this factor, due to the absence of the VHL protein, results in the uncontrolled production of factors promoting the formation of blood vessels such as vascular endothelial growth factor implicated in tumor development [28–31]. Germline *VHL* mutations have been characterized in more than 500 patients and have provided a wealth of data for genotype-phenotype correlations [32–34]. Among patients with VHL syndrome, about 40 % of mutations are genomic deletions and the rest are predominantly truncating or missense mutations [35]. VHL-associated tumors show somatic alteration of the remaining wild-type allele by allelic loss or, more rarely, by promoter hypermethylation [36]. Molecular profiling of VHL PanNETs compared to sporadic PanNETs has recently demonstrated that VHL PanNETs have specific genetic alterations; most striking are those related to angiogenesis and HIF signaling [37].

Neurofibromatosis type 1 and tuberous sclerosis are the two other inherited autosomal syndromes that are associated, albeit infrequently, with increased susceptibility to PanNETs (Table 20.1). Both NF1 and TS are disorders of unregulated progression through the cell cycle, in which causative genes behave as characteristic tumor suppressor genes. The pathogenesis of these familial syndromes is linked by the shared regulation of a common pathway, the protein kinase mammalian target of rapamycin (mTOR).

NF1 is caused by a germline mutation of the *NF1* gene at 17q11.2, which encodes the protein neurofibromin. Half of the mutations in the *NF1* gene occur de novo. Loss of function mutations in *NF1* therefore cause increased activation of ras and increased signaling via downstream pathways, including the mitogen-activated protein kinase (MAPK) pathway and mTOR pathway. Gastroenteropancreatic NETs that develop in the setting of NF1 include duodenal somatostatin-cell tumors and insulinomas (in up to 10 % of patients) [38].

TS is caused by mutations in one of two different genes: the *TSC1* gene located at 9q34 and the *TSC2* gene located at 16p13.3, which encode for the proteins hamartin and tuberin, respectively [39, 40]. The development of PanNETs in this syndrome is extremely rare, with only nine cases of TS-associated PanNETs reported in the literature [41]. The hamartin-tuberin complex functions as an inhibitor of downstream cellular signaling via mTOR pathway, and the development of tumors in patients with TS is the result of dysregulated signaling of mTOR to downstream targets [42].

20.2 Sporadic Pancreatic Neuroendocrine Tumors

Before the PanNETs exome was sequenced, much of the knowledge about the genetics of PanNETs arose from the studies of the above-mentioned hereditary syndromes and by applying these discoveries to sporadic lesions.

Somatic mutations of the *MEN1* gene have been found in roughly 30 % of sporadic PanNETs with frequent deletion of the wild-type allele in these cases [43–51]. Allelic deletion on 11q is frequently found in sporadic PanNETs, and by combining data from all the studies referred to, it appears that the LOH rate is usually two to three times higher than the frequency of mutations of the *MEN1* gene. This suggests that LOH at 11q13 per se is not an indicator of MEN1 mutations. Such findings can be explained by other mechanisms of *MEN1* gene inactivation, such as methylation of the promoter or the presence of mutations in unexamined noncoding regions. It also seems likely that the higher frequency of allelic deletions is an indicator for the inactivation of another tumor suppressor gene on 11q.

Compared to the *MEN1* gene, the *VHL* gene is only rarely mutated in sporadic PanNETs, mainly in a small proportion of nonfunctioning PanNETs [52]. Moreover, the *VHL* gene may be inactivated by alternative means, such as promoter hypermethylation or deletion, as has been reported for up to 25 % of PanNETs [53]. Allelic deletion on 3p was frequently found in sporadic PanNETs and a positive correlation between 3p loss and malignant tumor behavior was observed by different authors [54, 55]. Chung et al. [54] and Barghorn et al. [55] identified the smallest common region of allelic loss between 3p25.3-p25.1 and 3p23, suggesting the presence of another tumor suppressor gene centromeric to the *VHL* gene. Barghorn et al. [55] observed that most nonfunctioning tumors lost the entire chromosome 3 during progression to the metastatic phenotype, while functioning PanNETs lost only parts of chromosome 3p and rarely the entire chromosome 3p. Since the pattern of allelic deletions at 3p differs among PanNET subtypes and microsatellite markers at 3p25.3-p23 may have already been lost at an early tumor stage, caution was suggested with respect to the use of 3p markers in distinguishing clinically benign from potentially malignant PanNETs.

Finally, while no *NF1* mutations have been reported in sporadic PanNETs, recent evidence demonstrates that the *TSC2* gene may have a role in the development of these tumors. Thus, Missaglia et al. found *TSC2* expression was downregulated in a majority of sporadic PanNETs [56], and more recently Jiao et al. found the TSC2 gene to be mutated in 8.8 % of 68 sporadic PanNETs [57]. In this study, the complete exome of ten primary PanNETs was sequenced, followed by screening for mutations in the most commonly altered genes in an additional 58 tumors. As anticipated from prior studies, *MEN1* was found to be the most frequently mutated gene in PanNETs, as it was altered in 44 % of the tumors. In addition, genes in the mTOR signaling pathway were also mutated in about 16 % of PanNETs, with inactivating mutations in *TSC2* and *PTEN* genes, plus a single case showing an activating mutation in *PIK3CA* (Table 20.2). The most striking result from the exome sequencing

Table 20.2 Genetic mutations in sporadic PanNETs

Gene	Protein function	Mutation frequency (%)
MEN1	Histone remodeling	44
DAXX	Chromatin assembly	25
ATRX	Chromatin assembly	18
TSC2	GTPase-activating protein	9
PTEN	Protein tyrosine phosphatase	7
PIK3CA	Phosphoinositide 3-kinase	2
TP53	Cell-cycle arrest	5

was the identification of recurrent somatic mutations in two genes that had previously not been associated with cancer, namely, *DAXX* (death domain-associated protein; located on 6p21.3) and *ATRX* (alpha-thalassemia/mental retardation syndrome; located on Xq21.1). Intriguingly, mutations in *ATRX* or *DAXX* were mutually exclusive, occurring in a total of 43 % of PanNETs examined. Most of *ATRX* and *DAXX* mutations were of an inactivating type, and there was a significant positive correlation between gene mutation and loss of the nuclear protein, as assessed by immunostaining. Both of the proteins encoded by these genes participate in heterochromatin maintenance at telomeres, particularly in the incorporation of the histone variant H3.3 at the chromosome ends [58, 59]. Interestingly, tumors with loss of *ATRX or DAXX* proteins show the presence of a telomerase-independent telomere maintenance mechanism known as alternative lengthening of telomeres (ALT) [60]. ALT occurs in approximately 5 % of cancers [61] and is considered an alternative telomerase-independent telomere maintenance mechanism [62]. Recently, de Wilde and colleagues demonstrated that *ATRX* and *DAXX* mutations are relatively late events in PanNET tumorigenesis being associated both with higher grade (G2 versus G1) and with larger tumor size. Remarkably, patients with PanNETs exhibiting altered *ATRX* or *DAXX* genes have a significantly longer survival rate than patients with wild-type tumors [63]. In addition to gene mutation analyses, numerous cytogenetic and molecular studies have been performed to detect recurrent genetic changes in PanNETs. The primary techniques

used in these works have been loss of heterozygosity (LOH) analysis to identify genetic losses and comparative genome hybridization (CGH), including classical CGH and array-based CGH (aCGH), which provides information on both gains and losses of genetic material. Although these studies are diverse, featuring different (frequently small) tumor cohorts and a variety of techniques, some patterns emerge from the overall results. One frequent observation is that the quantity of genetic abnormalities is often positively correlated with indicators of tumor aggressive behavior [64–70]. Overall, these results indicate that neuroendocrine tumor progression is likely to be driven by ongoing chromosomal instability (CIN) leading to the accumulation of multiple genetic aberrations, with increasing numbers of alterations associated with more aggressive biological behavior and consequently worse patient prognosis. The alterations described are not randomly distributed on chromosomes but are particularly common in distinct chromosomal regions. In PanNETs, losses are common at chromosomes 1p, 1q, 3p, 6q, 10q, 11p, 11q, 22q, and Y, while frequent gains are observed on 7p, 7q, 9p, 9q, 14, 17q, and 20q [47, 54, 65, 66, 68, 69, 71–78]. Some differences have been reported among PanNETs considering both type and number of DNA alterations. Insulinomas exhibit a lower number of genomic alterations than other PanNETs and they frequently show gain of 9q32 and loss of 22q13.1, which appear to be early genetic events in these tumors [79]. By contrast, they rarely show 3p and 6q losses associated with malignancy [55, 77]. Malignant insulinomas, in contrast, harbor a large number of chromosomal alterations similar to those seen in other types of malignant PanNETs [79]. In pancreatic gastrinomas, only limited chromosomal imbalances are encountered. Losses at 3p and 18q21 occur in approximately 33 % and 22 % of cases, respectively [66, 74]. Nonfunctioning PanNETs (NF-PanNETs) in general harbor higher numbers of chromosomal gains and losses than functioning tumors [72].

To date very few studies have been published about DNA methylation changes in PanNETs, and there is scant information about the role of gene promoter-specific hypermethylation as well as global hypomethylation in the development and progression of these tumors. Using global analysis of the methylation status of LINE-1 and Alu repeat sequences that are widely distributed throughout the genome, it was found that these sequences were hypomethylated in the vast majority of cases, when compared to adjacent normal tissue and, when present, hypomethylation correlated with tumor aggressive behavior [80–82]. In addition, epigenetic silencing through promoter hypermethylation has also been assessed. Several specific CpG-island-associated genes are frequently methylated in PanNETs, namely, RASSF1A, CDKN2A, HIC1, RARß, APC, MGMT, and ER [83–88]. The cumulative methylation frequency ranges from only a few percent to more than 70 % for some of these genes. Among the genes examined, the methylation status of *MGMT* is of potential clinical importance because it may help in predicting the clinical efficacy of alkylating agents in these tumors [89, 90]. House et al. found that the *MGMT* promoter was methylated in 40 % of the 48 PanNETs examined, thus potentially explaining the decreased protein expression observed in up to 50 % of these tumors by other studies [86, 90]. The methylation status of the *MGMT* gene is of possible clinical importance because expression of this DNA repair enzyme is associated with poor clinical responses to alkylating agents [91]. The *RASSF1A* tumor suppressor gene, located on 3p21, is reportedly methylated in 75–83 % of lesions, where methylation is correlated with reduced RASSF1A mRNA expression, increased tumor size, and the presence of metastases [85, 87]. Although several authors suggested that *RASSF1A* methylation may provide prognostic information in PanNETs, there is evidence that this epigenetic marker is also observed in a significant fraction of tumor-adjacent normal pancreas tissue [92] and further studies are required to clarify this point. The *CDKN2A* gene codes for the p16 tumor suppressor protein, a member of the Rb cell-cycle regulatory pathway that modulates the arrest of the cell cycle at G1-S. Muscarella et al. [93] reported the presence of *CDKN2A* promoter hypermethyl-

ation or homozygous deletion in a limited number of pancreatic gastrinomas and in nonfunctioning PanNETs. These data were confirmed by Lubomierski et al. [94] who reported loss of expression of at least one of the tumor suppressor genes *CDKN2A*/p16, *CDKN2B*/p15, and *CDKN2D*/p14 localized as a gene cluster at 9p21. mRNA transcripts of these genes were lost more frequently in nonfunctioning PanNETs (57 %) than in insulinomas (30 %) and gastrinomas (22 %). Unlike *RASSF1A*, methylation of the *CDKN2A* in PanNETs displayed good specificity for tumor tissue versus adjacent normal tissue.

Overall, many DNA methylation changes have already been uncovered in these initial studies. With the increasing availability of whole genome methods, this list will undoubtedly grow in the near future, with the hope that some of these methylation marks will be useful as diagnostic and prognostic biomarkers.

20.3 Pancreatic Neuroendocrine Carcinomas

PanNECs are poorly differentiated neuroendocrine tumors of the pancreas, characterized by a very aggressive behavior and a dismal prognosis. These tumors are much rarer than PanNETs and at present there are very few reports on their genetic and molecular profiles [95–98].

In contrast to PanNETs, they are characterized by a high proliferation rate and this has allowed standard karyotypic analyses of metaphase chromosomes of PanNECs to be performed [95]. Specifically, Welborn at al. published karyotypic profiles of two PanNECs, and they concluded that they probably represent a genetically distinct entity compared with PanNETs, because of the very different spectra of chromosomal abnormalities observed in the two subsets of tumors. Strong support for this hypothesis comes from recent sequencing analysis of PanNECs [96]. In this study, Yachida et al. performed targeted exomic sequencing and immunohistochemical analyses, comparing high-grade PanNECs (both small cell and large cell subtypes) with PanNETs. Their results showed that small cell and large cell

NECs are genetically related entities, because mutations in *RB1* and *TP53* were very common in these tumors, while they were completely absent in PanNETs. Aberrant p53 and Rb staining occurred exclusively in PanNECs at a rate of 95 % and 74 %, respectively. Interestingly, aberrant p16 staining was not exclusive to PanNECs, but also occurred in a mutually exclusive manner with respect to Rb such that all PanNECs had disruption of the p16/Rb pathway. Related to this finding, inactivating mutations in *DAXX* and *ATRX* were exclusively found in PanNETs while they were completely absent in PanNECs. Moreover, BCL-2 overexpression was a more common feature of PanNECs (74 %) versus PanNETs (18 %).

Finally, the potential genetic relationship between PanNECs and pancreatic ductal carcinomas (PDACs) has been considered [99]. At present, available data demonstrates that their mutational spectra are significantly different, although PanNECs and PDACs share a high frequency of *TP53* alterations. Indeed, the genetic changes frequently observed in ductal adenocarcinomas, such as *KRAS* mutations and loss of *SMAD4/DPC4*, were observed infrequently in PanNECs [96]. These results seem to suggest that most panNECs do not arise from preexisting ductal lesions and that the possibility that some PDACs may coexist with panNECs may be a relatively uncommon occurrence [98]. Only in MANECs (mixed adenoneuroendocrine carcinomas) a close genetic relationship between the exocrine and the endocrine components has been demonstrated, suggesting a monoclonal origin of these rare cancers in all the gastroenteropancreatic tract [98, 100].

References

1. Jensen RT, Berna MJ, Bingham DB et al (2008) Inherited pancreatic endocrine tumor syndromes: advances in molecular pathogenesis, diagnosis, management, and controversies. Cancer 113:1807–1843
2. Chandrasekharappa SC, Guru SC, Manickam P et al (1997) Positional cloning of the gene for multiple endocrine neoplasia-type 1. Science 276:404–407
3. Lemmens I, Van de Ven WJ, Kas K et al (1997) Identification of the multiple endocrine neoplasia type 1 (MEN1) gene. The European Consortium on MEN1. Hum Mol Genet 6:1177–1183
4. Wu X, Hua X (2008) Menin, histone h3 methyltransferase, and regulation of cell proliferation: current knowledge and perspective. Curr Mol Med 8:805–815
5. Thakker RV, Newey PJ, Walls GV et al (2012) Clinical practice guidelines for multiple endocrine neoplasia type 1 (MEN1). J Clin Endocrinol Metab 97:2990–3011
6. Zhang H, Li W, Wang Q et al (2012) Glucose-mediated repression of menin promotes pancreatic β-cell proliferation. Endocrinology 153:602–611
7. Wang Y, Ozawa A, Zaman S et al (2011) The tumor suppressor protein menin inhibits AKT activation by regulating its cellular localization. Cancer Res 71:371–382
8. Bertolino P, Radovanovic I, Casse H et al (2003) Genetic ablation of the tumor suppressor menin causes lethality at mid-gestation with defects in multiple organs. Mech Dev 120:549–560
9. Bertolino P, Tong WM, Galendo D et al (2003) Heterozygous Men1 mutant mice develop a range of endocrine tumors mimicking multiple endocrine neoplasia type 1. Mol Endocrinol 17:1880–1892
10. Crabtree JS, Scacheri PC, Ward JM et al (2001) A mouse model of multiple endocrine neoplasia, type 1, develops multiple endocrine tumors. Proc Natl Acad Sci U S A 98:1118–1123
11. Crabtree JS, Scacheri PC, Ward JM et al (2003) Of mice and MEN1: insulinomas in a conditional mouse knockout. Mol Cell Biol 23:6075–6085
12. Agarwal SK, Guru SC, Heppner C et al (1999) Menin interacts with the AP1 transcription factor JunD and represses JunD-activated transcription. Cell 96:143–152
13. Hughes CM, Rozenblatt-Rosen O, Milne TA et al (2004) Menin associates with a trithorax family histone methyltransferase complex and with the hoxc8 locus. Mol Cell 13:587–597
14. Karnik SK, Hughes CM, Gu X et al (2005) Menin regulates pancreatic islet growth by promoting histone methylation and expression of genes encoding p27Kip1 and p18INK4c. Proc Natl Acad Sci U S A 102:14659–14664
15. Schnepp RW, Chen YX, Wang H et al (2006) Mutation of tumor suppressor gene Men1 acutely enhances proliferation of pancreatic islet cells. Cancer Res 66:5707–5715
16. Scacheri PC, Davis S, Odom DT et al (2006) Genome-wide analysis of menin binding provides insights into MEN1 tumorigenesis. PLoS Genet 2(4):e51
17. Agarwal SK, Impey S, McWeeney S et al (2007) Distribution of menin-occupied regions in chromatin specifies a broad role of menin in transcriptional regulation. Neoplasia 9:101–107
18. Francis J, Lin W, Rozenblatt-Rosen O et al (2011) The menin tumor suppressor protein is phosphorylated in response to DNA damage. PLoS One 6:e16119

19. Fang M, Xia F, Mahalingam M et al (2013) MEN1 is a melanoma tumor suppressor that preserves genomic integrity by stimulating transcription of genes that promote homologous recombination-directed DNA repair. Mol Cell Biol 33:2635–2647

20. Lonser RR, Glenn GM, Walther M et al (2003) von Hippel-Lindau disease. Lancet 361:2059–2067

21. Mukhopadhyay B, Sahdev A, Monson JP et al (2002) Pancreatic lesions in von Hippel-Lindau disease. Clin Endocrinol (Oxf) 57:603–608

22. Corcos O, Couvelard A, Giraud S et al (2008) Endocrine pancreatic tumors in von Hippel-Lindau disease: clinical, histological, and genetic features. Pancreas 37:85–93

23. Latif F, Tory K, Gnarra J et al (1993) Identification of the von Hippel-Lindau disease tumor suppressor gene. Science 260:1317–1320

24. Hoang MP, Hruban RH, Albores-Saavedra J (2001) Clear cell endocrine pancreatic tumor mimicking renal cell carcinoma: a distinctive neoplasm of von Hippel-Lindau disease. Am J Surg Pathol 125:602–609

25. Libutti SK, Choyke PL, Bartlett DL et al (1998) Pancreatic neuroendocrine tumors associated with von Hippel-Lindau disease: diagnostic and management recommendations. Surgery 124:1153–1159

26. Lee S, Chen DY, Humphrey JS et al (1996) Nuclear/cytoplasmic localization of the von Hippel-Lindau tumor suppressor gene product is determined by cell density. Proc Natl Acad Sci U S A 93:1770–1775

27. Pause A, Lee S, Worrell RA et al (1997) The von Hippel-Lindau tumor-suppressor gene product forms a stable complex with human CUL-2, a member of the Cdc53 family of proteins. Proc Natl Acad Sci U S A 94:2156–2161

28. Kaelin WG Jr (2002) Molecular basis of the VHL hereditary cancer syndrome. Nat Rev Cancer 2: 673–682

29. Maxwell PH, Wiesener MS, Chang GW et al (1999) The tumour suppressor protein VHL targets hypoxia-inducible factors for oxygen-dependent proteolysis. Nature 399:271–275

30. Carmeliet P, Dor Y, Herbert JM et al (1998) Role of HIF-1alpha in hypoxia-mediated apoptosis, cell proliferation and tumour angiogenesis. Nature 394: 485–490

31. Kim WY, Kaelin WG (2004) Role of VHL gene mutation in human cancer. J Clin Oncol 22:4991–5004

32. Crossey PA, Richards FM, Foster K et al (1994) Identification of intragenic mutations in the von Hippel-Lindau disease tumour suppressor gene and correlation with disease phenotype. Hum Mol Genet 3:1303–1308

33. Webster AR, Richards FM, MacRonald FE et al (1998) An analysis of phenotypic variation in the familial cancer syndrome von Hippel-Lindau disease: evidence for modifier effects. Am J Hum Genet 63:1025–1035

34. Sgambati MT, Stolle C, Choyke PL et al (2000) Mosaicism in von Hippel-Lindau disease: lessons from kindreds with germline mutations identified in offspring with mosaic parents. Am J Hum Genet 66:84–91

35. Brauch H, Kishida T, Glavac D et al (2005) Von Hippel-Lindau (VHL) disease with pheochromocytoma in the Black Forest region of Germany: evidence for a founder effect. Hum Genet 95:551–556

36. Prowse AH, Webster AR, Richard FM et al (1997) Somatic inactivation of the VHL gene in von Hippel-Lindau disease tumors. Am J Hum Genet 60: 765–771

37. Speisky D, Duces A, Bièche I et al (2012) Molecular profiling of pancreatic neuroendocrine tumors in sporadic and Von Hippel-Lindau patients. Clin Cancer Res 18:2838–2849

38. McClatchey AI (2007) Neurofibromatosis. Annu Rev Pathol 2:191–216

39. European Chromosome 16 Tuberous Sclerosis Consortium (1993) Identification and characterization of the tuberous sclerosis gene on chromosome 16. Cell 75:1305–1315

40. van Slegtenhorst M, de Hoogt R, Hermans C et al (1997) Identification of the tuberous sclerosis gene TSC1 on chromosome 9q34. Science 277:805–808

41. Arva NC, Pappas JG, Bhatla T et al (2012) Well-differentiated pancreatic neuroendocrine carcinoma in tuberous sclerosis–case report and review of the literature. Am J Surg Pathol 36:149–153

42. Tee AR, Fingar DC, Manning BD et al (2002) Tuberous sclerosis complex-1 and -2 gene products function together to inhibit mammalian target of rapamycin (mTOR)-mediated downstream signaling. Proc Natl Acad Sci U S A 99:13571–13576

43. Perren A, Anlauf M, Henopp T et al (2007) Multiple endocrine neoplasia type 1 (MEN1): loss of one MEN1 allele in tumors and monohormonal endocrine cell clusters but not in islet hyperplasia of the pancreas. J Clin Endocrinol Metab 92:1118–1128

44. Hessman O, Lindberg D, Einarsson A et al (1999) Genetic alterations on 3p, 11q13, and 18q in nonfamilial and MEN 1-associated pancreatic endocrine tumors. Genes Chromosomes Cancer 26:258–264

45. Corbo V, Dalai I, Scardoni M et al (2010) MEN1 in pancreatic endocrine tumors: analysis of gene and protein status in 169 sporadic neoplasms reveals alterations in the vast majority of cases. Endocr Relat Cancer 17:771–783

46. Görtz B, Roth J, Krähenmann A et al (1999) Mutations and allelic deletions of the MEN1 gene are associated with a subset of sporadic endocrine pancreatic and neuroendocrine tumors and not restricted to foregut neoplasms. Am J Pathol 154: 429–436

47. D'adda T, Pizzi S, Azzoni C et al (2002) Different patterns of 11q allelic losses in digestive endocrine tumors. Hum Pathol 33:322–329

48. Debelenko LV, Zhuang Z, Emmert-Buck MR et al (1997) Allelic deletions on chromosome 11q13 in multiple endocrine neoplasia type 1-associated and sporadic gastrinomas and pancreatic endocrine tumors. Cancer Res 57:2238–2243

49. Pizzi S, Azzoni C, Bassi D et al (2003) Genetic alterations in poorly differentiated endocrine carcinomas of the gastrointestinal tract. Cancer 98:1273–1282

50. Toliat MR, Berger W, Ropers HH et al (1997) Mutations in the MEN I gene in sporadic neuroendocrine tumours of gastroenteropancreatic system. Lancet 350:1223

51. Capelli P, Martignoni G, Pedica F et al (2009) Endocrine neoplasms of the pancreas: pathologic and genetic features. Arch Pathol Lab Med 133:350–364

52. Zhuang Z, Vortmeyer AO, Pack S et al (1997) Somatic mutations of the MEN1 tumor suppressor gene in sporadic gastrinomas and insulinomas. Cancer Res 57:4682–4686

53. Schmitt AM, Schmid S, Rudolph T et al (2009) VHL inactivation is an important pathway for the development of malignant sporadic pancreatic endocrine tumors. Endocr Relat Cancer 16:1219–1227

54. Chung DC, Smith AP, Louis DN et al (1997) A novel pancreatic endocrine tumor suppressor gene locus on chromosome 3p with clinical prognostic implications. J Clin Invest 100:404–410

55. Barghorn A, Komminoth P, Bachmann D et al (2001) Deletion at 3p25.3-p23 is frequently encountered in endocrine pancreatic tumors and is associated with metastatic progression. J Pathol 194:451–458

56. Missiaglia E, Dalai I, Barbi S et al (2010) Pancreatic endocrine tumors: expression profiling evidences a role for AKT-mTOR pathway. J Clin Oncol 28:245–255

57. Jiao Y, Shi C, Edil BH et al (2011) DAXX/ATRX, MEN1, and mTOR pathway genes are frequently altered in pancreatic neuroendocrine tumors. Science 331:1199–1203

58. Goldberg AD, Banaszynski LA, Noh KM et al (2010) Distinct factors control histone variant H3.3 localization at specific genomic regions. Cell 140: 678–691

59. Lewis PW, Elsaesser SJ, Noh KM et al (2010) Daxx is an H3.3-specific histone chaperone and cooperates with ATRX in replication-independent chromatin assembly at telomeres. Proc Natl Acad Sci U S A 107:14075–14080

60. Heaphy CM, de Wilde RF, Jiao Y et al (2011) Altered telomeres in tumors with ATRX and DAXX mutations. Science 333(6041):425

61. Heaphy CM, Subhawong AP, Hong SM et al (2011) Prevalence of the alternative lengthening of telomeres telomere maintenance mechanism in human cancer subtypes. Am J Pathol 179:1608–1615

62. Shay JW, Reddel RR, Wright WE (2012) Cancer. Cancer and telomeres-an ALTernative to telomerase. Science 336:1388–1390

63. de Wilde RF, Heaphy CM, Maitra A et al (2012) Loss of ATRX or DAXX expression and concomitant acquisition of the alternative lengthening of telomeres phenotype are late events in a small subset of MEN-1 syndrome pancreatic neuroendocrine tumors. Mod Pathol 25:1033–1039

64. Beghelli S, Pelosi G, Zamboni G et al (1998) Pancreatic endocrine tumours: evidence for a tumour suppressor pathogenesis and for a tumour suppressor gene on chromosome 17p. J Pathol 186:41–50

65. Speel EJ, Richter J, Moch H et al (1999) Genetic differences in endocrine pancreatic tumor subtypes detected by comparative genomic hybridization. Am J Pathol 155:1787–1794

66. Speel EJ, Scheidweiler AF, Zhao J et al (2001) Genetic evidence for early divergence of small functioning and nonfunctioning endocrine pancreatic tumors: gain of 9Q34 is an early event in insulinomas. Cancer Res 61:5186–5192

67. Zhao J, Moch H, Scheidweiler AF et al (2001) Genomic imbalances in the progression of endocrine pancreatic tumors. Genes Chromosomes Cancer 32:364–372

68. Rigaud G, Missiaglia E, Moore PS et al (2001) High resolution allelotype of nonfunctional pancreatic endocrine tumors: identification of two molecular subgroups with clinical implications. Cancer Res 61:285–292

69. Jonkers YM, Claessen SM, Perren A et al (2005) Chromosomal instability predicts metastatic disease in patients with insulinomas. Endocr Relat Cancer 12:435–447

70. Nagano Y, Kim do H, Zhang L et al (2007) Allelic alterations in pancreatic endocrine tumors identified by genome-wide single nucleotide polymorphism analysis. Endocr Relat Cancer 14:483–492

71. Kim do H, Nagano Y, Choi IS et al (2008) Allelic alterations in well-differentiated neuroendocrine tumors (carcinoid tumors) identified by genome-wide single nucleotide polymorphism analysis and comparison with pancreatic endocrine tumors. Genes Chromosomes Cancer 47:84–92

72. Floridia G, Grilli G, Salvatore M et al (2005) Chromosomal alterations detected by comparative genomic hybridization in nonfunctioning endocrine pancreatic tumors. Cancer Genet Cytogenet 156:23–30

73. Guo SS, Arora C, Shimoide AT et al (2002) Frequent deletion of chromosome 3 in malignant sporadic pancreatic endocrine tumors. Mol Cell Endocrinol 190:109–114

74. Ebrahimi SA, Wang EH, Wu A et al (1999) Deletion of chromosome 1 predicts prognosis in pancreatic endocrine tumors. Cancer Res 59:311–315

75. Chung DC, Brown SB, Graeme-Cook F et al (1998) Localization of putative tumor suppressor loci by genome-wide allelotyping in human pancreatic endocrine tumors. Cancer Res 58:3706–3711

76. Chen YJ, Vortmeyer A, Zhuang Z et al (2003) Loss of heterozygosity of chromosome 1q in gastrinomas: occurrence and prognostic significance. Cancer Res 63:817–823

77. Barghorn A, Speel EJ, Farspour B et al (2001) Putative tumor suppressor loci at 6q22 and 6q23-q24 are involved in the malignant progression of sporadic endocrine pancreatic tumors. Am J Pathol 158:1903–1911

78. Yang YM, Liu TH, Chen YJ et al (2005) Chromosome 1q loss of heterozygosity frequently occurs in

sporadic insulinomas and is associated with tumor malignancy. Int J Cancer 117:234–240

79. Jonkers YM, Claessen SM, Veltman JA et al (2006) Molecular parameters associated with insulinoma progression: chromosomal instability versus p53 and CK19 status. Cytogenet Genome Res 115:289–297

80. Stricker I, Tzivras D, Nambiar S et al (2012) Site- and grade-specific diversity of LINE1 methylation pattern in gastroenteropancreatic neuroendocrine tumours. Anticancer Res 32:3699–3706

81. Choi IS, Estecio MR, Nagano Y et al (2007) Hypomethylation of LINE-1 and Alu in well-differentiated neuroendocrine tumors (pancreatic endocrine tumors and carcinoid tumors). Mod Pathol 20:802–810

82. Stefanoli M, La Rosa S, Sahnane N et al (2014) Prognostic relevance of aberrant DNA methylation in G1 and G2 pancreatic neuroendocrine tumors. Neuroendocrinology 100:26–34

83. Pizzi S, Azzoni C, Bottarelli L et al (2005) RASSF1A promoter methylation and 3p21.3 loss of heterozygosity are features of foregut, but not midgut and hindgut, malignant endocrine tumours. J Pathol 206:409–416

84. Arnold CN, Nagasaka T, Goel A et al (2008) Molecular characteristics and predictors of survival in patients with malignant neuroendocrine tumors. Int J Cancer 123:1556–1564

85. Malpeli G, Amato E, Dandrea M et al (2011) Methylation-associated down-regulation of RASSF1A and up-regulation of RASSF1C in pancreatic endocrine tumors. BMC Cancer 11:351

86. House MG, Herman JG, Guo MZ et al (2003) Aberrant hypermethylation of tumor suppressor genes in pancreatic endocrine neoplasms. Ann Surg 238:423–431

87. Liu L, Broaddus RR, Yao JC et al (2005) Epigenetic alterations in neuroendocrine tumors: methylation of RAS-association domain family 1, isoform A and p16 genes are associated with metastasis. Mod Pathol 18:1632–1640

88. Arnold CN, Sosnowski A, Schmitt-Gräff A et al (2007) Analysis of molecular pathways in sporadic neuroendocrine tumors of the gastro-entero-pancreatic system. Int J Cancer 120:2157–2164

89. Strosberg JR, Cheema A, Kvols LK (2011) A review of systemic and liver-directed therapies for metastatic neuroendocrine tumors of the gastroenteropancreatic tract. Cancer Control 18:127–137

90. Kulke MH, Hornick JL, Frauenhoffer C et al (2009) O6-methylguanine DNA methyltransferase deficiency and response to temozolomide-based therapy in patients with neuroendocrine tumors. Clin Cancer Res 15:338–345

91. Schmitt AM, Pavel M, Rudolph T et al (2014) Prognostic and predictive roles of MGMT protein expression and promoter methylation in sporadic pancreatic neuroendocrine neoplasms. Neuroendocrinology 100:35–44

92. Furlan D, Sahnane N, Bernasconi B et al (2014) APC alterations are frequently involved in the pathogenesis of acinar cell carcinoma of the pancreas, mainly through gene loss and promoter hypermethylation. Virchows Arch 464:553–564

93. Muscarella P, Melvin WS, Fisher WE et al (1998) Genetic alterations in gastrinomas and nonfunctioning pancreatic neuroendocrine tumors: an analysis of p16/MTS1 tumor suppressor gene inactivation. Cancer Res 58:237–240

94. Lubomierski N, Kersting M, Bert T et al (2001) Tumor suppressor genes in the 9p21 gene cluster are selective targets of inactivation in neuroendocrine gastroenteropancreatic tumors. Cancer Res 61:5905–5910

95. Welborn J, Jenks H, Taplett J et al (2004) High-grade neuroendocrine carcinomas display unique cytogenetic aberrations. Cancer Genet Cytogenet 155:33–41

96. Yachida S, Vakiani E, White CM et al (2012) Small cell and large cell neuroendocrine carcinomas of the pancreas are genetically similar and distinct from well-differentiated pancreatic neuroendocrine tumors. Am J Surg Pathol 36:173–184

97. Iacobuzio-Donahue CA, Fu B, Yachida S et al (2009) DPC4 gene status of the primary carcinoma correlates with patterns of failure in patients with pancreatic cancer. J Clin Oncol 27:1806–1813

98. Scardoni M, Vittoria E, Volante M et al (2014) Mixed Adenoneuroendocrine Carcinomas (MANECs) of the gastrointestinal tract: targeted next generation sequencing suggests a monoclonal origin of the two components. Neuroendocrinology 100:310–316

99. Hruban RH, Fukushima N (2007) Pancreatic adenocarcinoma: update on the surgical pathology of carcinomas of ductal origin and PanINs. Mod Pathol Suppl 1:S61–S70

100. Furlan D, Cerutti R, Genasetti A et al (2003) Microallelotyping defines the monoclonal or the polyclonal origin of mixed and collision endocrine-exocrine tumors of the gut. Lab Invest 83:963–971

Surgical Therapy of Pancreatic Neuroendocrine Neoplasms

Angela Maurizi, Stefano Partelli, Francesca Muffatti,
Sara Nobile, and Massimo Falconi

21.1 Introduction

Pancreatic neuroendocrine tumors (PanNETs) are rare neoplasms, that have been increasing largely in incidence over the past few decades because of the diagnosis of pancreatic "incidentalomas" on cross-sectional imaging [1]. They consist of single or multiple benign or malignant neoplasms, and in 10–20 % of patients, they can be associated with inherited syndromes, such as multiple endocrine neoplasia type 1 (MEN1) [2]. They are clinically heterogeneous and classified into functioning (10–30 %) and nonfunctioning (70–90 %) tumors, depending on their ability to produce symptoms due to hormone production [3]. The hormones secreted by functioning tumors include gastrin, insulin, glucagon, somatostatin, vasoactive intestinal polypeptide (VIP), growth hormone-releasing factor, and adrenocorticotrophic hormone [4]. Diagnostic workup aims to assess the stage and grade of the disease as these parameters represent the main driver for treatment choice. The treatment of PanNET varies from conservative management to extensive surgical resection. Surgical resection is the only curative treatment and remains the cornerstone therapy for this patient group, even in patients with advanced disease [5, 6], in which it represents one of several therapeutic options. Radical surgery for PanNETs includes both typical and atypical pancreatic resections. Over the last decade, there has been a noticeable trend toward minimally invasive surgery in patients with PanNETs. This resulted in shorter length of hospital stay and comparable long-term outcomes in patients with limited disease treated minimally invasively.

21.2 Treatment

21.2.1 Surgery

Incidental diagnosis of PanNET is associated with a significant better survival after curative resection respective of patients with symptoms [7]. Moreover, Bettini et al. [8] demonstrated that patients with incidental diagnosis associated with a tumor size <2 cm had a 5-year overall survival of 100 % with a minimal risk of recurrence. On the basis of these experiences, the European Neuroendocrine Tumor Society (ENETS) guidelines now recommend a *wait-and-see* policy in selected patients with asymptomatic sporadic PanNET less than 2 cm in size [9]. Preliminary

A. Maurizi
Department of Surgery, Università Politecnica delle Marche, Via Conca, Ancona 60100, Italy
e-mail: angegiu@aesinet.it

S. Partelli • F. Muffatti • S. Nobile • M. Falconi (✉)
Pancreatic Surgery Unit, San Raffaele Hospital, Milan, Italy
e-mail: falconi.massimo@hsr.it

S. La Rosa, F. Sessa (eds.), *Pancreatic Neuroendocrine Neoplasms: Practical Approach to Diagnosis,
Classification, and Therapy*, DOI 10.1007/978-3-319-17235-4_21,
© Springer International Publishing Switzerland 2015

reports have demonstrated the safety of this conservative approach [7, 10, 11]. On the other hand, surgery still represents the treatment of choice for PanNET >2 cm and/or for symptomatic forms. There is a strict correlation between tumor size and malignancy in these tumors [8]. Tumors larger than 2 cm have an increased risk of malignancy [12].

21.2.2 Technical Aspects

21.2.2.1 Nonfunctioning PanNET

Nonfunctioning PanNETs represent 30–50 % of all PanNETs, malignancy occurs in 60–90 % [13–15], and long-term survival can be achieved in many patients [16]. Pancreatic resections differ according to tumor site: lesions of the pancreatic head are treated with a pancreaticoduodenectomy while lesions of the body and tail with a distal pancreatectomy. Functional impairment of the organ due to the loss of parenchyma is a general risk of major pancreatic resections, resulting in exocrine and/or endocrine insufficiency. When tumors occur in the neck, they can be removed through a parenchyma-sparing operation called "middle" or "central" pancreatectomy [17]. There is the possibility of leaks from both the closed-cut edge of the head and the pancreatico-jejunostomy, considering that in most patients, we are dealing with a normal soft pancreatic texture with a small Wirsung's duct. Enucleation is a feasible procedure for the radical treatment of benign and borderline pancreatic neoplasms [18] and is associated with long-term survival, despite a relatively high risk of pancreatic fistula formation [19, 20]. Before enucleating a PanNET, it is important to consider where the tumor is located in relation to the main pancreatic duct, as enucleations of tumors located very close to this may result in damage to the pancreatic duct and subsequent pancreatic leakage. Clear negative margins cannot be obtained after both enucleation and intermediate resection, and a standard lymphadenectomy is not usually performed [21]. On the other hand, tumor enucleation is associated with shorter operative time, less intraoperative blood loss, and shorter hospital stay compared to pancreaticoduodenectomy and distal pancreatectomy [18]. The main advantage for atypical resections is that they are associated with a lower risk of long-term endocrine/exocrine impairment when compared to standard resections [22]. In the presence of multifocal disease, a total pancreatectomy is the treatment of choice.

21.2.2.2 Functioning PanNET

Functioning PanNETs are often small in size, and localization may be difficult also due to their possible extra duodenal-pancreatic origin (for gastrinomas) as jejunum, stomach, mesentery, spleen, and ovaries. They primarily include insulinomas and gastrinomas, with an incidence of 70–80 % and 20–25 % of all PanNETs, and an incidence of malignancy of <10 % and 50–60 %, respectively [14]. Insulinoma is one of the most frequent functioning PanNET. It is generally solitary, benign, and curable with surgery [14, 23, 24]. Recurrence after resection occurs in about 3 % of cases [25]. The procedures of choice are enucleation for small and isolated insulinomas and partial pancreatectomy for large and potentially malignant insulinomas [26]. Besides enucleation, middle pancreatectomy is an alternative parenchyma-sparing technique for this tumor entity [27]. Also, laparoscopic management of insulinoma in the body and tail of the pancreas, with distal pancreatectomy or enucleation, is widely accepted and used [28]. In the case of occult insulinoma, blind distal pancreatectomy should be avoided [29]. However, explorative surgery with intraoperative ultrasound may be indicated in cases where preoperative diagnostics could not reveal any pancreatic lesion, as this is an excellent method for identifying occult insulinoma [30] (see also Chap. 2).

Most gastrinomas are located in the "gastrinoma triangle," which comprises the head of the pancreas and the first and second parts of the duodenum [31]. Gastrinoma is associated with gastric ulcerations due to overproduction of gastrin [32]. The clinical presentation of gastrinoma is referred to as Zollinger-Ellison syndrome. With the introduction of proton pump inhibitors, which prevent ulcer formation, surgery changed from being a symptomatic treatment to curative treatment in patients with Zollinger-Ellison syndrome [23]. All patients with Zollinger-Ellison syndrome without multiple neuroendocrine neoplasia type 1 or metastatic disease should be offered surgical exploration for possible cure [33]. The extent of surgery is a highly controversial issue in gastrinoma [34]. This is especially true for duodenal gastrinomas. Several groups suggested that duodenotomy with excision of duodenal wall gastrinomas, enucleation of any head gastrinomas, and peripancreatic lymph node dissection with or without distal pancreatic resection is the adequate procedure for duodenal gastrinoma [35]. Other groups, as well as the authors, choose pancreaticoduodenectomy as the first-line procedure for duodenal gastrinoma, because it is very likely that proliferative gastrin cells in the normal duodenal mucosa are the precursors of these tumors, and, for this reason, long-term cure is only possible if the organ of origin is removed. Moreover, a standard pancreaticoduodenectomy allows to perform a standard lymphadenectomy in a disease where lymph node metastases are very frequent. The incidences of other functioning PanNETs, such as vasoactive intestinal peptide-producing tumors (VIPoma), glucagonoma, and somatostatinoma, are very low. These patients should undergo tumor resection to correct the severe hormonally caused metabolic derangements [23].

21.2.3 Locally Advanced Disease

Hill et al. found that resection of the primary tumor in patients with PanNETs is associated with improved survival across all stages of disease [36]. Based on this, surgery of locally advanced PanNET without metastasis should be attempted. Interestingly, R1 resections of PanNET are not associated with a worse overall survival compared to R0 resections [37]. A proportion of patients with PanNETs have locally advanced disease at the diagnosis. Locally advanced disease extends beyond the limits of the pancreas directly into surrounding organs or tissue, involves regional lymph nodes, or fulfills both of these criteria [38]. The surgical removal of the tumor mass is associated with an improved survival for patients [31]. Criteria for surgical resection of PanNETs can also include the presence of nearby organ invasion (stomach, spleen, colon, kidney, adrenal gland) or the invasion of vascular structures. However, most patients will develop recurrence [39]. When not operated, patients with locally advanced PanNETs may suffer from complications related to local mass effect and infiltrative growth, including gastrointestinal bleeding, vascular/intestinal/biliary obstruction, and occlusion of the superior mesenteric (SMV) or portal vein (PV) [40].

21.2.4 Metastatic Disease

PanNETs commonly metastasize to the liver. At diagnosis, 25–93 % of patients with NET have synchronous neuroendocrine tumor liver metastases [41]. This is especially true for nonfunctioning tumors as these are generally diagnosed at a late stage. Whenever a resection leaves no residual disease, an aggressive approach, including liver resection, is recommended [42]. The conditions that have to be assessed preoperatively are the absence of extra-abdominal disease [43], the presence of low proliferative index (Ki67) by FNA [44], and the existence of somatostatin receptors in order to deliver radiolabeled therapies as they resulted effective after cytoreductive surgery [9, 45]. The type of hepatic resection depends on the number of liver metastases, site, and hepatic reserve itself. It can range from simple enucleation to segmental resection or to hepatectomy. In selected patients, resection of the primary PanNET in the setting of unresectable but limited hepatic metastases may be indicated [46] as this may prolong survival [47].

In those patients with bilobar metastases or more than 75 % of liver involvement, radical surgery can be rarely performed. In this light, medical, ablative, and embolization techniques can be provided in order to allow radical resection. There are valid palliative options in patients with PanNETs with liver metastases which are not candidates for surgical resection. These mainly include transarterial embolization (TAE), transarterial chemoembolization (TACE), and radiofrequency ablation (RFA). Such procedures can be used as locoregional ablative therapy per se or as an adjunct to palliative surgery. Liver transplantation has been proposed as a potentially curative treatment in patients free of extrahepatic metastases and with low proliferation rate, for whom standard surgical and medical therapies have failed [9].

21.2.5 Lymph Node Sampling

From studies performed on pancreatic ductal adenocarcinoma, it is known that lymph node status is an important prognostic factor in resectable disease [48]. Role of lymphadenectomy for patients with PanNET is still unclear [22]. Lymph node metastases occur only in 30 % of patients affected by these tumors, but the association between node metastases and poorer survival is still debated [22].

21.2.6 Open Versus Laparoscopic Surgery

Over the last decade, there has been a trend toward minimally invasive techniques in the management of PanNETs. This shift has not increased morbidity or compromised survival [49]. Laparoscopic surgery for small and solitary PanNETs is feasible and safe [50]. Advantages of the minimally invasive approach are less intraoperative bleeding [51], faster postoperative recovery [52], shorter hospital stay [53], and improved cosmesis, compared to the open approach. It has been demonstrated that laparoscopic distal pancreatectomy and enucleation are safe and feasible in patients with PanNETs [54]. Insulinomas in non-MEN1 patients are increasingly being treated by laparoscopic approach. In 85 % of patients, they are single tumors, almost always intrapancreatic, and if they can be localized preoperatively, they can be cured in 70–100 % of cases using a laparoscopic approach [44].

As for insulinomas the laparoscopic approach is adequate, the role of laparoscopic surgery for gastrinomas appears to be limited.

The procedure provides similar short- and long-term oncologic outcomes as open distal pancreatectomy [55], and a selective use of it also seems to be a cost-efficient alternative to open distal pancreatectomy [51]. Laparoscopic distal pancreatectomy with preservation of the spleen is feasible with a moderate risk of postoperative splenic infarction [56]. However, the significance of spleen preservation on oncologic outcome in patients with PanNET remains unclear. The laparoscopic procedure needs to be integrated with the use of intraoperative ultrasonography to correctly define the area of pancreatic transection during distal pancreatectomy.

If the tumor cannot be identified precisely by laparoscopic ultrasound, conversion to open surgery should be considered [57]. Laparoscopic pancreatic surgery demands a high level of surgical skills in minimally invasive surgery and should be performed in specialized centers [58].

References

1. Milan SA, Yeo CJ (2012) Neuroendocrine tumors of the pancreas. Curr Opin Oncol 24(1):46–55
2. Metz DC, Jensen RT (2008) Gastrointestinal neuroendocrine tumors: pancreatic endocrine tumors. Gastroenterology 135:1469–1492
3. Kulke MH, Bendell J, Kvols L, Picus J, Pommier R, Yao J (2011) Evolving diagnostic and treatment strategies for pancreatic neuroendocrine tumors. J Hematol Oncol 4: article no. 29
4. Kouvaraki MA, Ajani JA, Hoff P, Wolff R, Evans DB, Lozano R et al (2005) Fluorouracil, doxorubicin, and streptozocin in the treatment of patients with locally advanced and metastatic pancreatic endocrine carcinomas. J Clin Oncol 22(23):4762–4771
5. Liang H, Wang P, Wang XN, Wang JC, Hao XS (2004) Management of nonfunctioning islet cell tumors. World J Gastroenterol 10(12):1806–1809
6. Gomez-Rivera F, Stewart AE, Arnoletti JP, Vickers S, Bland KI, Heslin MJ (2007) Surgical treatment of pancreatic endocrine neoplasm. Am J Surg 193(4):460–465
7. Cheema A, Weber J, Strosberg JR (2012) Incidental detection of pancreatic neuroendocrine tumors: an analysis of incidence and outcomes. Ann Surg Oncol 19:2932–2936
8. Bettini R, Partelli S, Boninsegna L et al (2011) Tumor size correlates with malignancy in nonfunctioning pancreatic endocrine tumor. Surgery 150:75–82
9. Falconi M, Bartsch D, Eriksson B et al (2012) ENETS consensus guidelines for the management of patients with digestive neuroendocrine neoplasms of

the digestive system: well-differentiated pancreatic non-functioning tumors. Neuroendocrinology 95: 120–134

10. Lee LC, Grant CS, Salomao DR et al (2012) Small, nonfunctioning, asymptomatic pancreatic neuroendocrine tumors (PNETs): role for nonoperative management. Surgery 152:965–974

11. Gaujoux S, Partelli S, Maire F et al (2013) Observational study of natural history of small sporadic nonfunctioning pancreatic neuroendocrine tumors. J Clin Endocrinol Metab 98:4784–4789

12. Fernandez-Cruz L, Molina V, Vallejos R, Jimenez Chavarria E, Lopez-Boado MA, Ferrer J (2012) Outcome after laparoscopic enucleation for nonfunctional neuroendocrine pancreatic tumours. HBP 14(3):171–176

13. Dralle H, Krohn SL, Karges W, Boehm BO, Brauckhoff M, Gimm O (2004) Surgery of resectable nonfunctioning neuroendocrine pancreatic tumors. World J Surg 28(12):1248–1260

14. Fendrich V, Waldmann J, Bartsch DK, Langer P (2009) Surgical management of pancreatic endocrine tumors. Nat Rev Clin Oncol 6(7):419–428

15. Eckhauser FE, Cheung PS, Vinik AI (1986) Nonfunctioning malignant neuroendocrine tumors of the pancreas. Surgery 100(6):978–988

16. Rindi G, Kloppel G, Alhman H (2006) TNM staging of foregut (neuro)endocrine tumors: a consensus proposal including a grading system. Virchows Arch 449(4):395–401

17. Crippa S, Bassi C, Warshaw AL, Falconi M, Partelli S, Thayer SP, Pederzoli P, Fernández-del Castillo C (2007) Middle pancreatectomy: indications, short- and long-term operative outcomes. Ann Surg 246(1): 69–76, http://www.ncbi.nlm.nih.gov/pubmed?term= (Falconi%5BAuthor%5D)%20AND%20middle%20 pancreatectomy%5BTitle%5D

18. Hackert T, Hinz U, Fritz S et al (2011) Enucleation in pancreatic surgery: indications, technique, and outcome compared to standard pancreatic resections. Langenbecks Arch Surg 396:1197–1203

19. Crippa S, Bassi C, Salvia R, Falconi M, Butturini G, Pederzoli P (2007) Enucleation of pancreatic neoplasms. Br J Surg 94(10):1254–1259

20. Dedieu A, Rault A, Collet D, Masson B, Sa Chunha A (2011) Laparoscopic enucleation of pancreatic neoplasm. Surg Endosc Interv Tech 25(2):575–576

21. Heeger K, Falconi M, Partelli S, Waldmann J, Crippa S, Fendrich V, Bartsch DK (2014) Increased rate of clinically relevant pancreatic fistula after deep enucleation of small pancreatic tumors. Langenbecks Arch Surg 399(3):315–321

22. Partelli S, Gaujoux S, Boninsegna L, Cherif R, Crippa S, Couvelard A, Scarpa A, Ruszniewski P, Sauvanet A, Falconi M (2013) Pattern and clinical predictor of lymph node involvement in nonfunctioning pancreatic neuroendocrine tumors (NF-PanNETs). JAMA Surg 148(10):932–939

23. Grant CS (1993) Surgical management of malignant islet cell tumors. World J Surg 17(4):498–503

24. Grama D, Eriksson B, Martensson H et al (1992) Clinical characteristics, treatment and survival in patients with pancreatic tumors causing hormonal syndromes. World J Surg 16(4):632–639

25. Crippa S, Zerbi A, Boninsegna L et al (2012) Surgical management of insulinomas: short- and long-term outcomes after enucleations and pancreatic resections. Arch Surg 147(3):261–266

26. Vaidakis D, Karoubalis J, Pappa T, Piaditis G, Zografos GN (2010) Pancreatic insulinoma: current issues and trends. Hepatobiliary Pancreat Dis Inter 9(3):234–241

27. Falconi M, Zerbi A, Crippa S et al (2010) Parenchyma-preserving resections for small nonfunctioning pancreatic endocrine tumors. Ann Surg Oncol 17(6): 1621–1627

28. Zhao YP, Zhan HK, Zhang TP et al (2011) Surgical management of patients with insulinomas: result of 292 cases in a single institution. J Surg Oncol 103(2): 169–174

29. Hirshberg B, Libutti SK, Alexander HR et al (2002) Blind distal pancreatectomy for occult insulinoma, an inadvisable procedure. J Am Coll Surg 194(6): 761–764

30. Norton JA, Shawker TH, Doppman JL et al (1990) Localization and surgical treatment of occult insulinomas. Ann Surg 212(5):615–620

31. Rindi G, Falconi M, Klersy C, Albarello L, Boninsegna L, Buchler MW, Capella C, Caplin M, Couvelard A, Doglioni C, Delle Fave G, Fischer L, Fusai G, de Herder WW, Jann H, Komminoth P, de Krijger RR, La Rosa S, Luong TV, Pape U, Perren A, Ruszniewski P, Scarpa A, Schmitt A, Solcia E, Wiedenmann B (2012) TNM staging of neoplasms of the endocrine pancreas: results from a large international cohort study. J Natl Cancer Inst 104(10):764–777

32. Ellison EC, Sparks J, Verducci JS et al (2006) 50-year appraisal of gastrinoma: recommendations for staging and treatment. J Am Coll Surg 202(6):897–905

33. Norton JA, Fraker DL, Alexander HR et al (1999) Surgery to cure the Zollinger-Ellison syndrome. N Engl J Med 341(9):635–644

34. Lopez CL, Falconi M, Waldmann J, Boninsegna L, Fendrich V, Goretzki PK, Langer P, Kann PH, Partelli S, Bartsch DK (2013) Partial pancreaticoduodenectomy can provide cure for duodenal gastrinoma associated with multiple endocrine neoplasia type. Ann Surg 257(2):308–314

35. Norton JA, Alexander HR, Fraker DL et al (2004) Does the use of routine duodenotomy (DUODX) affect rate of cure, development of liver metastases, or survival in patients with Zollinger-Ellison syndrome? Ann Surg 239(5):617–626

36. Hill JS, McPhee JT, McDade TP et al (2009) Pancreatic neuroendocrine tumors. Cancer 115(4):741–751

37. Pomianowska E, Gladhaug IP, Grzyb K et al (2010) Survival following resection of pancreatic endocrine tumors: importance of R-status and the WHO and TNM classification systems. Scand J Gastroenterol 45(7–8):971–979

38. Yao JC, Hassan M, Phan A et al (2008) One hundred years after "carcinoid": epidemiology of and prognostic factors for neuroendocrine tumors in 35,825 cases in the United States. J Clin Oncol 26(18):3063–3072

39. Norton JA, Kivlen M, Li M et al (2003) Morbidity and mortality of aggressive resection in patients with advanced neuroendocrine tumors. Arch Surg 138(8): 859–866

40. Hellman P, Andersson M, Rastad J et al (2000) Surgical strategy for large or malignant endocrine pancreatic tumors. World J Surg 24(11):1353–1360

41. Touzios JG, Kiely JM, Pitt SC, Rilling WS, Quebbeman EJ, Wilson SD, Pitt HA (2005) Neuroendocrine hepatic metastases: does aggressive management improve survival? Ann Surg 241(5):776–783

42. Cho CS, Labow DM, Tang L et al (2008) Histologic grade is correlated with outcome after resection of hepatic neuroendocrine neoplasms. Cancer 113(1):126–134

43. Lawrence B, Gustafsson BI, Chan A et al (2011) The epidemiology of gastroenteropancreatic neuroendocrine tumors. Endocrinol Metab Clin North Am 40:1–18, vii

44. Kulke MH, Anthony LB, Bushnell DL, de Herder WW, Goldsmith SJ, Klimstra DS, Marx SJ, Pasieka JL, Pommier RF, Yao JC, Jensen RT (2010) NANETS treatment guidelines: well-differentiated neuroendocrine tumors of the stomach and pancreas. Pancreas 39:735–752

45. Niederle MB, Hackl M, Kaserer K, Niederle B (2010) Gastroenteropancreatic neuroendocrine tumours: the current incidence and staging based on the WHO and European Neuroendocrine Tumour Society classification: an analysis based on prospectively collected parameters. Endocr Relat Cancer 17:909–918

46. Bruzoni M, Parikh P, Celis R et al (2009) Management of the primary tumor in patients with metastatic pancreatic neuroendocrine tumor: a contemporary single-institution review. Am J Surg 197(3):376–381

47. Musunuru S, Chen H, Rajpal S et al (2006) Metastatic neuroendocrine hepatic tumors: resection improves survival. Arch Surg 141(10):1000–1004

48. Boninsegna L, Panzuto F, Partelli S et al (2012) Malignant pancreatic neuroendocrine tumour: lymph node ratio and Ki67 are predictors of recurrence after curative resections. Eur J Cancer 48(11):1608–1615

49. DiNorcia J, Lee MK, Reavey PL et al (2010) One hundred thirty resections for pancreatic neuroendocrine tumor: evaluating the impact of minimally invasive and parenchyma-sparing techniques. J Gastrointest Surg 14(10):1536–1546

50. Assalia A, Gagner M (2004) Laparoscopic pancreatic surgery for islet cell tumors of the pancreas. World J Surg 28(12):1239–1247

51. Limongelli P, Belli A, Russo G et al (2012) Laparoscopic and open surgical treatment of left-sided pancreatic lesions: clinical outcomes and cost-effectiveness analysis. Surg Endosc Interv Tech 26(7): 1830–1836

52. Kim SC, Park KT, Hwang JW et al (2008) Comparative analysis of clinical outcomes for laparoscopic distal pancreatic resection and open distal pancreatic resection at a single institution. Surg Endosc Interv Tech 22(10):2261–2268

53. Baker MS, Bentrem DJ, Ujiki MB, Stocker S, Talamonti MS (2009) A prospective single institution comparison of peri-operative outcomes for laparoscopic and open distal pancreatectomy. Surgery 146(4):635–645

54. Fernández-Cruz L, Blanco L, Cosa R, Rendón H (2008) Is laparoscopic resection adequate in patients with neuroendocrine pancreatic tumors? World J Surg 32(5):904–917

55. Kooby DA, Hawkins WG, Schmidt CM et al (2010) Curative laparoscopic resection for pancreatic neoplasms: a critical analysis from a single institution. J Am Coll Surg 210(5):779–785

56. Butturini G, Inama M, Malleo G et al (2012) Perioperative and long-term results of laparoscopic spleen-preserving distal pancreatectomy with or without splenic vessels conservation: a retrospective analysis. J Surg Oncol 105(4):387–392

57. Fernandez-Cruz L, Cesar-Borges G (2006) Laparoscopic strategies for resection of insulinomas. J Gastrointest Surg 10(5):752–760

58. Toniato A, Meduri F, Foletto M, Avogaro A, Pelizzo M (2006) Laparoscopic treatment of benign insulinomas localized in the body and tail of the pancreas: a single-center experience. World J Surg 30(10): 1916–1919

Medical Therapy of Pancreatic Neuroendocrine Neoplasms

Nicola Fazio

22.1 Introduction

Generally, medical therapy of patients with pancreatic neuroendocrine neoplasms (PNENs) has a role in the metastatic and unresectable locally advanced stage.

Among nonsurgical treatments, several different therapies can be proposed, including chemotherapy, targeted therapies, biological therapies, and locoregional treatments. More specifically, chemotherapy can be performed with various agents, regimens, and schedules; targeted therapy can be directed toward different molecular targets, with several drugs and techniques; biological therapies include several agents and approaches, and finally, locoregional treatments can be performed with various procedures, mainly liver directed.

Although medical therapeutic options for PNENs have been increasing over the years, very few therapies were approved, including streptozotocin in 1970s, somatostatin analogs and IFN in 80s-90s, and finally everolimus and sunitinib in 2011 (Fig. 22.1).

N. Fazio, MD, PhD
Unit of Gastrointestinal Medical Oncology
and Neuroendocrine Tumors, European Institute
of Oncology, Via Ripamonti 435, Milan 20141, Italy
e-mail: nicola.fazio@ieo.it

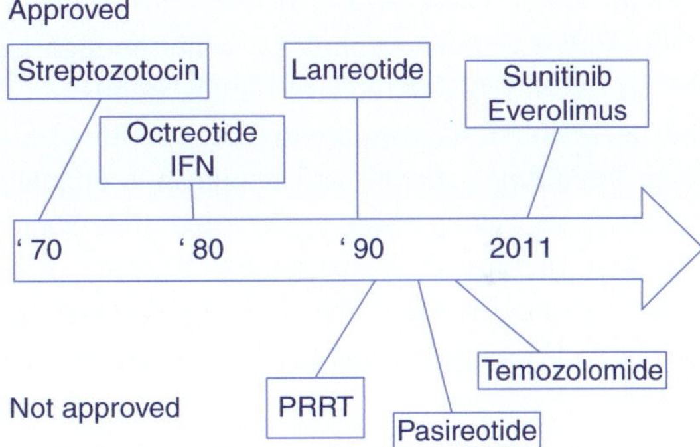

Fig. 22.1 Approved and not approved therapies in NENs. *IFN* interferon, *PRRT* peptide radioreceptor therapy

22.2 General Approach

Therapeutic approach can change according to the functioning/nonfunctioning status of the neoplasm. In functioning PNENs, the therapeutic priority is the syndrome control. Diazoxide in insulinomas and proton pump inhibitors (PPIs) in gastrinomas represent two medical therapies to be considered upfront. Somatostatin analogs (SSAs) are indicated in VIPoma, in glucagonoma, rarely in gastrinoma and insulinoma, and in very rare functioning PNENs, like ACTHomas, carcinoid syndrome-related PNENs, or hypercalcemia-related PNENs (PTHrp-omas) [1].

As for antiproliferative treatment, therapeutic approach varies according to the grade of malignancy and clinical behavior of the neoplasm.

S. La Rosa, F. Sessa (eds.), *Pancreatic Neuroendocrine Neoplasms: Practical Approach to Diagnosis,*
Classification, and Therapy, DOI 10.1007/978-3-319-17235-4_22,
© Springer International Publishing Switzerland 2015

More in general for advanced fast-growing PNENs, chemotherapy is usually the only option, whereas for advanced slow-growing PNENs, many other options can be considered (Fig. 22.2).

Therefore, it is crucial differentiating between the two categories. An important help comes from the 2010 pathology classification that distinguishes G1/G2 from G3 PNENs [2]; in other words, G1/G2 would correspond to low/intermediate grade of malignancy and G3 to the high grade. The first group is also the most numerous that means that in our clinical practice, it is most common to run into G1/G2 than into G3 PNENs. On the other hand, Ki-67 and/or mitotic index (MI) and/or tumor morphology is not enough to be sure to have understood the clinical behavior of the neoplasm or its response to therapy. Other factors, including patient's and neoplasm's characteristics, are usually necessary to better understand the best therapy to be proposed. Except for a minority of cases where the clinical picture of the tumor and/or patient is particularly severe or rap-

idly worsening, the vast majority of cases can be faced applying an algorithm including confirmation of diagnosis, definition of prognostic characteristics, performing an adequate staging, and discussing therapy and therapeutic strategy within a multidisciplinary dedicated team (Table 22.1). It is essential to be sure that the patient really has a "pure" PNEN (neither a mixed tumor nor an adenocarcinoma with neuroendocrine differentiation); sometimes, it requires a second opinion by a pathologist particularly skilled in NEN.

22.3 Fast-Growing PNENs

This category is represented mainly by high-grade PNENs, which are named carcinomas (PNECs) according to the 2010 WHO classification. Basically for this category, chemotherapy represents the only therapeutic option. Historically in advanced stage NECs, platinum/etoposide has been the most used chemotherapy; it represents a sort of standard of care, although it is based on old and small-size studies [3–5]. It is based on the assumption that a NEC is clinically similar to the small cell lung cancer (SCLC). However, increasing clinical knowledge seems to support different categories of PNECs.

Probably, a small cell neuroendocrine carcinoma (SCNEC), with a high Ki-67 (>70 %), will be directly related with a fast growth, and in that case, an approach similar to that of the SCLC is shared within the clinical community. However, some data reported a different response rate (RR) and survival between patients with gastroenteropancreatic (GEP) NECs with >55 % and <55 % Ki-67 [6]. Furthermore, some authors reported that among patients with GEP NECs (all with >20 % Ki-67),

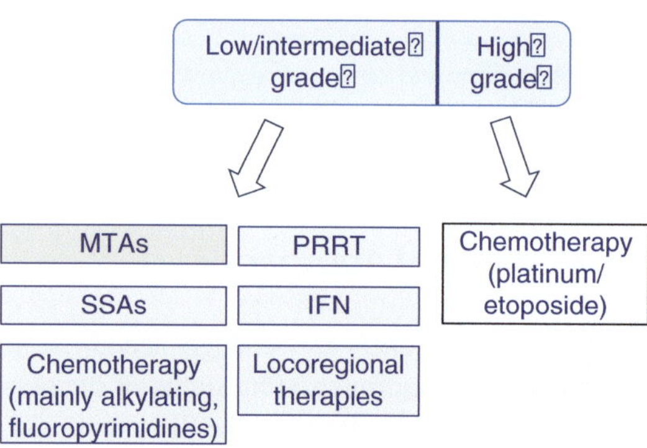

Fig. 22.2 PNENs: therapeutic options related to the grade of malignancy. *MTAs* molecular-targeted agents, *SSAs* somatostatin analogs, *IFN* interferon, *PRRT* peptide radioreceptor therapy

Table 22.1 Algorithm for diagnosis, characterization, and prognosis estimate of the disease

Steps	Key point	Specialist
Right diagnosis	"Pure" PNEN	Pathologist
Histological prognostic factors	Tumor differentiation, Ki-67/MI	Pathologist
Morphological imaging	CT scan/MRI	Radiologist
Functional imaging	SRS/^{68}Ga-DOTA-octreotide PET-CT	Nuclear medicine expert
	^{18}FDG PET-CT	
Clinical picture	Syndrome/symptoms/P.S.	Clinician

Table 22.2 Randomized phase III trials with SSAs and MTAs in PNETs

	Experimental arm	Control arm	Target	Tumors	N° of pts	Author
Clarinet	Lanreotide autogel	Placebo	sstr-2	Nonfunctioning enteropancreatic	204	Caplin, ENETS, 2014 [9]
Radiant-3	Everolimus +/− octreotide LAR	Placebo +/− octreotide LAR	mTORC1	PNET	410	Yao, NEJM, 2011 [11]
A6181111	Sunitinib	Placebo	VEGFR, PDGFR, KIT, FLT3	PNET	171	Raymond, NEJM, 2011 [10]

LAR long-acting repeatable, *SSTR* somatostatin receptor, *mTORC* mammalian target of rapamycin, *PNET* pancreatic neuroendocrine tumor, *VEGFR* vascular endothelial growth factor receptor, *PDGFR* platelet-derived growth factor receptor, *KIT* stem cell factor receptor, *FLT* FLT ligand, *MTAs* molecular-targeted agents, *SSAs* somatostatin analogs

those with a well-moderately differentiated tumor morphology did not respond to platinum-based chemotherapy although their survival was better compared with that of patients with poorly differentiated tumor morphology [7]. Therefore, in the "low" Ki-67 PNECs, chemotherapies different from platinum/etoposide could be considered, like alkylating-based regimens, and even biological therapies, like everolimus (EVE) or sunitinib (SUN) or peptide receptor radionuclide therapy (PRRT), could be discussed for "well-differentiated PNEC."

22.4 Slow-Growing PNENs

This category is represented mainly by low-/intermediate-grade PNENs, which are named tumors (PNETs) according to the 2010 WHO classification. It is known that this category is clinically heterogenous. It includes different clinical histories, from advanced PNETs radiologically stable even for months without any antitumor therapy to PNETS with a pronounced radiological progression of disease within 2–3 months. Usually the former group has a very low Ki-67 (<5 %), well-differentiated tumor morphology, and high functional expression of somatostatin receptors (sstrs) at somatostatin receptor scintigraphy (SRS) or ⁶⁸gallium-DOTA-octreotide positron emission tomography-computed tomography (⁶⁸Ga-DOTA-octreotide PET-CT), with a patient in a very good clinical condition.

A number of different nonsurgical therapies can be considered in PNETs, including SSAs, interferon (IFN), several chemotherapeutics, molecular-targeted agents (MTAs), peptide receptor radionuclide therapy (PRRT), and liver-directed interventional radiology procedures (Fig. 22.2).

The role of SSAs as antiproliferative agents in GEP NETs has been debated for several years. Based on retrospective and prospective evidence [8, 9], octreotide (OCT) or lanreotide (LAN) now can be effective in functioning or nonfunctioning PNETs, radiologically stable or slowly progressing, G1 or G2 (better if <10 % Ki-67), preferably with high sstr functional expression, independently from the tumor burden, with an asymptomatic patient.

In PNETs progressing on or after SSAs, EVE or SUN can be considered. These two MTAs were approved on the basis of results of two placebo-controlled phase 3 trials in patients with pancreatic well/moderately differentiated, advanced NENs, with a baseline radiological progression [10, 11] (Table 22.2).

The EVE trial was completed, with 410 patients, whereas the SUN trial was prematurely stopped due to a positive interim analysis. Both trials showed a PFS advantage of around 6 months (5 vs. 11 months in favor of the experimental arm). In very selected cases, EVE or SUN can be considered upfront. Interferon alfa-2b can be considered in selected cases progressing on SSA, especially if associated with carcinoid syndrome, with an indolent course, when other therapies cannot be used.

The most common all-grade EVE toxicity was stomatitis, in more than 60 % of cases; anemia (6 %), stomatitis (7 %), and hyperglycemia (5 %) were the grade 3 toxicities observed in >5 % of patients. Noninfectious pneumonitis is a rare and typical toxicity from EVE.

The most common adverse event (AE) associated with SUN was diarrhea (60 %). The most common treatment-related grade 3–4 AEs reported in >5 % of patients were neutropenia (12 %), hypertension (10 %), palmar-plantar erythrodysesthesia (6 %), diarrhea (5 %), asthenia (5 %), and abdominal pain (5 %).

Peptide receptor radionuclide therapy is an interesting investigational therapy for NENs. It has been reported to be active and potentially effective in low-/intermediate-grade sstr-positive NENs. It was not yet approved in any setting, and a regulatory phase 3 randomized trial is ongoing comparing ^{177}Lu-Dotatate with OCT LAR 60 mg/4 weeks in advanced small bowel NENs progressing on OCT LAR 30 mg/4 weeks.

More than 200 patients have been treated in the three largest series of PNENs so far reported [12–14].

The largest one is a subgroup of 91 patients with advanced pretreated PNEN included in the retrospective Dutch analysis of 310 GEP NENs published in the JCO in 2010. Noteworthy 40 months of time to progression (TTP) (although related to the global population) and more than 40 % of partial response (PR). However, it should be considered that the tumor status at study entry, the proliferation index, and the concomitant use of SSA were unknown for many patients. Therefore, a possible bias related to a spontaneous selection of better prognosis population cannot be excluded.

The second published series is that of a phase II trial, with 52 patients treated with two schedules of ^{177}Lu-Dotatate, and better results were observed in ^{18}FDG-PET/CT-negative tumors. A disease control rate (complete response, CR + PR + stable disease, SD) of 80 % with 88 % of tumors progressing at study entry is interesting although also in this case, a bias of selection of better prognosis population should be considered.

The third published series is that of a retrospective analysis of 68 patients with advanced PNEN treated with ^{177}Lu-octreotate. Sixty-eight percent of them had a baseline tumor progression during the 12 months before initiation of treatment, and PRRT was the first-line systemic treatment in 51 % of patients. A 60 % PR and 34 month PFS were observed.

The two main types of toxicity related to PRRT are renal and bone marrow toxicities. All-grade nephrotoxicity can occur in around 30 % of patients with ^{90}yttrium-based PRRT and in around 10 % with ^{177}lutetium based. Bone marrow toxicity can be acute (around 10 % of G3–4) and very late (myelodysplastic syndrome, 2 %, and leukemia, 1 %) [15].

In slow-growing PNENs, chemotherapy can be considered, particularly in G2 with "high" Ki-67. Alkylating-based regimen is the most proposed. Temozolomide (TMZ) is an oral alkylating agent that represents the evolution of the parenteral and more toxic streptozotocin (STZ). Literature data have been progressively accumulating over the last years, both as single agent and in combination. Combined with capecitabine, it has been reported highly active in PNENs [16]. So far around 150 patients were treated in several different studies. O(6)-Methylguanine-DNA methyltransferase (MGMT) is the enzyme that can repair the DNA damage produced by TMZ, therefore creating resistance to the drug. Due to problems of reproducibility, the detection of MGMT is still investigational. Oxaliplatin-based chemotherapy is another active studied option. Unfortunately, the number of patients with PNENs treated with this therapy included in different studies is quite low (<100) so far.

A number of liver-directed treatments have been performed in patients with liver metastases from PNETs. Some of them are intravascular and some others ablative. Among the intravascular treatments, trans-arterial chemoembolization (TACE) is probably the oldest one, and then there are the trans-arterial embolization (TAE) and selective internal ^{90}Y radioembolization therapy (^{90}Y SIRT). These treatments can have a role in different settings, more often including metastases debulking within a global therapeutic strategy, syndrome control, and monofocal tumor progression. The radiofrequency ablation (RFA) is an ablative technique that can be considered for small liver metastases with curative intent when surgery has been excluded.

References

1. Jensen RT, Berna MJ, Bingham DB, Norton JA (2008) Inherited pancreatic endocrine tumor syndromes: advances in molecular pathogenesis, diagnosis, management, and controversies. Cancer 113:1807–1843
2. Bosman (2010) WHO classification of tumor of the digestive system. IARC Press, Lyon
3. Moertel CG, Kvols LK, O'Connel MJ (1991) Treatment of neuroendocrine carcinomas with combined etoposide and cisplatin. Cancer 68:227–232
4. Mitry E, Baudin E, Ducreaux M et al (1999) Treatment of poorly differentiated neuroendocrine tumours with etoposide and cisplatin. Br J Cancer 81:1351–1355
5. Fjallskog MLH, Granberg DPH, Welin SLW et al (2001) Treatment with cisplatin and etoposide in patients with neuroendocrine tumors. Cancer 92(5):1101–1107
6. Sorbye H, Welin S, Langer SW et al (2013) Predictive and prognostic factors for treatment and survival in 305 patients with advanced gastrointestinal neuroendocrine carcinoma (WHO G3): the NORDIC NEC study. Ann Oncol 24:152–160
7. Vélayoudom-Céphise FL, Duvillard P, Foucan L, Hadoux J, Chougnet CN, Leboulleux S, Malka D, Guigay J, Goere D, Debaere T, Caramella C, Schlumberger M, Planchard D, Elias D, Ducreux M, Scoazec JY, Baudin E (2013) Are G3 ENETS neuroendocrine neoplasms heterogeneous? Endocr Relat Cancer 20:649–657
8. Rinke A, Müller H-H, Schade-Brittinger C et al (2009) Placebo-controlled, double-blind, prospective, randomized study on the effect of octreotide LAR in the control of tumor growth in patients with metastatic neuroendocrine midgut tumors: a report from the PROMID Study Group. J Clin Oncol 27:4656–4663
9. Caplin ME, Pavel M, Cwikla JB et al (2014) Lanreotide in metastatic enteropancreatic neuroendocrine tumors. N Engl J Med 371:224–233
10. Raymond E, Dahan L, Raoul JL, Bang YJ, Borbath I, Lombard-Bohas C et al (2011) Sunitinib malate for the treatment of pancreatic neuroendocrine tumors. N Engl J Med 364(6):501–513
11. Yao JC, Shah MH, Ito T, Bohas CL, Wolin EM, Van Cutsem E et al (2011) Everolimus for advanced pancreatic neuroendocrine tumors. N Engl J Med 364(6): 514–523
12. Kwekkeboom DJ et al (2008) Treatment with the radiolabeled somatostatin analog [177 Lu-DOTA 0, Tyr3]octreotate: toxicity, efficacy, and survival. J Clin Oncol 26(13):2124–2130
13. Sansovini M, Severi S, Ambrosetti A, Monti M, Nanni O, Sarnelli A, Bodei L, Garaboldi L, Bartolomei M, Paganelli G (2013) Treatment with the radiolabelled somatostatin analog Lu-DOTATATE for advanced differentiated neuroendocrine tumors. Neuroendocrinology 97(4):347–354. doi:10.1159/000348394, Epub 2013 May 22
14. Ezziddin S, Khalaf F, Vanezi M, Haslerud T, Mayer K, Al Zreiqat A, Willinek W, Biersack HJ, Sabet A (2014) Outcome of peptide receptor radionuclide therapy with 177Lu-octreotate in advanced grade 1/2 pancreatic neuroendocrine tumours. Eur J Nucl Med Mol Imaging 41(5):925–933. doi:10.1007/s00259-013-2677-3
15. Bodei L, Kidd M, Paganelli G, Grana C, Drozdov I, Cremonesi M, Lepenski C, Kwekkeboom D, Baum R, Krenning E, Modlin IM (2015) Long-term tolerability of PRRT in 807 patients with neuroendocrine tumours: the value and limitations of clinical factors. Eur J Nucl Med Mol Imaging 42(1):5–19
16. Strosberg JR, Fine RL, Choi J et al (2011) First-line chemotherapy with capecitabine and temozolomide in patients with metastatic pancreatic endocrine carcinomas. Cancer 117:268–275

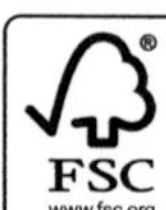